Current Topics on Renal Dysfunction: From Basics to Clinic

Edited by

Rafael Valdez-Ortiz
Department of Nephrology
Hospital General de México
Dr. Eduardo Liceaga, Mexico City
Mexico

Katy Sánchez-Pozos
Research Division, Hospital Juárez de México
Mexico City, Mexico

Ana Carolina Ariza
Center for Nutrition and Health Research
National Institute of Public Health
Cuernavaca, Morelos, Mexico

&

Enzo C. Vásquez-Jiménez
Department of Nephrology
Hospital Juárez de México
Mexico City, Mexico

Current Topics on Renal Dysfunction: From Basics to Clinic

Editors: Rafael Valdez-Ortiz, Katy Sánchez-Pozos, Ana Carolina Ariza & Enzo C. Vásquez-Jiménez

ISBN (Online): 978-981-5305-69-2

ISBN (Print): 978-981-5305-70-8

ISBN (Paperback): 978-981-5305-71-5

First published in 2025.

need for a court order if at any point you breach any terms of this License Agreement. In no event will any delay or failure by Bentham Science Publishers in enforcing your compliance with this License Agreement constitute a waiver of any of its rights.

3. You acknowledge that you have read this License Agreement, and agree to be bound by its terms and conditions. To the extent that any other terms and conditions presented on any website of Bentham Science Publishers conflict with, or are inconsistent with, the terms and conditions set out in this License Agreement, you acknowledge that the terms and conditions set out in this License Agreement shall prevail.

Bentham Science Publishers Pte. Ltd.
No. 9 Raffles Place
Office No. 26-01
Singapore 048619
Singapore
Email: subscriptions@benthamscience.net

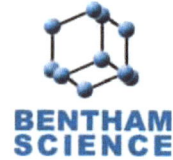

BENTHAM SCIENCE

CONTENTS

FOREWORD

I want to start this chapter by telling you a story: how and why I have been continually amazed and enthusiastic about learning every day a new issue about kidney physiology and pathophysiology and how this book starts a new era in Mexico by demonstrating how basic science can improve from using the laboratory results in our understanding of Kidney's health and the earliest identification and effective treatment of kidney diseases.

My interest in the kidneys started in my early days at medical school 53 years ago, since 1979, during and after my postdoctoral studies at the laboratory of nephrology and Mineral Metabolism at Washington University School of Medicine in Saint Louis, Missouri, where two outstanding professors Dr. Saulo Klahr and Eduardo Slatopolsky involved me under the tutorial of Kevin Martin and Ezequiel Bellorin-Font in the development of the area on mineral, bone metabolism and the intracellular pathways of action of parathyroid hormone throughout their proximal tubular receptors and intracellular signaling. After returning to the Nephrology and Mineral Metabolism at the National Institute of Nutrition, I coordinated and developed the mineral metabolism laboratory and clinical services.

A lifetime perspective of the last 5 decades in Mexico

Let me start a journey remembering some examples of the teaching strategies of my mentors, Dr. José Carlos Peña and Jaime Herrera, in the nephrology specialty training in the late 1970s: for example, to have a precise determination of glomerular filtration rate (GFR), we did use the inulin clearance rate if the clinical decision making needed such precision. The urinary collection during a 24-hour interval was used in several decision-making processes, including the Creatinine Clearance, to not only determine GFR but to define the fractional excretion of different substances or the metabolic balance of several substances in specific protocols conducted in an excellent clinical research service. Except for inulin determination, most tests performed lacked specificity, and their scientific basis was derived mainly from observational and metabolic studies. Looking at the conclusions we derived from their results in those days, I feel that they allowed us to use very intuitive reasoning due to their design. Their precision and reproducibility were difficult to standardize and, therefore, to perform in any clinical setting. Nonetheless, we made an excellent diagnosis, mainly with respect to the physiology and metabolic aspects of KD.

The characterization of the immune system was also in its very early years. Therefore, its role in CKD etiology and evolution was suspected, and the evidence was merely observational. During these decades, an enormous change has been achieved, and it is a consequence of basic research translated to clinical nephrology under the leadership of Dr. Donato Alarcon, Federico Chavez Peon, coworkers, and many groups in the transplant community.

In the early 1980s, the science of membrane receptors, membrane channels, transporters, and co-transporters was another considerable progress when applied to clinical nephrology. The mineral and bone metabolism system, the acidification system, and arterial hypertension, among other areas, greatly benefited from this research, and there are important groups around Mexico developing this area.

From 1990 to date, another big area of development in nephrology was the genomic, transcriptional, metabolomic, and microbiome research areas.

In this route of more than half a century, nephrology as a specialty of internal medicine was started around the world, and in Mexico, it happened in 1972. Not to forget are the advances in dialysis procedures and the quality-of-life improvements made possible since 1979 by fundamental scientific research on peritoneal membrane physiology and its adaptations to the procedure. The hemodialysis efficacy was also improved due to the development of biocompatible membranes, up-to-date purification of water, and better dialysates.

This book comes together as an example of the collaboration and enthusiasm of at least 10 different institutional groups around the country; they work as a community where CKD, AKD, ESRD, and transplantation are potent stimuli for their work.

The renal circulatory system is pivotal for these mechanisms to act in precise coordination

Over these decades, the kidneys have always been a great laboratory where the multiple functions covered by the two kidneys are paramount to the whole-body economy and health. The anatomic place where nature allocated them is strategic. Humans, a species that stands on two feet and in a vertical position and walks as a bipod, need a barometric sensor system and a unique propulsion of blood. This peculiarity, combined with the non-permeable characteristics of our skin, is also related to the volume control of the intra and extracellular compartments. In a few words, the Kidney, the central nervous system, and the heart have evolved in the human species with a very complex system for precisely regulating fluid and volume control. The strategic position of the kidneys in the retroperitoneum and under the diaphragm allows them to have an excellent mechanism for sensing and adjusting both fluid and volume, with a super specialized mechanism: a. the renin-angiotensin; b. the vasopressin; and c. renal innervation is also an essential component.

Another consequence of humans is having non-permeable skin, which obligates the body to have precise water and mineral homeostasis conservation mechanisms. The role of the kidneys in this area is of great importance; a precise balance between ingestion, metabolic needs, and excretion depends on the coordinated function of many different systems for secretion, reabsorption, transport, and cotransport of the monovalent and divalent ions coordinated with glucose, nitrogen, and ammonium either in the proximal or distal tubule where acidification is also regulated and, therefore, the metabolic acid-base balance of the whole body.

The urine concentration and sodium/chloride balance are coordinated in the renal medulla where the loops of Henle and distal /collecting ducts are to be studied.

Also, the kidney interstitium was elucidated and understood in the last two decades, along with the role of erythropoietin and anemia of CKD, inflammation, fibrosis , and tissue death.

Hence, this book is a unique opportunity to invite you to focus our attention on the great opportunity that the contemporary clinical practice of nephrology already has in several areas, namely earliest detection of Kidney Diseases (KD) and the mechanisms involved in the damage of kidney tissues, acute kidney injuries, the effect of different toxic exposures on kidney function, the mechanisms of tissue death and fibrosis as well as the mechanisms of action of specific treatments/therapeutic interventions among others, thanks to the advances generated by the results of very well focused basic scientific research.

The kidneys are bright organs; they play a role in the human body's health

You will enjoy analyzing the contributions of my co-authors, which can be addressed considering the focus of their interest in some of the issues summarized in the contents table.

A group of chapters are focused on genomic sciences and the Kidney, namely the pleiotropic aspects of CKD, the genetic influence on cell differentiation, kidney/urinary tract cancers, epigenetics of CKD, and their relationships with microbiota. A fascinating area related to stem cell science is the integration of new organs, including functional kidneys, and forecasting a new era in successful organ transplantation.

Examples of how inflammation and metabolic syndromes affect energy utilization are exemplified by the chapters analyzing mitochondria and oxidative stress (oxygen and ROS), for example, in diabetic kidney damage.

Arterial hypertension, sodium balance, acid-base metabolism, and nephrolithiasis are also areas where co-authors had incursion and generated new insights into the pathophysiology and treatment options.

An emerging area regarding mechanisms of kidney damage is related to the toxic effects of different chemicals to which people are exposed, either due to the natural contamination of the habitat or anthropogenic activities.

Regarding clinical nephrology, this book discusses the science related to the diagnosis and association of CKD with metabolic syndrome, type 2 diabetes mellitus, systemic arterial hypertension, nephrolithiasis, renal tubular acidosis, polycystic kidney disease, and acute kidney injuries.

CKD in Mexico and the world;A global burden lacking fundamental strategies to be controlled, diminished, or ideally avoided

When getting accurate data on the number of Mexican citizens living with CKD, we will face the results of small population studies from which only a gross estimation can be done. This latter is explained by the complexity of our fragmented health system, which makes it almost impossible to adopt a uniform policy for early detection, classification, and, very importantly, successful intervention of this disease.

Therefore, the Mexican scenario shows late identification and ineffective intervention of CKD, leading to a growing and uncontrolled number of patients facing the irreversible end stage of kidney disease (ESKD) and the need for the high cost of dialysis treatment to survive. This resource does not cover the whole ESKD population.

There is enough international evidence of the catastrophic costs implied of the yearly expenses of the different options to treat ESKD when hemo and peritoneal dialysis are unavoidable treatments for survival.

In Mexico, these data are available only for the significant health provider system: the Mexican Institute of Social Security (IMSS), where formal workers are covered, and a significant percentage of ESKD patients receive either hemo and/or peritoneal dialysis. Note that there is a significant and underestimated ESKD population of IMSS beneficiaries who do not receive dialysis.

The direct and indirect expenses of such programs are catastrophic for the IMSS. If they are extrapolated to the estimated ESKD population not covered by IMSS, it is easy to realize that they are catastrophic for the whole country. What do we mean when considering a cost catastrophic for any health system? There is an example for you to analyze before you go through this publication. In 2020, the direct cost of the IMSS dialysis programs, just the costs related to the treatment session or the peritoneal supplies for approximately 60,000 ESKD patients, equals the expenses to attend all the millions of births attended at IMSS facilities in the whole IMSS population. In addition, there are indirect costs bearableby this population, namely of the complications of treatment, hospitalizations, and death. They almost cost three times more than the direct cost just described.

I hope these examples provide enough reasons to be enthusiastic about fostering the kind of scientific research presented throughout this book, which is focused on the early identification of renal tissue damage, the options to prevent it and stop deterioration, and lastly, avoiding fibrosis and tissue death.

In the last three decades, a significant effort has been made to identify the presence of CKD in high-risk populations; there are many worldwide spread programs with this purpose, one of which has been active in Mexico, the Kidney Early Evaluation Program (KEEP) of the International Kidney Foundation which allows estimating the "remnant glomerular reserve." This program is well designed to identify clinical antecedents correctly to establish the kind of risk present, correlating with clinical anthropometry, classifying the stage of CKD estimating glomerular filtration rate using standardized determination of serum creatinine and different validated formulas as well as glomerular integrity through the albumin/creatinine ratio in one sporadic urine sample.

Although it is very "glomerulocentric," it has been demonstrated to be very useful as a clinical tool to conscientize the patient and, in very few cases, to provide a photograph of the size of the CKD problem to a specific health system, which ultimately is responsible for providing access to effective treatment options; all oriented to stop the deterioration of such glomerular remnant function and to slow the need of dialysis, ideally to recover functional glomerulus.

Using this model in the year 2010 in the Mexican state of Jalisco, it became evident that we were able to screen nearly 8000 citizens with type 2 diabetes (DM2) covered by the public health state services in only two weeks, adapting a validated version of the KEEP protocol. As a result of this campaign, we did generate consciousness of the kind of care that the individual patient needs to have according to the CKD remnant "kidney" reserve, as well as those that did not have CKD; in this case, the patients became aware that they can develop this undesirable complication of DM2 if they do not adhere to appropriate medical care and control of their disease.

We also established and finished a course online designed to train general practitioners (GPs) in taking medical care of this DM2 population in their primary care clinics; the course was peer-reviewed, and the intervention protocol was validated to treat each deterioration stage. These GPs identified approximately 100 CKD patients in their own DM2 registry. We also asked for the nephrologist evaluation online in a very well-programmed schedule.

The Health Care Authorities of Jalisco stopped the program because there were several logistical problems regarding accessibility to laboratory testing and medications. Nonetheless, the program yielded a model to be pursued at the non-IMSS covered population affected by DM2, which is most of the population in the country, nearly 60% of the adult population older than 20 years old.

These results were compared with those obtained in other Mexican States where the Mexican Kidney Foundation (FMR) openly invited the public to participate in KEEP testing events. Those with known risk factors for developing CKD were accepted, regardless of whether they have IMSS or other insurance coverage. The results were significantly similar, if not almost identical, to those we obtained in the Jalisco scenario.

With these data, it is easy to speculate on how many people are affected by one or more of the Metabolic Syndrome components identified by the Nationwide Health and Nutrition Survey conducted by the National Institute of Public Health (INSP, ENSANUT), which may have developed CKD and classify them according to the KDOQUI/EPI criteria in the whole country.

Although imprecise, the figure is of millions of cases with CKD in the 20-year and older adult group, which are affected by CKD, of which 96% are in the early stages of the disease. Therefore, a significant opportunity exists to establish a fundamental public policy to face this challenge through systematic early identification, classification, and protocolized interventions, briefly a cost-efficient policy that should decrease the burden to the nation represented by CKD and ESKD.

Let us finish this section by mentioning that many new biomarkers identified and understood by recent scientific research can identify when a kidney starts deteriorating its integrity; KEEP accepts a patient as having CKD.

Which will be the best-case scenario for CKD in Mexico?

As we have reviewed in this chapter, I hope you became aware of the significant avenues opened today for the research community regarding the importance of kidney integrity in the health sustainability of anyone, with a large emphasis on people with one or more components of metabolic syndrome as several chapters of this book endorse.

Let's drive the route on the contemporary issues that syndemic entities like metabolic syndrome present to an integrated science community to develop effective and sustainable public policies to solve these problems; it is mandatory to acknowledge that they have conditionings that are not only related to a specific disease state but also include many socio-economic, ambient, and geographical factors. Therefore, the research on these multifactorial human conditions needs to establish a compelling inter- and transdisciplinary approach .

The interinstitutional and interdisciplinary nature of the present publications must encourage their institutions to promote transdisciplinary involvement; this is more feasible in universities where many disciplines and specialties are available. Recent efforts by the National Council of Science and Technology (CONACyT) have encouraged this approach, which has been demonstrated to be particularly cumbersome but necessary if feasible; long-term policies are to be implemented.

Meanwhile, the example given in this publication is excellent; basic scientists working on specific mechanisms of CKD and AKD and interacting with nephrology specialists have made a tremendous effort that is unique to my knowledge in Mexico.

Juan Alfredo Tamayo y Orozco
Accessalud, Mexico City, Mexico

PREFACE

Renal dysfunction includes a wide range of diseases affecting kidney function. But what are the common factors in development and disease progression? What do we know so far? and what are the most recent discoveries in this matter? One thing we know is that the common outcome is chronic kidney disease, end-stage renal disease, and finally the need for a transplant.

The kidney is a multifaceted organ, with its main function being the removal of excess water and toxins from the body as urine. Among the other functions are, the production of hormones, the regulation of fluid and mineral levels, the production of vitamin D, the regulation of blood pressure and the maintenance of the acid-base balance. Structured by a complex network of cellular interactions such as mesangial, parietals, podocytes and endothelial cells. Thus, any imbalance in whichever of their functions will have a detrimental effect on the systemic physiology.

Also, kidney failure can reach other organs, such as the heart, circulatory system, mineral balance, bones, muscles and joints, the gastrointestinal system as well as the immune system, at least in part through the suggested crosstalk between renal dendritic cells and T cells as suggested by some authors, causing maintained systemic inflammation and immunodeficiency.

Lately, new available approaches like the next generation sequencing, microbiota analysis, and epigenetics, are contributing to novel perspectives on physiological and pathological conditions of the kidney.

This e-book aims to address the current studies in kidney diseases, from basics to clinic, and from environmental factors to genetics, integrating the convoluted systems involved in kidney disease.

Rafael Valdez-Ortiz
Department of Nephrology
Hospital General de México
Dr. Eduardo Liceaga, Mexico City
Mexico

Katy Sánchez-Pozos
Research Division, Hospital Juárez de México
Mexico City, Mexico

Ana Carolina Ariza
Center for Nutrition and Health Research
National Institute of Public Health
Cuernavaca, Morelos, Mexico

&

Enzo C. Vásquez-Jiménez
Department of Nephrology
Hospital Juárez de México
Mexico City, Mexico

List of Contributors

Ana Carolina Ariza	Center for Nutrition and Health Research, National Institute of Public Health Mexico, Cuernavaca, Morelos, Mexico
Ana Laura Calderón-Garcidueñas	Neuropathology Department, Research Direction, Instituto Nacional de Neurologia y Neurocirugía, Manuel Velasco Suarez, Tlalpan 14269, Mexico City, Mexico
Ana Ligia Gutiérrez-Solís	Research Division, Hospital Regional de Alta Especialidad de la Península de Yucatán IMSS-Bienestar, Mérida, Yucatán, Mexico Centro de Investigación y de Estudios Avanzados del IPN (CINVESTAV-IPN) Mérida, Yucatán, Mexico
Azalia Ávila-Nava	Research Division, Hospital Regional De Alta Especialidad De la Península De Yucatán IMSS-Bienestar, Mérida, Yucatán, Mexico
Claudia J. Bautista	Department of Reproduction Biology, Instituto Nacional de Ciencias Médicas y Nutrición" Salvador Zubirán", Mexico City, Mexico
Consuelo Plata	Department of Nephrology and Mineral Metabolism, Instituto Nacional de Ciencias Médicas y Nutrición Salvador Zubirán, Mexico City, Mexico
Cristino Cruz	Department of Nephrology, Instituto Nacional de Ciencias Médicas y Nutrición" Salvador Zubirán", Mexico City, Mexico
Enzo C. Vásquez-Jiménez	Department of Nephrology, Hospital Juárez de México, Gustavo A. Madero 07760, Mexico City, Mexico
Estefani Yaquelin Hernández-Cruz	Chemistry School, Department of Biology, Universidad Nacional Autónoma de México (UNAM), Mexico City, Mexico Posgrado en Ciencias Biológicas, Universidad Nacional Autónoma de México (UNAM), Mexico City, Mexico
Estefany Ingrid Medina-Reyes	Chemistry School, Department of Biology, Universidad Nacional Autónoma de México (UNAM), Mexico City, Mexico
Fabio Solis-Jiménez	Instituto Nacional de Cardiología Ignacio Chávez, Tlalpan 14080, Mexico City, Mexico
Guadalupe Ortiz-López	Research Division, Hospital Juárez de México, Gustavo A. Madero 07760, Mexico City, Mexico
Isabel Medina-Vera	Methodology of Investigation, Instituto Nacional de Pediatría, Mexico City, Mexico
Iván Calderón-Lojero	Research Division, Hospital Juárez de México, Mexico City, Mexico
Jazmin Marlen Pérez-Rojas	Research Division, Instituto Nacional De Cancerología, Tlalpan 14080, Mexico City, Mexico
José Pedraza-Chaverri	Chemistry School, Department of Biology, Universidad Nacional Autónoma de México (UNAM), Mexico City, Mexico
Joyce Trujillo	Secretaría de Ciencia, Humanidades, Tecnología e Innovación (SECIHTI) - División de Materiales Avanzados-Instituto Potosino de Investigación Científica y Tecnológica - (SECIHTI-IPICYT), San Luis Potosí, Mexico

Juan Carlos Diaz Núñez	Department of Nephrology, Hospital General de México Dr. Eduardo Liceaga, Mexico City, Mexico
Juan Reyna-Blanco	Department of Nephrology, Hospital General de México Dr. Eduardo Liceaga, Mexico City, Mexico
Karina Robledo-Márquez	Facultad de Ingeniería, Universidad Autónoma de San Luis Potosí, San Luis Potosí, México
Katy Sánchez-Pozos	Research Division, Hospital Juárez de México, Gustavo A. Madero 07760, Mexico City, Mexico
Laura Elena Zamora- Cervantes	Department of Nephrology, Hospital Juárez de México, Gustavo A. Madero 07760, Mexico City, Mexico
María De Los Ángeles Granados-Silvestre	Research Division, Hospital Juárez de México, Gustavo A. Madero 07760, Mexico City, Mexico
Martha Medina-Escobedo	Research Division, Hospital Regional de Alta Especialidad de la Península de Yucatán IMSS-Bienestar, Mérida, Yucatán, Mexico
Mercedes Aguilar-Soto	Instituto Nacional de Ciencias Médicas y Nutrición" Salvador Zubirán", Mexico City, Mexico
Nayeli Goreti Nieto-Velázquez	Research Division, Hospital Juárez de México, Mexico City, Mexico
Nina Mendez-Domínguez	Research Division, Hospital Regional de Alta Especialidad de la Península de Yucatán IMSS-Bienestar, Mérida, Yucatán, Mexico
Rafael Valdez Ortiz	Department of Nephrology, Hospital General de México Dr. Eduardo Liceaga, Mexico City, Mexico
Roberto Lugo	Research Division, Hospital Regional de Alta Especialidad de la Península de Yucatán IMSS-Bienestar, Mérida, Yucatán, Mexico
Victoria Ramírez	Department of Experimental Surgery, Instituto Nacional de Ciencias Médicas y Nutrición" Salvador Zubirán", Mexico City, Mexico
Yadira Ramírez	División de Materiales Avanzados, Instituto Potosino de Investigación Científica y Tecnológica (IPICYT), San Luis Potosí, Mexico

CHAPTER 1

Metabolism in Kidney Disease

Azalia Ávila-Nava[1], Isabel Medina-Vera[2] and Consuelo Plata[3,*]

[1] *Research Division, Hospital Regional De Alta Especialidad De la Península De Yucatán IMSS-Bienestar, Mérida, Yucatán, Mexico*

[2] *Methodology of Investigation, Instituto Nacional de Pediatría, Mexico City, Mexico*

[3] *Department of Nephrology and Mineral Metabolism, Instituto Nacional de Ciencias Médicas y Nutrición Salvador Zubirán, Mexico City, Mexico*

Abstract: The kidney contains numerous types of cells; this cellular heterogeneity and functional diversity make the kidney an organ with great metabolic activity. Most solute reabsorption occurs in the proximal tubules, so much energy is used to recover them. The proximal tubules use fatty acid oxidation as their preferred metabolic pathway to carry out this process. The kidney plays a central role in glucose reabsorption, production, and utilization. However, it is important to note that the proximal tubules of the nephron prefer fatty acids as energy. Much of the glucose in the glomerular filtrate is reabsorbed in the proximal tubules by the two isoforms of glucose/Na+ transporters (SGLT1 and SGLT2) located in the apical zone of the tubular epithelium. It is well known that the human kidney is a key organ for maintaining systemic glucose homeostasis through gluconeogenesis. The only organs that can synthesize and release glucose into the bloodstream are the kidney and the liver because both synthesize glucose 6-phosphatase, which is necessary to form glucose from glucose-6-phosphate. Remarkably, the kidney produces approximately 25% of all glucose delivered into the blood. Several studies have demonstrated that lactate is the primary substrate of gluconeogenesis in the kidney. However, after kidney injury, metabolism is impaired, resulting in increased lactic acid generation and decreased fatty acid oxidation.

Keywords: Amino acid metabolism, Fatty acid oxidation, Gluconeogenesis, Glycolysis, Metabolic activity.

INTRODUCTION

To successfully carry out their functions, the kidney contains numerous types of cells that constitute the functional units known as nephrons, which react to diverse

---

* **Corresponding author Consuelo Plata:** Nephrology and Mineral Metabolism, Instituto Nacional de Ciencias Médicas y Nutrición Salvador Zubirán, Mexico City, Mexico; E-mail: consueloplata@hotmail.com.

Rafael Valdez-Ortiz, Katy Sánchez-Pozos, Ana Carolina Ariza & Enzo C. Vásquez-Jiménez (Eds.)

hormonal, neuronal, inflammatory, and intra- and intercellular stimuli. Various cell populations are in well-defined and specific microenvironments, such as hypoxic and hypersaline areas, where they perform many functions to maintain kidney homeostasis and, in turn, systemic balance. The communication and functional coordination between the nephron cells is responsible for the three important functional processes of the kidney: filtration, reabsorption, and secretion [1]. This cellular heterogeneity and functional diversity make the kidney an organ with great metabolic activity that depends on 20 highly specialized epithelial cells in charge of reabsorbing almost all the solutes and water infiltrated [2]. The proximal tubules of the nephron reabsorb more than 70% of the glomerular filtrate, so the cells need a large amount of energy to facilitate the absorption of different solutes. Under physiological conditions, the cells of the proximal tubules obtain this energy mainly through the oxidation of fatty acids since they produce a more significant amount of adenosine triphosphate (ATP) molecules than glycolysis. Nonetheless, after kidney injury occurs, energy metabolism is modified, favoring an increase in lactate due to the activity of anaerobic glycolysis and a decrease in the oxidation of fatty acids [3].

Kidney damage or injury is caused by various situations, such as ischemia, infections, or the consumption of various substances, such as toxins and drugs, or by secondary damage to chronic diseases, such as diabetes, hypertension, glomerulonephritis, autoimmune diseases (systemic lupus erythematosus, rheumatoid arthritis) and a history of cardiovascular disease. In general, renal tubules are susceptible to acute kidney injury (AKI) and chronic kidney disease, though specifically proximal tubules, which are more sensitive to injury. Therefore, it has been hypothesized that metabolic disturbances observed during AKI or CKD can be corrected, attenuating injury or improving recovery. Below, we briefly discuss general aspects of renal tubular metabolism under physiological conditions and the metabolic changes reported during kidney damage [4].

FATTY ACID OXIDATION (FAO)

As previously mentioned, the proximal tubules in the nephrons recover most of the glomerular filtration (70%). Various solutes and water transport systems are present in this zone, and many ATP molecules are needed to accomplish their functions. The cells of the proximal tubules are rich in mitochondria that generate the necessary ATP in a very similar way to that of cardiomyocytes. Therefore, the proximal tubules depend on the oxidation of fatty acids to produce a greater quantity of ATP than glucose. In this sense, the kidney consumes most of the oxygen it receives to generate energy through the oxidation of fatty acids [4].

The reabsorption of long-chain fatty acids (LCFAs) in the renal tubules occurs through fatty acid transport proteins (FATPs), the membrane CD36 receptor, and fatty acid binding proteins (FABPs) [5 - 7]. Fatty acids are used for energy or other metabolic requirements and are obtained from the diet. Some are obtained from phospholipids through phospholipase A2, and others are synthesized by the enzyme fatty acid synthase in the cytosol. The catabolism of LCFAs, such as palmitate, occurs in the mitochondria through beta-oxidation for the synthesis of ATP. In order to cross the mitochondrial membrane, fatty acids must bind to carnitine [3]. The fatty acid is linked to CoA by Acyl-CoA-synthetase, forming an acyl-CoA to interact with carnitine palmitoyl transferase 1 (CPT1) in the outer mitochondrial membrane. This enzyme will exchange CoA for carnitine; that is, CPT1 transforms acyl CoA to acyl-carnitine, which allows the movement of the molecule toward the internal mitochondrial membrane where acyl-CoA is reconstituted with the enzyme carnitine palmitoyltransferase-2 (CPT2), allowing the entry of acyl-CoA into the mitochondrial matrix for oxidation. The acetyl-CoA resulting from beta-oxidation is oxidized in the tricarboxylic acid (TCA) cycle; in both metabolic pathways, reduced coenzymes (NADH and $FADH_2$) are obtained, which are responsible for donating electrons in the electron transport chain to form the proton gradient necessary for the synthesis of ATP molecules [8]. CPT-1 is the rate-limiting enzyme in fatty acid oxidation in mitochondria. CPT-1 deficiency results in energy failure and kidney disease. Three isoforms of CPT1 have been described (a, b, and c). The three isoforms are mainly expressed in the organs with high metabolic rates, such as the kidney and liver (CPT1a); skeletal muscle, heart, and adipose tissue (CPT1b); and brain and testes (CPT1c) [9].

In eukaryotes, principally in mammals, peroxisomes in conjunction with mitochondria constitute a tactical collaboration in the interplay of energy metabolism in cells. Usually, short- and medium-chain fatty acids are transformed mainly by mitochondria, while very long-chain fatty acids (VLCFAs) with more than 22 carbons are metabolized by peroxisomes. The VLCFAs in the peroxisomes are shortened and later transported to mitochondria, where they are oxidized to acetyl-CoA. Fatty acid oxidation in peroxisomes generates H_2O_2, a byproduct of oxidative reactions. In peroxisomes, the energy is released as heat because these organelles do not contain respiratory chain enzymes coupled to the generation of ATP. Fatty acid oxidation enzymes differ between peroxisomes and mitochondria. The first reaction in peroxisomal fatty acid oxidation is catalyzed by an acyl-CoA oxidase (ACOX), followed by reactions catalyzed by a bifunctional enzyme and 3-ketoacyl-CoA thiolase. The impaired activity of peroxisomal enzymes, mainly the rate-limiting enzyme ACOX, is responsible for unmetabolized fatty acids that promote lipoperoxidation and cellular damage, increasing oxidative stress and apoptosis [10].

GLUCOSE METABOLISM

Although the proximal tubules of the nephron prefer fatty acids as energy substrates, the kidney is a key organ for the reabsorption, production, and utilization of glucose. The kidney maintains glucose homeostasis through gluconeogenesis and uses glucose as a metabolic substrate. Almost all glucose in the glomerular filtrate is reabsorbed in the proximal tubule by the two isoforms of glucose/Na^+ transporters (SGLT1 and SGLT2) located in the apical zone of the tubular epithelium. Ninety percent of the filtered glucose is reabsorbed by SGLT2, which is a transporter with low affinity for its substrates and high transport capacity; SGLT2 is located mainly in the segments S1 and S2 of the proximal tubule, and its solute stoichiometry is one Na^+ per glucose (1:1). The remaining ~10% of glucose reabsorption is glucose, which SGLT1 facilitates. SGLT1 is a transporter with a high affinity for its substrates and low transport capacity. It is located in segment S3 of the proximal tubule. Its stoichiometry is two ions, $Na+$ per glucose (2:1) [11]. Na^+ gradients are primarily maintained by the principal active Na^+/K^+-pump, or Na^+/K^+-ATPase, and by SGLT1 through sugar cotransport as a secondary active transport. Therefore, glucose transport directly depends on the magnitude of the Na gradients across the plasma membrane. In normal cells, the Na^+/K^+-pump determines the direction and magnitude of the sodium gradient [12]. Despite the large amount of glucose entering the proximal tubules, only a small quantity of glucose is metabolized in the undamaged proximal tubules, so the reabsorbed glucose returns to the bloodstream through glucose transporters (GLUTs) that are in the basolateral tubular epithelial cell region. GLUT2 is found in the S1 and S2 segments, whereas GLUT1 is present in the S3 segment [13, 14].

Research on renal metabolism using *in vivo* radioactive isotope techniques, such as [3H] glucose, has enabled detailed glucose production and utilization assessments. Findings from these studies indicate that the kidneys significantly contribute to overall glucose production and utilization [15]. Currently, the human kidney is recognized for its role in regulating glucose homeostasis. It produces glucose through gluconeogenesis, releases it into the bloodstream, and reabsorbs it from the glomerular filtrate. During fasting, the liver and kidneys release comparable amounts of glucose synthesized during gluconeogenesis. However, in the postprandial state, renal gluconeogenesis approximately doubles as the endogenous release of glucose significantly diminishes. The liver and kidneys are the only organs that can synthesize and release glucose into the bloodstream because they contain glucose 6-phosphatase, which is essential for converting glucose-6-phosphate into glucose. Glucose production can occur through glycogenolysis or gluconeogenesis. However, since the kidneys lack glycogen reserves, they do not utilize the glycogenolysis pathway [16]. Substrates in gluconeogenesis like lactate, glycerol, alanine, and glutamine are the principal sources of glucose-6-phosphate. Studies have shown that lactate is the primary precursor for gluconeogenesis in the kidneys [17].

The kidneys produce approximately 25% of the glucose released into the bloodstream [15]. The production and consumption of glucose in the kidney occur in different areas of renal tubules. Gluconeogenesis occurs in the proximal tubules because the cells contain regulatory enzymes of this pathway, including glucose-6-phosphatase, phosphoenolpyruvate carboxykinase (PEPCK), and fructose-1,--bisphosphatase. In contrast, distal tubules use glucose to obtain energy. Enzymes that regulate glycolysis, such as hexokinase, phosphofructokinase, and pyruvate kinase, are expressed in the thick ascending loops of Henle and the distal and collecting tubules [3]. Many studies have shown that distal tubules convert glucose into lactate, even when oxygen is present. Conversely, the amount of lactate derived from glucose in proximal tubules is negligible, suggesting that proximal tubules possess a restricted ability to transform glucose into lactate [18]. Hence, in the renal tubules, both anabolism and catabolism of glucose occur localized. Proximal tubules produce glucose through gluconeogenesis, whereas distal nephron segments metabolize this glucose *via* glycolysis.

Notably, renal glucose release and uptake are under hormonal control. Insulin and catecholamines are part of acute glucoregulatory mechanisms that activate/deactivate the key enzymes of glycolysis or gluconeogenesis to regulate plasma glucose levels [14]. Insulin suppresses the release of glucose in the liver and the kidney, reduces the disposal of gluconeogenic substrates, and reduces gluconeogenic activator activity [19].

Catecholamines are also implicated in controlling glucose homeostasis in the kidney, with several acute effects, including stimulating renal glucose release, inhibiting insulin secretion, increasing the supply of gluconeogenic substrates, stimulating lipolysis, and reducing glucose uptake in tissues [20]. Hence, the kidney is important in controlling blood glucose because it can improve impaired hepatic glucose release and manage the increased glucose release observed in people with diabetes.

AMINO ACID METABOLISM

Under physiological conditions, the kidneys are involved in various amino acids' biosynthesis, reabsorption, and catabolism. Approximately 70 grams of free amino acids are filtered daily by the glomerulus. In the proximal tubule, the reabsorption of these amino acids is facilitated through diffusion, facilitated diffusion, and sodium-dependent active transport. This process involves various transporters on the apical membrane of proximal tubule cells, ensuring the maintenance of amino acid homeostasis in the plasma [21]. The HUGO Gene Nomenclature Committee (HGNC) has classified amino acid transporters into distinct SLC families according to sequence identity. Currently, 65 different SLC (Solute Carrier Transporters) families with high phylogenetic diversity have been identified. Most amino acid transporters in the kidney are members of the SLC1, SLC3, SLC6, SLC7, SLC36, SLC38, and SLC43 families. The amino acids reabsorbed by these transporters may serve as substrates for gluconeogenesis to produce glucose or substrates at different points of the TCA cycle and be oxidized. Generally, amino acids are categorized as glucogenic or ketogenic based on the type of products produced from their metabolism. For example, glycine, glutamine, glutamic acid, cysteine, aspartic acid, asparagine, arginine, and alanine are known as glucogenic amino acids because they are converted into either pyruvate or one of the intermediates in the TCA cycle. In the case of leucine and lysine, these are strictly ketogenic amino acids since they are catabolized only to acetyl-CoA [22, 23].

Leucine, isoleucine, and valine are considered branched-chain amino acids (BCAAs), an essential energy source. The kidneys reabsorb these amino acids after they consume a protein-rich meal. Accordingly, the kidneys contribute a substantial fraction of the circulating BCAAs (one-third of whole-body leucine production) by regulating their uptake, oxidation, and proteolysis. The first product of BAACs catabolism is branched-chain ketoacid, obtained from a limiting reaction catalyzed by branched-chain aminotransferases (BCAT) through transamination of BCAAs. Later, the branched-chain alpha-keto acid dehydrogenase (BCKDH) complex oxidatively decarboxylates the produced ketoacids. As a result, the end products of BCAA metabolism enter the tricarboxylic acid cycle (TCA) as acetyl-CoA or succinyl-CoA, where they are further oxidized [24]. It has been estimated that almost 8–13% of human BCAA metabolism occurs in the kidney [25]. Elevated plasma concentrations of BCAAs have been associated with insulin resistance and related metabolic disturbances, as well as with pancreatic cancer and heart disease [26, 27]. There has been reported an association between elevated BCAA levels and the risk of progression to end-stage renal failure in patients with type 2 diabetes, suggesting that the role of amino acids in the kidney is complex and can impact the progression of CKD. However, the mechanisms involved are unclear [28, 29].

Dietary proteins and circulating amino acids have been shown to regulate kidney function. High-protein diets can increase amino acid exposure in the proximal tubules, increase hyperfiltration, and possibly stimulate the development of CKD [30, 31]. Indeed, patients affected with diabetes and rodents exposed to a protein-rich diet or amino acid infusion progress to renal failure *via* increased glomerular hyperfiltration, which may directly impact the different kinds of kidney cells. Additionally, dietary proteins and circulating amino acids can indirectly impact glucagon, nitric oxide, and angiotensin II pathways [32, 33].

Conversely, independent of their capacity to generate energy, proteins, and amino acids can also regulate acid-base balance through the acid load (NH_4^+) produced during their metabolism. In this context, urinary ammonia excretion comprises approximately 50% to 70% of the net basal acid excretion in humans and rodents. Glutamine is the primary amino acid used during renal ammonia genesis to preserve acid/base equilibrium in the body because its metabolism in proximal tubules produces equal concentrations of ammonia and bicarbonate. Glutamine is metabolized in the proximal tubule to glutamate, converted to alfa-ketoglutarate, a TCA cycle intermediary, and oxidized to CO2 in the TCA cycle. A portion of this ammonia enters the urine *via* the sodium-hydrogen exchanger-3 (NHE3), and bicarbonate. This latter is returned to circulation through the basolateral sodium-coupled bicarbonate cotransporter, isoform 1A (NBCe-1A) [34]. Hence, during acidosis, in order to maintain acid-base balance, glutamine metabolism in the proximal tubule has to increase. This latter is achieved through the upregulation of glutaminase and the increased expression of basolateral glutamine transporters, which boosts the uptake of this amino acid into the tubules [35]. Glutamine is the primary source of ammonia production, while the metabolism of other amino acids can only contribute with a minor fraction [36].

Amino acids play crucial roles in the kidney's biological functions. For example, citrulline, a byproduct of the urea cycle produced by enterocytes in the small intestine, is converted into arginine in the kidneys' proximal convoluted tubules. Arginine, an amino acid precursor to nitric oxide (NO), is vital for endothelial function and has significant implications for blood properties, including the immune response and protein synthesis [37, 38].

Additionally, tyrosine is produced in the kidney through the hydroxylation of phenylalanine by phenylalanine hydroxylase, an active enzyme in the kidney and liver. Tyrosine is important for synthesizing neurotransmitters (such as epinephrine, norepinephrine, and dopamine) and producing thyroid hormones. Notably, patients with end-stage renal disease (ESRD) exhibit a 50% decrease in the conversion rate of phenylalanine to tyrosine compared with individuals with normal renal function [39, 40]. Although in the healthy kidney, the most significant energy contribution to metabolism is obtained from glucose and fatty acids, the metabolism of amino acids is crucial for the homeostasis of an organism.

METABOLIC CHANGES IN KIDNEY DISEASE

As previously stated, the cells of the renal tubules, particularly those in the proximal tubules, distal convoluted tubules, and connecting segments, are abundant in the mitochondria. Consequently, the substantial oxygen demand of these tubules increases their susceptibility to kidney injury when exposed to hypoxic conditions. The proximal tubule S3 segment is particularly vulnerable to damage because of its high expression of transporters and movement of solutes, making it susceptible to toxins such as mercury and lead or drugs such as aminoglycosides. Additionally, inadequate oxygen supply resulting from compromised hemodynamics, as observed in conditions such as sepsis, ischemia, or cardiopulmonary bypass, is a primary cause of kidney injury. This latter is due to significant disruptions in renal tubules, leading to damage progression. Consequently, such injury can progress to acute kidney injury (AKI) or chronic kidney disease (CKD). Clinically, patients with AKI are at a substantially increased risk of developing CKD [41].

In AKI, there are evident changes in mitochondrial structure and function. These changes are associated with decreased mitochondrial quantity in proximal tubule cells, organelle swelling, and disrupted cristae. Such mitochondrial disturbances contribute to the pathophysiology of kidney damage in AKI and its progression to CKD. Moreover, disruption in mitochondrial fusion and fission results in mitochondrial fragmentation, initiating the release of cytochrome c and mitochondrial DNA, which may trigger apoptosis and lead to impairments in energy metabolism [42, 43].

There is compelling evidence indicating that fatty acid oxidation is suppressed in AKI, favoring the metabolism of anaerobic glycolysis, which leads to the production of lactic acid. During ischemia-reperfusion injury, there is an increase in lactate and pyruvate levels in the affected kidney, along with an increase in the expression of glycolytic enzymes such as hexokinase 2, indicating the activation of anaerobic glycolysis [44]. It remains uncertain whether anaerobic glycolysis aids in the recovery of tubular damage or merely reflects the persistence of injury [3].

In addition, concerning the changes observed in FAO in renal injury caused by ischemia, a reduction in the fatty acid oxidation limiting enzyme carnitine palmitoyl-transferase 1 (CPT1) contributes to the deterioration of this metabolism after ischemic renal failure. The administration of C75, a synthetic compound (α-methylene-γ-butyrolactone) that upregulates CPT1 activity and is a fatty acid synthase inhibitor, ameliorated kidney function, reduced renal injury, and suppressed proinflammatory cytokine production and neutrophil infiltration after

IR insult. Therefore, enhancing metabolic pathways for energy production may provide a novel modality for treating renal injury [45].

Another significant aspect of altered fatty acid metabolism is the intracellular accumulation of fatty acid caused by decreased oxidation of these molecules, potentially leading to lipotoxicity. During ischemia, an imbalance occurs between the hydrolysis and removal of membrane phospholipids due to a disparity in re-esterification and the oxidation of mitochondrial fatty acids. This disruption leads to the accumulation of no-esterified fatty acids (NEFAs), which can function as detergents, increasing membrane permeability and ultimately inducing apoptosis. The activation of metabolic pathways that favor the reduction of NEFAs (for example, the application of substrates of the citric acid cycle) protects proximal tubules from injury caused by hypoxia-reoxygenation. It restores the normal production of ATP [46 - 48]. The sequestration of harmful fatty acids such as triglycerides may represent an innate adaptive response to injury. The presence of triglycerides in the cortical and medullary segments of nephrons is increasingly recognized as a characteristic of several types of kidney injuries, such as acute obstruction, experimental sepsis, and ischemia-reperfusion injury [49].

Endothelial nitric oxide synthase (eNOS) is known to protect against kidney injury, although the underlying molecular mechanisms have not been fully characterized; it is known that cell signaling by nitric oxide is generally mediated by S-nitrosylation of proteins through the oxidation of cysteine residues to form S-nitrosothiols. This mechanism regulates the function of several proteins, including S-nitrosylases and denitrosylases, which add and remove S-nitrosothiols from proteins, respectively [50]. A study by Zhou *et al.* showed inhibitory S-nitrosylation of the enzyme pyruvate kinase M2 (PKM2) inhibits glycolysis; as a consequence, the PKM2 enzyme becomes less functional when S-nitrosylated, which protects against IR. It has been proposed that the protective mechanism is due to the pentose phosphate pathway being preferred by blocking glycolysis, which increases the generation of NADPH, increasing the amount of glutathione and the activity of antioxidant enzymes. Therefore, directing glucose from glycolysis toward energy generation through the pentose phosphate pathway may protect the kidneys from ischemic damage by reducing oxidative stress [51]. On the contrary, other studies have reported that glycolysis is suppressed in AKI transiently. However, tubular cells can be protected from ischemia-reperfusion injury (IR), promoting glycolysis in AKI. In the renal outer medullary proximal straight tubules, the proteins poly(ADP–ribose) polymerase-1 (PARP-1) and Tp53-induced glycolysis and apoptosis regulator (TIGAR) are induced and activated after an event of IR, promoting a reduction in glycolysis [52, 53]. PARP-1 reduces glycolysis by inhibiting glyceraldehyde-3-phosphate dehydrogenase (GAPDH) during IR. Inhibition of PARP-1 function was found to be cytoprotective by restoring GAPDH activity and ATP levels and decreasing tubular cell death in an *in vitro* hypoxia/reperfusion model [52]. Conversely, TIGAR can regulate phosphofructokinase-1 and glucose 6-phosphate dehydrogenase (G6PD) activities and glycolytic pathway, inducing ATP depletion, oxidative stress, autophagy, and apoptosis, promoting damage. If G6PD activity and NADPH levels are restored, TIGAR activation can redirect the glycolytic pathway to gluconeogenesis or the pentose phosphate pathway to produce NADPH in mild ischemia. Hence, increasing the NADPH level reduces the glutathione (GSH) level and, consequently, the reactive oxygen species (ROS), which results in less injury to the proximal tubule cells. In severe ischemia, G6PD activity and NADPH levels are reduced during reperfusion. Therefore, blocking TIGAR increase during severe ischemia reduced oxidative stress and apoptosis, protecting proximal tubule cells from severe IR injury. When a low ischemic load was produced, the pentose phosphate pathway and autophagy were activated by TIGAR as a defensive mechanism [53].

Complete glucose oxidation has a protective role in AKI. In hypoxia, the enzyme pyruvate dehydrogenase (PDH), which connects glycolysis to the TAC cycle, is inhibited by phosphorylation processes regulated by pyruvate dehydrogenase kinase (PDK). Consequently, an increase in PDH phosphorylation accompanied by tubular atrophy and increased expression of glycolytic enzymes and lactate accumulation in AKI has been observed [54, 55]. This increase in PDH phosphorylation and decrease in renal function have also been observed in patients treated with cisplatin, a chemotherapeutic agent whose use is often limited owing to its nephrotoxicity (as mentioned in chapter 11).

Other cellular organelles that may participate in the development of AKI are peroxisomes. As mentioned above, peroxisomes preferentially oxidize VLCFAs, and this metabolic process generates hydrogen peroxide (H_2O_2), which needs a large amount of catalase to metabolize the H_2O_2 produced without generating cellular damage due to the production of reactive oxygen species (ROS) [56]. Therefore, peroxisomes and supporting mitochondria eliminate ROS by completely oxidizing fatty acids, a process deregulated in AKI. Sirtuin 5 (Sirt5) may play an important role in regulating fatty acid oxidation. Studies involving wild-type and Sirt5 knockout mice showed a significant increase in renal function, which diminished damage following ischemia or cisplatin treatment. The authors suggested that deletion of Sirt5 reversed the posttranslational acylation of lysine in several enzymes implicated in FAO. Therefore, the protection of Sirt5 deficiency is mediated by the reduction of mitochondrial-derived ROS and driving peroxisomal FAO. Hence, blocking Sirt5 can be a potential treatment for treating AKI [56, 57].

Current drug therapies cannot wholly treat or prevent kidney disease, leaving the management of associated complications as the only option [58, 59]. Clinical trials have demonstrated that the use of hypoxia-inducible factor (HIF)-prolyl hydroxylase domain inhibitors improve anemia derived from CKD and that sodium-glucose cotransporter 2 (SGLT2) inhibitors help to prevent kidney failure in patients with type 2 diabetes and CKD [60, 61]. The clinical advantages are believed to stem from the modulation of cellular metabolism [62]. The kidneys are remarkable for housing a variety of distinct epithelial, vascular, and stromal cells, along with tissue-resident immune cells, whose functions can be influenced by the availability of nutrients and energy metabolism.

CONCLUSION

These data suggest that AKI reduces fatty acid oxidation and glucose oxidation *via* mitochondrial dysfunction, leading to increased anaerobic glycolysis and lactic acid production. Knowledge of these metabolic changes has made it possible to propose targets or therapeutic strategies to restore the normal metabolism of the renal tubules, such as increasing biogenesis and mitochondrial function and promoting the oxidation of fatty acids and glucose. As mentioned, procedures or therapies can improve tubular injury and kidney function. On the other hand, the regulation of protein expression involved in physiological changes in kidney disease has aroused interest as a therapeutic target that could allow the restoration of renal homeostasis, as is the case for sirtuins.

REFERENCES

[1]   Wessely O, Cerqueira DM, Tran U, Kumar V, Hassey JM, Romaker D. The bigger the better: determining nephron size in kidney. Pediatr Nephrol 2014; 29(4): 525-30.
[http://dx.doi.org/10.1007/s00467-013-2581-x] [PMID: 23974984]

[2]   Quatredeniers M, Serafin AS, Benmerah A, Rausell A, Saunier S, Viau A. Meta-analysis of single-cell and single-nucleus transcriptomics reveals kidney cell type consensus signatures. Sci Data 2023; 10(1): 361.
[http://dx.doi.org/10.1038/s41597-023-02209-9] [PMID: 37280226]

[3]   Gewin LS. Sugar or fat? Renal tubular metabolism reviewed in health and disease. Nutrients 2021; 13(5): 1580.
[http://dx.doi.org/10.3390/nu13051580] [PMID: 34065078]

[4]   Simon N, Hertig A. Alteration of fatty acid oxidation in tubular epithelial cells: From acute kidney injury to renal fibrogenesis. Front Med (Lausanne) 2015; 2: 52.
[http://dx.doi.org/10.3389/fmed.2015.00052] [PMID: 26301223]

[5]   Yang X, Okamura DM, Lu X, *et al.* CD36 in chronic kidney disease: novel insights and therapeutic opportunities. Nat Rev Nephrol 2017; 13(12): 769-81.
[http://dx.doi.org/10.1038/nrneph.2017.126] [PMID: 28919632]

[6]   Jin R, Hao J, Yi Y, Sauter E, Li B. Regulation of macrophage functions by FABP-mediated inflammatory and metabolic pathways. Biochim Biophys Acta Mol Cell Biol Lipids 2021; 1866(8): 158964.
[http://dx.doi.org/10.1016/j.bbalip.2021.158964] [PMID: 33984518]

[7]   Gai Z, Wang T, Visentin M, Kullak-Ublick G, Fu X, Wang Z. Lipid accumulation and chronic kidney disease. Nutrients 2019; 11(4): 722.
[http://dx.doi.org/10.3390/nu11040722] [PMID: 30925738]

[8]   Houten SM, Violante S, Ventura FV, Wanders RJA. The Biochemistry and Physiology of Mitochondrial Fatty Acid β-Oxidation and Its Genetic Disorders. Annu Rev Physiol 2016; 78(1): 23-44.
[http://dx.doi.org/10.1146/annurev-physiol-021115-105045] [PMID: 26474213]

[9]   Szeto HH. Pharmacologic approaches to improve mitochondrial function in AKI and CKD. J Am Soc Nephrol 2017; 28(10): 2856-65.
[http://dx.doi.org/10.1681/ASN.2017030247] [PMID: 28778860]

[10]   Visko R. Peroxisomes and kidney injury. Antioxid Redox Signal 2016; 25: 217-31.
[http://dx.doi.org/10.1089/ars.2016.6666] [PMID: 26972522]

[11]   Wright EM, Ghezzi C, Loo DDF. Novel and unexpected functions of SGLTs. Physiology (Bethesda) 2017; 32(6): 435-43.
[http://dx.doi.org/10.1152/physiol.00021.2017] [PMID: 29021363]

[12]   Wright EM, Hirayama BA, Loo DF. Active sugar transport in health and disease. J Intern Med 2007; 261(1): 32-43.
[http://dx.doi.org/10.1111/j.1365-2796.2006.01746.x] [PMID: 17222166]

[13]   Szablewski L. Distribution of glucose transporters in renal diseases. J Biomed Sci 2017; 24(1): 64.
[http://dx.doi.org/10.1186/s12929-017-0371-7] [PMID: 28854935]

[14]   Mitrakou A. Kidney: Its impact on glucose homeostasis and hormonal regulation. Diabetes Res Clin Pract 2011; 93 (Suppl. 1): S66-72.
[http://dx.doi.org/10.1016/S0168-8227(11)70016-X] [PMID: 21864754]

[15]   Stumvoll M, Chintalapudi U, Perriello G, Welle S, Gutierrez O, Gerich J. Uptake and release of glucose by the human kidney. Postabsorptive rates and responses to epinephrine. J Clin Invest 1995; 96(5): 2528-33.
[http://dx.doi.org/10.1172/JCI118314] [PMID: 7593645]

[16]   Stumvoll M, Meyer C, Mitrakou A, Nadkarni V, Gerich JE. Renal glucose production and utilization: new aspects in humans. Diabetologia 1997; 40(7): 749-57.
[http://dx.doi.org/10.1007/s001250050745] [PMID: 9243094]

[17]   Meyer C, Stumvoll M, Dostou J, Welle S, Haymond M, Gerich J. Renal substrate exchange and gluconeogenesis in normal postabsorptive humans. Am J Physiol Endocrinol Metab 2002; 282(2): E428-34.
[http://dx.doi.org/10.1152/ajpendo.00116.2001] [PMID: 11788376]

[18]   Bagnasco S, Good D, Balaban R, Burg M. Lactate production in isolated segments of the rat nephron. Am J Physiol Renal Physiol 1985; 248(4): F522-6. Epub ahead of print
[http://dx.doi.org/10.1152/ajprenal.1985.248.4.F522] [PMID: 3985159]

[19]   Sahoo B, Srivastava M, Katiyar A, Ecelbarger C, Tiwari S. Liver or kidney: Who has the oar in the gluconeogenesis boat and when? World J Diabetes 2023; 14(7): 1049-56.
[http://dx.doi.org/10.4239/wjd.v14.i7.1049] [PMID: 37547592]

[20]   Lelou E, Corlu A, Nesseler N, *et al.* The Role of Catecholamines in Pathophysiological Liver Processes. Cells 2022; 11(6): 1021. Epub ahead of print
[http://dx.doi.org/10.3390/cells11061021] [PMID: 35326472]

[21]   Verrey F, Singer D, Ramadan T, Vuille-dit-Bille RN, Mariotta L, Camargo SMR. Kidney amino acid transport. Pflugers Arch 2009; 458(1): 53-60.
[http://dx.doi.org/10.1007/s00424-009-0638-2] [PMID: 19184091]

[22]   Kandasamy P, Gyimesi G, Kanai Y, Hediger MA. Amino acid transporters revisited: New views in

health and disease. Trends Biochem Sci 2018; 43(10): 752-89.
[http://dx.doi.org/10.1016/j.tibs.2018.05.003] [PMID: 30177408]

[23]   Hinden L, Kogot-Levin A, Tam J, *et al.* Pathogenesis of diabesity-induced kidney disease: role of kidney nutrient sensing. FEBS J 2022; 289(4): 901-21.
[http://dx.doi.org/10.1111/febs.15790] [PMID: 33630415]

[24]   Neinast MD, Jang C, Hui S, *et al.* Quantitative Analysis of the Whole-Body Metabolic Fate of Branched-Chain Amino Acids. Cell Metab 2019; 29(2): 417-429.e4.
[http://dx.doi.org/10.1016/j.cmet.2018.10.013] [PMID: 30449684]

[25]   Karlsson KR, Ko R, Blomstrand E. Branched-Chain Amino Acids: Metabolism, Physiological Function, and Application Branched-Chain Amino Acids Activate Key Enzymes in Protein Synthesis. J Nutr 2006; 136: 269-73.
[http://dx.doi.org/10.1093/jn/136.1.269S]

[26]   Mayers JR, Wu C, Clish CB, *et al.* Elevation of circulating branched-chain amino acids is an early event in human pancreatic adenocarcinoma development. Nat Med 2014; 20(10): 1193-8.
[http://dx.doi.org/10.1038/nm.3686] [PMID: 25261994]

[27]   Huang Y, Zhou M, Sun H, Wang Y. Branched-chain amino acid metabolism in heart disease: an epiphenomenon or a real culprit? Cardiovasc Res 2011; 90(2): 220-3.
[http://dx.doi.org/10.1093/cvr/cvr070] [PMID: 21502372]

[28]   Niewczas MA, Sirich TL, Mathew AV, *et al.* Uremic solutes and risk of end-stage renal disease in type 2 diabetes: metabolomic study. Kidney Int 2014; 85(5): 1214-24.
[http://dx.doi.org/10.1038/ki.2013.497] [PMID: 24429397]

[29]   Welsh P, Rankin N, Li Q, *et al.* Circulating amino acids and the risk of macrovascular, microvascular and mortality outcomes in individuals with type 2 diabetes: results from the ADVANCE trial. Diabetologia 2018; 61(7): 1581-91.
[http://dx.doi.org/10.1007/s00125-018-4619-x] [PMID: 29728717]

[30]   Jhee JH, Kee YK, Park S, *et al.* High-protein diet with renal hyperfiltration is associated with rapid decline rate of renal function: a community-based prospective cohort study. Nephrol Dial Transplant 2019; 35(1): gfz115.
[http://dx.doi.org/10.1093/ndt/gfz115] [PMID: 31172186]

[31]   Malhotra R, Lipworth L, Cavanaugh KL, *et al.* Protein Intake and Long-term Change in Glomerular Filtration Rate in the Jackson Heart Study. J Ren Nutr 2018; 28(4): 245-50.
[http://dx.doi.org/10.1053/j.jrn.2017.11.008] [PMID: 29452887]

[32]   Tuttle KR, Puhlman ME, Cooney SK, Short RA. Effects of amino acids and glucagon on renal hemodynamics in type 1 diabetes. Am J Physiol Renal Physiol 2002; 282(1): F103-12. Epub ahead of print
[http://dx.doi.org/10.1152/ajprenal.00155.2001] [PMID: 11739118]

[33]   Ko GJ, Rhee CM, Kalantar-Zadeh K, Joshi S. The Effects of High-Protein Diets on Kidney Health and Longevity. J Am Soc Nephrol 2020; 31(8): 1667-79.
[http://dx.doi.org/10.1681/ASN.2020010028] [PMID: 32669325]

[34]   Weiner ID, Verlander JW. Renal ammonia metabolism and transport. Compr Physiol 2013; 3(1): 201-20.
[http://dx.doi.org/10.1002/cphy.c120010] [PMID: 23720285]

[35]   Moret C, Dave MH, Schulz N, Jiang JX, Verrey F, Wagner CA. Regulation of renal amino acid transporters during metabolic acidosis. Am J Physiol Renal Physiol 2007; 292(2): F555-66.
[http://dx.doi.org/10.1152/ajprenal.00113.2006] [PMID: 17003226]

[36]   Weiner ID, Mitch WE, Sands JM. Urea and ammonia metabolism and the control of renal nitrogen excretion. Clin J Am Soc Nephrol 2015; 10(8): 1444-58.
[http://dx.doi.org/10.2215/CJN.10311013] [PMID: 25078422]

[37]   Wu G, Bazer FW, Davis TA, *et al.* Arginine metabolism and nutrition in growth, health and disease. Amino Acids 2009; 37(1): 153-68.
[http://dx.doi.org/10.1007/s00726-008-0210-y] [PMID: 19030957]

[38]   Bahadoran Z, Mirmiran P, Kashfi K, *et al.* Endogenous flux of nitric oxide: Citrulline is preferred to arginine. Acta Physiol 2021; 231: 0–1.
[http://dx.doi.org/10.1111/apha.13572]

[39]   van de Poll MCG, Soeters PB, Deutz NEP, Fearon KCH, Dejong CHC. Renal metabolism of amino acids: its role in interorgan amino acid exchange. Am J Clin Nutr 2004; 79(2): 185-97.
[http://dx.doi.org/10.1093/ajcn/79.2.185] [PMID: 14749222]

[40]   Kopple JD. Phenylalanine and tyrosine metabolism in chronic kidney failure. J Nutr 2007; 137(6) (Suppl. 1): 1586S-90S.
[http://dx.doi.org/10.1093/jn/137.6.1586S] [PMID: 17513431]

[41]   Coca SG, Singanamala S, Parikh CR. Chronic kidney disease after acute kidney injury: a systematic review and meta-analysis. Kidney Int 2012; 81(5): 442-8.
[http://dx.doi.org/10.1038/ki.2011.379] [PMID: 22113526]

[42]   Zhang X, Agborbesong E, Li X. The Role of Mitochondria in Acute Kidney Injury and Chronic Kidney Disease and Its Therapeutic Potential. Int J Mol Sci 2021; 22(20): 11253. Epub ahead of print [http://dx.doi.org/10.3390/ijms222011253] [PMID: 34681922]

[43]   Tang C, Cai J, Yin XM, Weinberg JM, Venkatachalam MA, Dong Z. Mitochondrial quality control in kidney injury and repair. Nat Rev Nephrol 2021; 17(5): 299-318.
[http://dx.doi.org/10.1038/s41581-020-00369-0] [PMID: 33235391]

[44]   Lan R, Geng H, Singha PK, *et al.* Mitochondrial pathology and glycolytic shift during proximal tubule atrophy after ischemic AKI. J Am Soc Nephrol 2016; 27(11): 3356-67.
[http://dx.doi.org/10.1681/ASN.2015020177] [PMID: 27000065]

[45]   Idrovo JP, Yang WL, Nicastro J, Coppa GF, Wang P. Stimulation of carnitine palmitoyltransferase 1 improves renal function and attenuates tissue damage after ischemia/reperfusion. J Surg Res 2012; 177(1): 157-64.
[http://dx.doi.org/10.1016/j.jss.2012.05.053] [PMID: 22698429]

[46]   Feldkamp T, Kribben A, Roeser NF, *et al.* Accumulation of nonesterified fatty acids causes the sustained energetic deficit in kidney proximal tubules after hypoxia-reoxygenation. Am J Physiol Renal Physiol 2021; 0676: 465-77.
[http://dx.doi.org/10.1152/ajprenal.00305.2005] [PMID: 16159894]

[47]   Weinberg JM, Venkatachalam MA, Roeser NF, Nissim I. Mitochondrial dysfunction during hypoxia/reoxygenation and its correction by anaerobic metabolism of citric acid cycle intermediates. Proc Natl Acad Sci USA 2000; 97(6): 2826-31.
[http://dx.doi.org/10.1073/pnas.97.6.2826] [PMID: 10717001]

[48]   Bienholz A, Al-Taweel A, Roeser NF, Kribben A, Feldkamp T, Weinberg JM. Substrate modulation of fatty acid effects on energization and respiration of kidney proximal tubules during hypoxia/reoxygenation. PLoS One 2014; 9(4): e94584. Epub ahead of print [http://dx.doi.org/10.1371/journal.pone.0094584] [PMID: 24728405]

[49]   Zager RA, Johnson ACM, Hanson SY. Renal tubular triglyercide accumulation following endotoxic, toxic, and ischemic injury. Kidney Int 2005; 67(1): 111-21.
[http://dx.doi.org/10.1111/j.1523-1755.2005.00061.x] [PMID: 15610234]

[50]   Seth D, Hess DT, Hausladen A, Wang L, Wang Y, Stamler JS. A Multiplex Enzymatic Machinery for Cellular Protein S-nitrosylation. Mol Cell 2018; 69(3): 451-464.e6.
[http://dx.doi.org/10.1016/j.molcel.2017.12.025] [PMID: 29358078]

[51]   Zhou H, Zhang R, Anand P, *et al.* Metabolic Reprogramming by the S-nitroso-CoA Reductase System Protects Against Kidney Injury. Nature 2019; 570.

[http://dx.doi.org/10.1038/s41586-018-0749-z]

[52]   Devalaraja-Narashimha K, Padanilam BJ. PARP-1 inhibits glycolysis in ischemic kidneys. J Am Soc Nephrol 2009; 20(1): 95-103.
[http://dx.doi.org/10.1681/ASN.2008030325] [PMID: 19056868]

[53]   Kim J, Devalaraja-Narashimha K, Padanilam BJ. TIGAR regulates glycolysis in ischemic kidney proximal tubules. Am J Physiol Renal Physiol 2015; 308(4): F298-308.
[http://dx.doi.org/10.1152/ajprenal.00459.2014] [PMID: 25503731]

[54]   Lu CW, Lin SC, Chen KF, Lai YY, Tsai SJ. Induction of pyruvate dehydrogenase kinase-3 by hypoxia-inducible factor-1 promotes metabolic switch and drug resistance. J Biol Chem 2008; 283(42): 28106-14.
[http://dx.doi.org/10.1074/jbc.M803508200] [PMID: 18718909]

[55]   Kim J, Tchernyshyov I, Semenza GL, Dang CV. HIF-1-mediated expression of pyruvate dehydrogenase kinase: A metabolic switch required for cellular adaptation to hypoxia. Cell Metab 2006; 3(3): 177-85.
[http://dx.doi.org/10.1016/j.cmet.2006.02.002] [PMID: 16517405]

[56]   Peasley K, Chiba T, Goetzman E, Sims-Lucas S. Sirtuins play critical and diverse roles in acute kidney injury. Pediatr Nephrol 2021; 36(11): 3539-46. Epub ahead of print
[http://dx.doi.org/10.1007/s00467-020-04866-z] [PMID: 33411071]

[57]   Chiba T, Peasley KD, Cargill KR, *et al.* Sirtuin 5 regulates proximal tubule fatty acid oxidation to protect against AKI. J Am Soc Nephrol 2019; 30(12): 2384-98.
[http://dx.doi.org/10.1681/ASN.2019020163] [PMID: 31575700]

[58]   Chen TK, Knicely DH, Grams ME. Chronic Kidney Disease Diagnosis and Management. JAMA 2019; 322(13): 1294-304.
[http://dx.doi.org/10.1001/jama.2019.14745] [PMID: 31573641]

[59]   Basso PJ, Andrade-Oliveira V, Câmara NOS. Targeting immune cell metabolism in kidney diseases. Nat Rev Nephrol 2021; 17(7): 465-80.
[http://dx.doi.org/10.1038/s41581-021-00413-7] [PMID: 33828286]

[60]   Gupta N, Wish JB. Hypoxia-Inducible Factor Prolyl Hydroxylase Inhibitors: A Potential New Treatment for Anemia in Patients With CKD. Am J Kidney Dis 2017; 69(6): 815-26.
[http://dx.doi.org/10.1053/j.ajkd.2016.12.011] [PMID: 28242135]

[61]   Perkovic V, Jardine MJ, Neal B, *et al.* Canagliflozin and Renal Outcomes in Type 2 Diabetes and Nephropathy. N Engl J Med 2019; 380(24): 2295-306.
[http://dx.doi.org/10.1056/NEJMoa1811744] [PMID: 30990260]

[62]   Marton A, Kaneko T, Kovalik JP, *et al.* Organ protection by SGLT2 inhibitors: role of metabolic energy and water conservation. Nat Rev Nephrol 2021; 17(1): 65-77.
[http://dx.doi.org/10.1038/s41581-020-00350-x] [PMID: 33005037]

CHAPTER 2

The Role of Mitochondria and Oxidative Stress in Renal Disease

Ana Carolina Ariza[1] and **Consuelo Plata**[2,*]

[1] *Center for Nutrition and Health Research, National Institute of Public Health Mexico, Cuernavaca, Morelos, Mexico*

[2] *Department of Nephrology & Mineral Metabolism, Instituto Nacional de Ciencias Médicas y Nutrición Salvador Zubirán, Tlalpan 14080, Mexico City, Mexico*

Abstract: The role of mitochondrial disorders in kidney diseases is receiving increasing attention since evidence indicates that mitochondrial structure, dynamics, and crosstalk within the local environment are related to physiological homeostasis for adequate kidney function. In particular, in acute kidney disease (AKI), there are well-established alterations in mitochondrial structure and function. These changes included decreased mitochondrial abundance in proximal tubule cells, swelling of individual organelles, and disturbance of tightly stacked cristae. In this chapter, we discuss how disturbances in mitochondria exacerbate the production of reactive oxygen species (ROS), aggravating renal dysfunction, particularly AKI, and increasing the risk of developing chronic kidney disease (CKD). In this context, this review of the role of mitochondria in renal disease revealed that knowledge concerning changes in the redox ratio caused by NADH/NAD in renal cells and cellular compartments is limited and needs further investigation.

Keywords: Amino acid metabolism, Chronic kidney disease, Mitochondrial dysfunction, NOX, Renal dysfunction.

INTRODUCTION

Renal disorders, like many other diseases that share some underlying metabolic mechanisms, are usually treated when the clinical manifestations are evident. However, a better prognosis could be achieved by preventing or ameliorating unsighted first signs such as inflammation and oxidative stress. The role of mitochondrial disorders in kidney diseases is gaining attention since evidence relates mitochondrial structure, dynamics, and crosstalk within the local environment to physiological homeostasis for adequate kidney function. In this

---

* **Corresponding author Consuelo Plata:** Department of Nephrology & Mineral Metabolism, Instituto Nacional de Ciencias Médicas y Nutrición Salvador Zubirán, Tlalpan 14080, Mexico City, Mexico; E-mail: consueloplata@hotmail.com.

Rafael Valdez-Ortiz, Katy Sánchez-Pozos, Ana Carolina Ariza & Enzo C. Vásquez-Jiménez (Eds.)

chapter, we discuss how disturbances in mitochondrial function and, consequently, the augmented generation of reactive oxygen species (ROS) can cause renal dysfunction, particularly acute kidney disease (AKI), which in turn increases the risk of developing chronic kidney disease (CKD). Understanding the cellular mechanisms that lead to increased ROS production, including mitochondrial dysfunction, with the subsequent establishment of systemic inflammation and oxidative stress, unlocks a novel era for advancing new drugs for treating kidney disorders.

MITOCHONDRIA AND OXIDATIVE STRESS

Mitochondria are bilayer-membrane-bound organelles that differ in morphology, quantity, and targeted functions among mammalian cells [1]. Since the late 1940s, mitochondria have been recognized as the "microscopic power plants" of cells due to their vital function in energy production [2]. These organelles possess their DNA (mtDNA), and besides ATP generation, they actively participate in other physiological processes such as ROS and heat production, cytosolic calcium homeostasis, and apoptosis regulation. Each mitochondrion has two membranes: an outer membrane (MOM) and an inner membrane (MIM). The outer membrane is porous since it contains VDACs (voltage-dependent anion channels).

In contrast, the inner membrane is tightly folded into structures called cristae, which increase the surface area and make energy production more efficient. The mitochondrial membranes create two main spaces: the matrix, which is inside the inner membrane and where important chemical reactions occur, and the intermembrane space (IMS), located between the inner and outer membranes. The shape and folds of the cristae are important because they help control the diffusion dynamics along the mitochondria, affecting their function [3, 4]. Therefore, alterations in the local or external cell environment or mitochondrial external and internal structures due to impaired physiological mechanisms can profoundly affect the functional state of these organelles and their surroundings. Regarding cellular stress, microenvironment plays an important role in mitochondrial dynamics, particularly the redox state achieved by substrate availability. Conditions such as hypoxia and hyperglycemia modify healthy adenosine triphosphate production to exacerbate ROS production, which in turn contributes to cell damage [5].

In the early 1980s, Professor Helmut Sies introduced the term oxidative stress to describe the effects on animal cells and tissues produced by altering the balance between cellular defense mechanisms and various conditions that promote oxidation reactions. After over 30 years, oxidative stress has been described as a disequilibrium between oxidant and antioxidant molecules in favor of the former, promoting a disorder in redox control and signaling and/or generating molecular damage [6]. ROS are highly reactive molecules that are produced physiologically as part of redox metabolism and include radical anions (O_2^*), nitric oxide (*NO), radical anion superoxide (HO*), and hydrogen peroxide (H_2O_2) [7]. ROS react with lipids, proteins, DNA, RNA, and even carbohydrates when generated excessively, causing cell damage. The body has an antioxidant system composed of various enzymes to counteract the damage, such as catalase (CAT), superoxide dismutase (SOD), glutathione peroxidase (GPx), and glutathione reductase (Gr), as well as cofactors (vitamins or inorganic nutrients) that inactivate ROS or transform them into inert metabolites [8]. Several biomarkers for assessing an individual's redox or oxidative stress status include ROS, intermediate metabolites, final metabolites, and damaged molecules from diverse compartments. The quantification of free radicals or ROS is complicated due to their high reactivity and short half-life. Thus, NO can be measured only indirectly by quantifying nitrates and nitrites. Currently, the most internationally accepted biomarkers include isoprostanes, 8-hydroxy-deoxyguanosine, protein carbonyls, lipid hydroperoxides, and malondialdehyde (MDA), the latter of which are thiobarbituric acid reactive species (TBARS). Similarly, the quantification of antioxidant enzymes (SOD, CAT, and GPx), inorganic nutrients, and vitamins with antioxidant functions (mainly retinol, tocopherols, magnesium, and ascorbic acid) or the total antioxidant capacity can be used to assess the state of the antioxidant system. Using two or more biomarkers is recommended due to their high intra- and inter-variability, obtaining a more accurate picture of the state of systemic oxidative stress [9].

Along with ROS production, cells produce cytokines and tissue-specific hormones that promote the attraction and activation of macrophages, generating a state of underlying chronic inflammation. This state of inflammation, in turn, promotes the generation of ROS, establishing a continuous cycle with chronic detrimental consequences to the tissue if not disrupted. Furthermore, oxidative stress activates multiple intracellular signaling pathways, which induces apoptosis, cell overgrowth, and endothelial dysfunction. Overall, oxidative stress contributes to heart failure and pancreatic, pulmonary, and renal dysfunction, causing hypertension, glucose intolerance/diabetes mellitus, pulmonary disorders, and CKD [10]. Importantly, once oxidative stress is established, a cascade of events that predict the rapid progression of damage and the development of complications occurs; this suggests that oxidative stress can be an initial risk marker of kidney disease.

MECHANISMS LEADING TO OXIDATIVE STRESS IN AKI AND CKD

As mentioned in the previous chapter, kidneys use a large amount of energy from different sources, such as glucose, fatty acids, and ketone bodies. They also have one of the highest metabolic and vascularization rates in the body, with a high content of mitochondria, to perform their functions, particularly urine production. A lack of regulation of mitochondrial function promotes ROS and decreases energy production, contributing to the development and progression of kidney diseases, particularly AKI and CKD [11].

The primary sources of ROS generated in the kidney are mitochondria and the nicotinamide adenine dinucleotide phosphate (NADPH) oxidase family of enzymes (NOXs) [12]. All NOX enzymes transfer an electron from NADPH to O_2. Eleven sites within the chain of mitochondrial electron transport and redox enzymes are capable of leaking electrons and causing one or two electron reductions of oxygen to produce O_2 and H_2O_2 [13]. These redox centers become locations of electron leakage when induced in a maximally reduced state due to either disturbance of electron flux or redistribution of electrons due to disorders in downstream catalytic subunits [14]. The NOX1 and NOX2 enzymatic systems require the assembly of a membrane subunit, two cytosolic subunits, and ras-related C3 botulinum toxin substrate 1 (Rac1).

In contrast, NOX4, which is highly expressed in the mitochondrial membranes of renal cells, does not require cytosolic subunits and produces H_2O_2 [15 - 17]. It has been demonstrated that NOX levels increase in different AKI and CKD models, causing ROS overproduction [18]. The production of mitochondrial ROS and ROS generated by NOXs also injures phospholipids and mitochondrial DNA [19]. Therefore, regulating the redox state is crucial for cell viability, activation, proliferation, and organ function. Hence, a disturbance in the redox balance leads to increased ROS concentrations, which can cause adverse changes in cell components, and if this disequilibrium persists, injury progresses to irreversible damage. Hence, AKI and CKD are characterized by hypoxia and oxidative stress, typically involved in renal fibrosis development [20, 21].

During kidney injury, hypoxia-inducible factor 1 (HIF-1) facilitates hypoxia. Under these circumstances, HIF-1 can regulate the expression of vascular endothelial growth factor (VEGF), glucose transporters, erythropoietin, and endothelin-1, which are involved in angiogenesis, energy metabolism, and erythropoiesis. Hence, HIF-1 allows cellular adaptation to hypoxia, preventing deleterious effects. Furthermore, it has also been demonstrated that HIF-1 is associated with inflammation, epithelial-mesenchymal transition (EMT), and extracellular matrix (ECM) deposition, all of which contribute to profibrotic changes, which, along with oxidative stress, lead to damage progression [22 - 24].

HIF-1 is a transcriptional regulator of oxygen homeostasis, in addition to the expression of erythropoietin, endothelin-1, and glucose transporters, among other genes. The role of HIF-1 is dual, depending on the circumstances. Hence, although HIF-1 can diminish hypoxia-related injury under short-term hypoxia, recent studies have proposed that HIF-1 may be involved in the progression of kidney disease [25 - 28]. Wang *et al.* demonstrated that long-term overactivation of HIF-1α in chronic ischemia in the kidney mediates chronic renal damage [29]. These findings suggest that HIF-1 is involved in developing fibrosis during kidney injury. During hypoxia, mitochondria augment the production of ROS and subsequently stabilize the HIF-1α protein [30]. It has also been demonstrated that angiotensin II stimulates H_2O_2 production, which in turn upregulates HIF-1α levels and subsequently stimulates tissue inhibitors of metalloproteinases, causing the accumulation of collagen I/III in cultured renal medullary interstitial cells [31]. Other studies have shown that the transcription of HIF-1α increases under hypoxia through the PI-3K/AKT and ERK pathways, which are related to apoptosis and cell proliferation [32, 33].

Oxidative stress and ROS production in the kidney alter the water-electrolyte and acid-base balance, which affects kidney homeostasis through disturbances in tubular glomerular feedback, the myogenic reflex in the supplying arteriole, and the renin-angiotensin-aldosterone system [34]. In addition, oxidative stress is directly connected to podocyte injury, a decreased glomerular filtration rate, proteinuria, and tubulointerstitial fibrosis [35, 36]. Damaging effects due to both reperfusion and ischemia are additive. In general, ischemia/reperfusion injury produces functional and structural changes. Some molecular mechanisms have been suggested to explain this injury; nonetheless, oxidative stress and reactive oxygen species (ROS) production are the principal factors in this pathogenesis [37]. The first ischemia signal is edema, characterized by pallor and a rise in turgor and organ weight. The promotion of systemic inflammation and, in turn, ischemic injury is due to increased cytokine production and augmented expression of adhesion molecules by hypoxic parenchymal and endothelial cells. A sudden supply of O_2 in reperfusion to hypoxic tissue results in a particular kind of damage, which is not present in the ischemic phase [38].

Since the early phases of injury, oxidative stress accompanies the worsening of renal function, which is exacerbated by hemodialysis [39 - 41]. Consequently, patients with impaired homeostasis undergo kidney transplantation due to oxidative imbalance [42].

Likewise, in patients undergoing hemodialysis, cardiovascular complications are aggravated by oxidative disequilibrium. As kidney function decreases, the risk of cardiovascular complications increases. In support of this, approximately half of the patients with CKD (stages 4-5) die from cardiovascular disease [43]. Endothelial dysfunction comprises both atherosclerosis and vascular stiffness, increasing the risk of cardiovascular death [44]. The endothelial barrier becomes dysfunctional and loses its integrity when permeability increases, and low-density lipoprotein (LDL) accumulates within the vessel wall. When LDL is oxidized, an inflammatory process is initiated [45]. Chemokine secretion and the expression of adhesion molecules by endothelial cells promote the recruitment of leukocytes, which adhere to endothelial cells and migrate into vessel walls [46, 47].

Furthermore, increased oxidative stress and ROS production reduce NO bioavailability, causing a reduction in endothelial cell-dependent vasodilation and increasing vascular stiffness [47]. Several studies have indicated that CKD-associated factors, such as systemic chronic low-grade inflammation, enhanced oxidative stress, and uremic toxins, accelerate atherosclerosis [48 - 50]. It is widely established that during systemic inflammation, elevated levels of inflammatory proteins such as C-reactive protein (CRP) and interleukin-6 (IL-6) and oxidative stress biomarkers are observed [49]. Hence, the progression of CKD strongly depends on oxidative stress levels [50].

Different uremic toxins, such as indoxyl sulfate, phosphate, cyanate, advanced glycation end products (AGEs), and uric acid, lead to diminished endothelial nitric oxide synthase (eNOS) expression and activity. This latter reduces the production of the potent vasodilator nitric oxide (NO) and, consequently, a reduction in vasorelaxation [51 - 55].

MITOCHONDRIAL FUNCTION AND RENAL DAMAGE

Mitochondrial dysfunction plays a pivotal role in the pathophysiology of AKI, increasing the risk for CKD. Key mechanisms of mitochondrial dysfunction in AKI include impaired oxidative phosphorylation, excessive production of reactive oxygen species (ROS), disrupted mitochondrial dynamics (fission and fusion), and alterations in mitophagy and biogenesis. These processes compromise cellular energy supply and exacerbate kidney injury by promoting cell death pathways, inflammation, and fibrosis [56]. Understanding these mechanisms provides critical insights into potential therapeutic targets for mitigating AKI and preserving renal function. In AKI, there are notable changes in mitochondrial structure and function. These changes involved a decrease in the number of mitochondria in the proximal tubule cells, swelling of individual organelles, and disturbance of the tightly stacked cristae. Mitochondrial dysfunction is crucial in the physiopathology of AKI. Among the metabolic pathways that cause mitochondrial injury is the reduction of NAD^+, which is necessary for the continuous production of ATP from fatty acid oxidation. Dysfunctional mitochondria deprive cells of ATP and amplify injury by generating molecules that promote cell death and induce inflammation. The release of ROS from injured mitochondria causes oxidative stress in AKI. Additionally, the balance between mitochondrial fusion and fission is disrupted, leading to mitochondrial fragmentation, which can sensitize cells to apoptosis by releasing cytochrome c and triggering apoptosis, as well as mitochondrial DNA, all of which can function as proinflammatory danger signals [57].

In murine sepsis models of AKI, a significant reduction in the expression of PPAR coactivator-1 (PGC-1), an inducer of mitochondrial biogenesis, was shown. This PGC-1 suppression was associated with reduced renal function and increased mitochondrial injury. Additionally, tubular cells reduced PGC-1α expression and oxygen consumption; interestingly, PGC-1 suppression was proportional to the degree of renal impairment. This finding was consistent with findings in global and tubule-specific PGC-1α–knockout mice; both types of mice presented normal renal function but experienced persistent injury following endotoxemia, while overexpression of PGC-1 protected against ischemic renal injury [58]. In addition, signaling from innate inflammatory pathways may result in the downregulation of PGC-1-α during infection [59]. In summary, the hypoxic environment of AKI results in impaired mitochondrial function, but restoring mitochondrial biogenesis through overexpression of PGC-1 may improve the response to AKI. Alternative treatments that focus on mitochondrial dysfunction or promote mitochondrial regeneration are being developed to delay the progression of AKI and promote the repair of damaged tissue [57, 60].

Conversely, the overexpression of PGC-1 favors the biosynthesis of NAD^+, which suggests that the alteration of PGC-1 in AKI promotes more significant injury by reducing the levels of NAD^+ due to the alteration of fatty acid oxidation (FAO) [61]. Regarding the changes observed in FAO in renal injury caused by ischemia, it was observed that the reduction in the FAO-limiting enzyme CPT1 contributes to the deterioration of this metabolism after ischemic renal failure. In contrast, the administration of C75, a synthetic compound (α-methyl-lene-γ-butyrolactone) that is an inhibitor of fatty acid synthase, upregulated CPT1 activity, ameliorated renal function, diminished tissue injury, and inhibited proinflammatory cytokine production and neutrophil infiltration after renal ischemia-reperfusion injury. Hence, increasing metabolic pathway activity for energy production could be a new alternative for treating renal injury [62].

Marked mitochondrial fragmentation is characteristic of AKI caused by toxins or ischemia. Fragmented mitochondria are rich sources of ROS, cytochrome c, mitochondrial DNA, and other cell-damaging molecules. Inhibition of mitochondrial fission through blockade of dynamin-related protein 1 (DRP1), a protein that mediates mitochondrial and peroxisomal division, has been shown to protect cultured renal tubular cells from apoptosis and mitigate AKI after ischemia-reperfusion or exposure to cisplatin [63, 64]. Moreover, in murine genetic models, deletion of DRP1 in the proximal tubule prevents renal damage, inflammation, and apoptosis induced by renal ischemia-reperfusion and promotes epithelial recovery. Loss of DRP1 preserves mitochondrial structure and reduces oxidative stress in injured kidneys. In addition, progressive kidney injury and fibrosis are attenuated [65]. These findings implicate both DRP1 and mitochondrial dynamics as important intermediaries of AKI and fibrosis progression, suggesting that DRP1 might be a potential therapeutic alternative for AKI. Consistent with this theory, experimental evidence suggests that the NAD-dependent sirtuin three deacetylase protein can reduce cisplatin-induced mitochondrial fragmentation and defend against AKI [66].

Another cellular process that is altered in AKI is mitochondrial turnover or mitophagy, which is closely connected with autophagy; the latter is a cellular process of 'self-feeding,' which is the sequestration of cytoplasmic components in vesicles or autophagic vacuoles (called autophagosomes) that are sent to lysosomes for degradation. This cellular mechanism is important for cells to break down and recycle cellular proteins and eliminate damaged organelles to protect cells from genotoxic stress, oxidative stress, the accumulation of misfolded proteins, and nutrient deprivation [67 - 69]. The elimination of damaged mitochondrial components is achieved through mitophagy; in this process, the subset of mitochondria that produces the most significant amount of ROS is mainly eliminated to reduce the oxidative load. The molecular machinery of autophagy has been identified; this machinery comprises a particular class of genes or proteins termed autophagy-related genes (Atgs). These Atgs are interrelated and interact with other regulatory proteins to form protein complexes for autophagosome initiation, expansion, and maturation. A lack of a specific Atg leads to the inhibition of relevant autophagic events. Renal ischemia-reperfusion injury induces mitophagy in renal tubules to protect against cell damage. Additionally, mice lacking the autophagy regulator Atg7 exhibited increased sensitivity to nephrotoxicity induced by cisplatin [70, 71]. Hence, drugs that induce mitophagy, such as rapamycin, could be good therapeutic strategies for improving the elimination of fragmented mitochondria that propagate lesions and accelerate recovery after AKI [57].

It has been proposed that the peroxisome is another cellular organelle involved in the development of AKI. As mentioned above, peroxisomes preferentially oxidize VLCFAs; this metabolic process generates H_2O_2, so large amounts of catalase are needed to metabolize H_2O_2 produced without generating cellular damage due to the production of ROS [72]. Therefore, peroxisomes and supporting mitochondria in the complete oxidation of fatty acids eliminate ROS, which are deregulated in AKI (Fig. **1**).

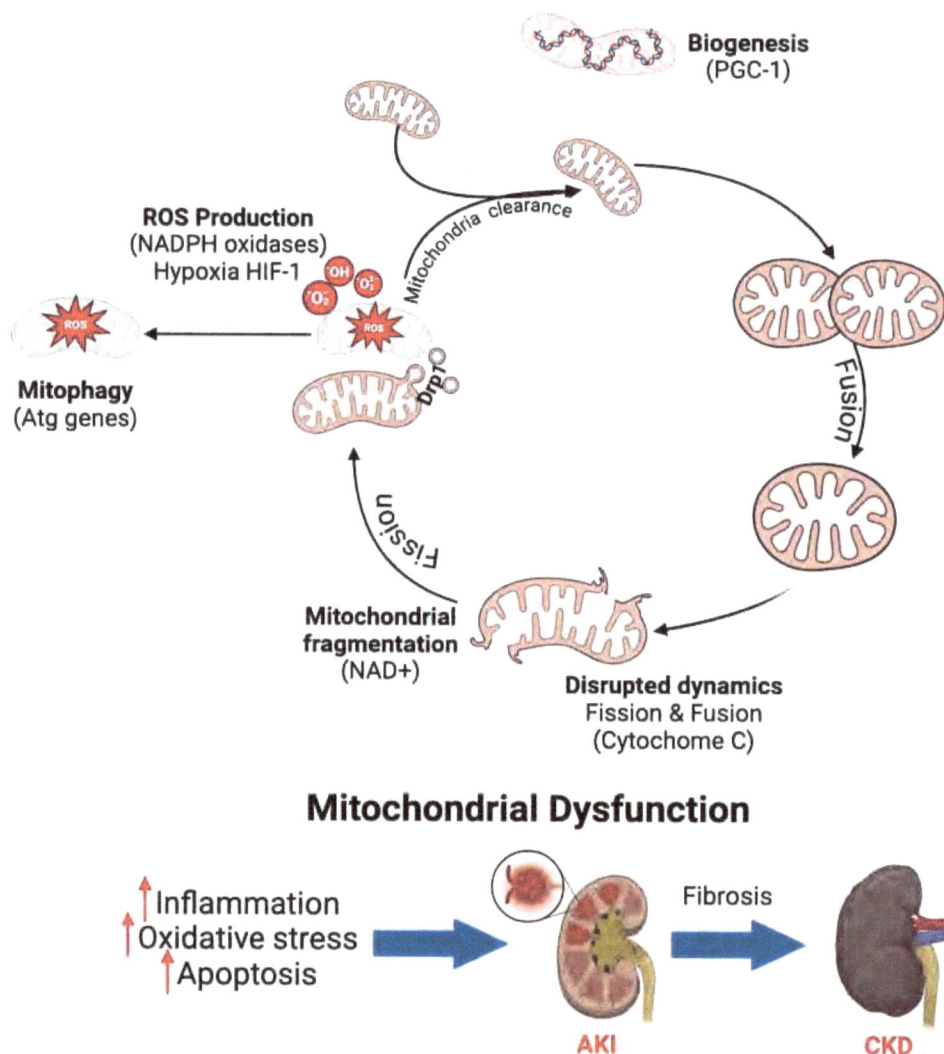

Fig. (1). Mitochondrial dysfunction triggers pathways such as inflammation, oxidative stress, and apoptosis, which contribute to pathophysiological processes like AKI. The sustained activation of these pathways promotes fibrosis, which leads to CKD.

SIRTUINS AND OTHER THERAPEUTIC TARGETS IN AKI

Sirtuin 5 (Sirt5) may play an important role in regulating FAO. Recently, renal function improved in Sirt5 knockout mice, in which AKI was induced by ischemia or by cisplatin treatment, and there was less tissue damage in these mice than in wild-type mice. This latter could be because the deletion of Sirt5 reverses the posttranslational lysine acylation of various enzymes implicated in FAO. These findings suggest that SIRT5 deficiency is protective through the reduction of mitochondrial-derived ROS and the drive of peroxisomal FAO. Disturbances or alterations to this mitochondrial-peroxisomal axis are key to the pathogenesis of AKI. These findings suggest a new mechanism with potential implications for AKI treatment [72 - 74].

Several sirtuins (including Sirt2, Sirt3, Sirt6, and SIRT7) have been shown to recruit inflammatory/fibrotic factors to the kidney after injury. In mammals, seven sirtuins (SIRT1– SIRT7) are expressed. These enzymes constitute an enzyme family in different cell compartments with broad enzymatic activity, such as deacetylases, mono-ADP ribosyl transferases, demalonilases, deglutarillases, and desuccinylases. Sirtuins regulate cellular energy metabolism and various physiological processes. In addition to the classical enzymatic activity of sirtuins as histone deacetylases in the nucleus, a set of proteins have also been recognized in the cytoplasm and mitochondria. Although sirtuins have been investigated for their contribution to caloric-restrictive vascular disease and diabetes, their substrates and role as sensors of cellular energy equilibrium suggest that these enzymes' functions are fundamental for restoring cellular homeostasis after tissue injury. In the kidney, sirtuins are involved in the pathophysiology of acute and chronic kidney diseases [72, 75].

Sirtuin 2 (SIRT2), an NAD^+-dependent deacetylase, modulates proinflammatory immune responses. SIRT2 deficiency decreases renal neutrophil and macrophage infiltration, ameliorates LPS-induced acute tubular injury, and reduces renal function and the expression of inflammatory chemokines such as CXCL2 and CCL2 [76]. Furthermore, SIRT2 positively regulates mitogen-activated protein kinase 1 (MAPK-1). Activation of MAPKs is related to drug-induced apoptosis and cisplatin-induced renal injury. Compared with wild-type mice, renal function and tubular damage were improved, apoptosis, necrosis, and inflammation were reduced, and acute kidney damage caused by cisplatin treatment was improved in the murine Sirt2 knockout and Sirt2 transgenic models. These findings suggest that the regulation of MAPK-1 expression by SIRT2 may be a new therapeutic target for improving cisplatin-induced kidney injury [77].

In the case of SIRT3, in a mouse model of cecal ligation and puncture, the overexpression of SIRT3 promoted autophagy and attenuated sepsis-induced kidney damage. It reduced apoptosis and inflammation, and overexpression of SIRT3 promoted increased phosphorylation of AMPK (p-AMPK) and decreased TOR (p-mTOR) phosphorylation. Blocking autophagy with 3-methyladenine (3-MA) suppressed the protective effect of SIRT3 on sepsis-induced AKI. These results suggest that SIRT3 protects against sepsis-induced AKI by promoting autophagy through regulation of the AMPK/mTOR pathway [78].

SIRT6 is a nuclear protein that plays an important role in the stability and repair of genomic DNA through its association with chromatin, which promotes resistance to DNA damage and suppresses genomic instability. SIRT6 deacetylates histone H3 to preserve genome integrity and telomere function [79]. In mammalian cells subjected to oxidative stress, SIRT6 is recruited at the sites of DNA double helix breaks and stimulates its repair through association with poly [adenosine diphosphate (ADP)-ribose] polymerase 1 (PARP1). This interaction stimulates the poly-ADP-ribosylase activity of PARP1, improving DNA double helix repair [80]. At the renal level, mice deficient in Sirt6 exhibit hypertrophy and glomerular enlargement, chronic inflammation, and renal fibrosis, as well as proteinuria and podocyte depletion in SIRT6-mutant mice, which indicates that the function of Sirt6 is important for podocyte homeostasis and the maintenance of kidney function [81]. Furthermore, the overexpression of the SIRT6 gene in HK-2 renal epithelial cells inhibited the LPS-induced apoptosis, negatively regulated cytokine secretion, tumor necrosis factor α (TNF-α), and interleukin-6 (IL-6), and induced autophagy [82]. These findings, taken together, suggest that SIRT6 is a new therapeutic target for treating renal damage caused by stress.

SIRT7 is another nuclear deacetylase and the only deacetylase detected in the nucleolus. The expression of SIRT7 is positively correlated with cell growth and is abundant in metabolically active tissues such as the liver. Among the functions of SIRT7 that have been studied are the activation of RNA polymerase I (RNA Pol I) through the deacetylation of upstream binding factor (UBF) [83] and the regulation of RNA Pol I transcription by the deacetylation of PAD53, a component of RNA Pol I [84]. Interestingly, SIRT7 knockout mice were found to have protection against cisplatin-induced AKI by controlling the nuclear expression of nuclear factor kappa B (NF-κB), a powerful catalyst of the immune system and the inflammatory response. SIRT7 deficiency improved cisplatin-induced AKI [85]. In addition, it was shown that inhibition of NF-κB can modulate the inflammatory response and reduce the amount of AKI damage [86]. Notably, both the innate and adaptive immune systems are implicated in the pathogenesis of AKI, and practically all immune cells are involved in this disease [87]. Therefore, the protective phenomenon observed in mice deficient in SIRT7 may be due to the reduction in the expression of tumor necrosis factor-α (TNF-α) caused by SIRT7 deficiency, which increases oxidative stress through the production of ROS through the NADPH oxidase complex [85]. Overall, the fact that SIRT7 is a key molecule in the development of AKI induced by cisplatin suggests that SIRT7 may be a new therapeutic target for nephrotoxicity [72].

Due to the multifaceted and important role of mitochondrial dysfunction in AKI and CDK, many potential therapeutic targets have emerged during the last twenty years. These can be categorized based on their effects on specific mitochondrial processes. Here are some examples of the most relevant ones [11].

Structure

Elamipretide: This peptide stabilizes mitochondrial membranes by interacting with cardiolipin, preserving mitochondrial structure and preventing cristae disorganization, particularly in ischemia-reperfusion injury models [88].

Cyclosporine A: Known to stabilize mitochondrial membranes by inhibiting cyclophilin D, reducing mitochondrial permeability transition pore (mPTP) opening [89].

Dynamics

P110: This small molecule inhibits the Drp1-Fis1 interaction. Drp1 is a protein responsible for mitochondrial fission. Promoting mitochondrial fusion protects against excessive fragmentation and reduces injury in AKI [90].

Biogenesis

Resveratrol: A natural polyphenol that activates PGC-1α, a key regulator of mitochondrial biogenesis. It has been shown to improve mitochondrial function and energy metabolism in CKD [91].

Nicotinamide Riboside: A precursor of NAD+, this compound supports mitochondrial biogenesis and improves renal outcomes by enhancing energy production [92].

Reactive Oxygen Species (ROS)

MitoQ: A mitochondria-targeted antioxidant that reduces ROS directly within mitochondria, protecting renal cells from oxidative damage [93, 94].

N-acetylcysteine (NAC) is a precursor to glutathione, enhancing mitochondrial antioxidant capacity [95].

Mitochondrial Permeability Transition Pore (mPTP)

Melatonin: Inhibits mPTP opening, reducing mitochondrial swelling and preventing cell death in models of renal ischemia and AKI [96, 97].

Sanglifehrin A: This compound has shown potential in inhibiting mPTP formation, protecting against mitochondrial-driven apoptosis [98].

These targeted therapies represent promising avenues for addressing mitochondrial dysfunction in AKI and CKD, though many remain in experimental stages or preclinical studies.

CONCLUSION

It is widely documented that mitochondrial defects are associated with many disturbances in cell metabolism and abnormalities, energy deficits, and oxidative stress. Impaired mitochondrial function impacts various cells, metabolic pathways, and organs. Thus, knowledge about variations in the NADH/NAD redox ratio in kidney cells and cellular compartments, together with the role of mitochondria in kidney diseases, is mainly limited and needs further investigation.

ACKNOWLEDGMENTS

Research conducted for this publication was supported by grants from "Consejo Nacional de Humanidades, Ciencia y Tecnología" CONAHCYT No. 290275. Ariza AC received a postdoctoral fellowship from "Consejo Nacional de Humanidades, Ciencia y Tecnología (CONAHCYT)".

REFERENCES

[1]   Milner JO. The functional development of mammalian mitochondria. Biol Rev Camb Philos Soc 1976; 51(2): 181-209.
[http://dx.doi.org/10.1111/j.1469-185X.1976.tb01124.x] [PMID: 179627]

[2]   Schatz G. The magic garden. Annu Rev Biochem 2007; 76(1): 673-8.
[http://dx.doi.org/10.1146/annurev.biochem.76.060806.091141] [PMID: 17313357]

[3]   Koopman WJH, Nijtmans LGJ, Dieteren CEJ, *et al.* Mammalian mitochondrial complex I: biogenesis, regulation, and reactive oxygen species generation. Antioxid Redox Signal 2010; 12(12): 1431-70.
[http://dx.doi.org/10.1089/ars.2009.2743] [PMID: 19803744]

[4]   Martínez-Revelles S, García-Redondo AB, Avendaño MS, *et al.* Lysyl Oxidase Induces Vascular Oxidative Stress and Contributes to Arterial Stiffness and Abnormal Elastin Structure in Hypertension: Role of p38MAPK. Antioxid Redox Signal 2017; 27(7): 379-97.
[http://dx.doi.org/10.1089/ars.2016.6642] [PMID: 28010122]

[5]   Thomas LW, Ashcroft M. Exploring the molecular interface between hypoxia-inducible factor signalling and mitochondria. Cell Mol Life Sci 2019; 76(9): 1759-77.
[http://dx.doi.org/10.1007/s00018-019-03039-y] [PMID: 30767037]

[6]   Lushchak VI, Storey KB. Oxidative stress concept updated: Definitions, classifications, and regulatory

pathways implicated. EXCLI J 2021; 20: 956-67.
[http://dx.doi.org/10.17179/excli2021-3596] [PMID: 34267608]

[7]   Lushchak VI. Free radicals, reactive oxygen species, oxidative stress and its classification. Chem Biol Interact 2014; 224: 164-75.
[http://dx.doi.org/10.1016/j.cbi.2014.10.016] [PMID: 25452175]

[8]   Nita M, Grzybowski A. The Role of the Reactive Oxygen Species and Oxidative Stress in the Pathomechanism of the Age□Related Ocular Diseases and Other Pathologies of the Anterior and Posterior Eye Segments in Adults. Oxid Med Cell Longev 2016; 2016(1): 3164734.
[http://dx.doi.org/10.1155/2016/3164734] [PMID: 26881021]

[9]   Vona R, Pallotta L, Cappelletti M, Severi C, Matarrese P. The Impact of Oxidative Stress in Human Pathology: Focus on Gastrointestinal Disorders. Antioxidants 2021; 10(2): 201. Epub ahead of print
[http://dx.doi.org/10.3390/antiox10020201] [PMID: 33573222]

[10]   Mittal M, Siddiqui MR, Tran K, Reddy SP, Malik AB. Reactive oxygen species in inflammation and tissue injury. Antioxid Redox Signal 2014; 20(7): 1126-67.
[http://dx.doi.org/10.1089/ars.2012.5149] [PMID: 23991888]

[11]   Zhang X, Agborbesong E, Li X. The Role of Mitochondria in Acute Kidney Injury and Chronic Kidney Disease and Its Therapeutic Potential. Int J Mol Sci 2021; 22(20): 11253. Epub ahead of print
[http://dx.doi.org/10.3390/ijms222011253] [PMID: 34681922]

[12]   Aranda-Rivera AK, Cruz-Gregorio A, Aparicio-Trejo OE, Pedraza-Chaverri J. Mitochondrial Redox Signaling and Oxidative Stress in Kidney Diseases. Biomolecules 2021; 11(8): 1144. Epub ahead of print
[http://dx.doi.org/10.3390/biom11081144] [PMID: 34439810]

[13]   Wong HS, Dighe PA, Mezera V, Monternier PA, Brand MD. Production of superoxide and hydrogen peroxide from specific mitochondrial sites under different bioenergetic conditions. J Biol Chem 2017; 292(41): 16804-9.
[http://dx.doi.org/10.1074/jbc.R117.789271] [PMID: 28842493]

[14]   Ahmad AA, Draves SO, Rosca M. Mitochondria in Diabetic Kidney Disease. Cells 2021; 10(11): 2945. Epub ahead of print
[http://dx.doi.org/10.3390/cells10112945] [PMID: 34831168]

[15]   Babelova A, Avaniadi D, Jung O, *et al.* Role of Nox4 in murine models of kidney disease. Free Radic Biol Med 2012; 53(4): 842-53.
[http://dx.doi.org/10.1016/j.freeradbiomed.2012.06.027] [PMID: 22749956]

[16]   Serrander L, Cartier L, Bedard K, *et al.* NOX4 activity is determined by mRNA levels and reveals a unique pattern of ROS generation. Biochem J 2007; 406(1): 105-14.
[http://dx.doi.org/10.1042/BJ20061903] [PMID: 17501721]

[17]   Lee H, Jose PA. Coordinated Contribution of NADPH Oxidase- and Mitochondria-Derived Reactive Oxygen Species in Metabolic Syndrome and Its Implication in Renal Dysfunction. Front Pharmacol 2021; 12: 670076.
[http://dx.doi.org/10.3389/fphar.2021.670076] [PMID: 34017260]

[18]   Molina-Jijón E, Aparicio-Trejo OE, Rodríguez-Muñoz R, *et al.* The nephroprotection exerted by curcumin in maleate□induced renal damage is associated with decreased mitochondrial fission and autophagy. Biofactors 2016; 42(6): 686-702.
[http://dx.doi.org/10.1002/biof.1313] [PMID: 27412471]

[19]   Hahn A, Zuryn S. Mitochondrial Genome (mtDNA) Mutations that Generate Reactive Oxygen Species. Antioxidants 2019; 8(9): 392. Epub ahead of print
[http://dx.doi.org/10.3390/antiox8090392] [PMID: 31514455]

[20]   Bernhardt WM, Câmpean V, Kany S, *et al.* Preconditional activation of hypoxia-inducible factors ameliorates ischemic acute renal failure. J Am Soc Nephrol 2006; 17(7): 1970-8.

[http://dx.doi.org/10.1681/ASN.2005121302] [PMID: 16762988]

[21]   Li ZL, Liu BC. Hypoxia and Renal Tubulointerstitial Fibrosis. Adv Exp Med Biol 2019; 1165: 467-85.
       [http://dx.doi.org/10.1007/978-981-13-8871-2_23] [PMID: 31399980]

[22]   Agarwal A, Nick HS. Renal response to tissue injury: lessons from heme oxygenase-1 Gene Ablation
       and expression. J Am Soc Nephrol 2000; 11(5): 965-73.
       [http://dx.doi.org/10.1681/ASN.V115965] [PMID: 10770977]

[23]   Warnecke C, Zaborowska Z, Kurreck J, et al. Differentiating the functional role of hypoxia□inducible
       factor (HIF)□1α and HIF□2α (EPAS□1) by the use of RNA interference: erythropoietin is a HIF□2α
       target gene in Hep3B and Kelly cells. FASEB J 2004; 18(12): 1462-4.
       [http://dx.doi.org/10.1096/fj.04-1640fje] [PMID: 15240563]

[24]   Honda T, Hirakawa Y, Nangaku M. The role of oxidative stress and hypoxia in renal disease. Kidney
       Res Clin Pract 2019; 38(4): 414-26.
       [http://dx.doi.org/10.23876/j.krcp.19.063] [PMID: 31558011]

[25]   Schietke R, Warnecke C, Wacker I, et al. The lysyl oxidases LOX and LOXL2 are necessary and
       sufficient to repress E-cadherin in hypoxia: insights into cellular transformation processes mediated by
       HIF-1. J Biol Chem 2010; 285(9): 6658-69.
       [http://dx.doi.org/10.1074/jbc.M109.042424] [PMID: 20026874]

[26]   Baumann B, Hayashida T, Liang X, Schnaper HW. Hypoxia-inducible factor-1α promotes
       glomerulosclerosis and regulates COL1A2 expression through interactions with Smad3. Kidney Int
       2016; 90(4): 797-808.
       [http://dx.doi.org/10.1016/j.kint.2016.05.026] [PMID: 27503806]

[27]   Zhao H, Jiang N, Han Y, et al. Aristolochic acid induces renal fibrosis by arresting proximal tubular
       cells in G2/M phase mediated by HIF□1α. FASEB J 2020; 34(9): 12599-614.
       [http://dx.doi.org/10.1096/fj.202000949R] [PMID: 32706145]

[28]   Nangaku M, Rosenberger C, Heyman SN, Eckardt KU. Regulation of hypoxia□inducible factor in
       kidney disease. Clin Exp Pharmacol Physiol 2013; 40(2): 148-57.
       [http://dx.doi.org/10.1111/1440-1681.12005] [PMID: 22905709]

[29]   Wang Z, Zhu Q, Li PL, et al. Silencing of hypoxia-inducible factor-1α gene attenuates chronic
       ischemic renal injury in two-kidney, one-clip rats. Am J Physiol Renal Physiol 2014; 306(10): F1236-
       42.
       [http://dx.doi.org/10.1152/ajprenal.00673.2013] [PMID: 24623146]

[30]   Louis K, Hertig A. How tubular epithelial cells dictate the rate of renal fibrogenesis? World J Nephrol
       2015; 4(3): 367-73.
       [http://dx.doi.org/10.5527/wjn.v4.i3.367] [PMID: 26167460]

[31]   Wang Z, Tang L, Zhu Q, et al. Hypoxia-inducible factor-1α contributes to the profibrotic action of
       angiotensin II in renal medullary interstitial cells. Kidney Int 2011; 79(3): 300-10.
       [http://dx.doi.org/10.1038/ki.2010.326] [PMID: 20881940]

[32]   Koshikawa N, Hayashi JI, Nakagawara A, Takenaga K. Reactive oxygen species-generating
       mitochondrial DNA mutation up-regulates hypoxia-inducible factor-1alpha gene transcription via
       phosphatidylinositol 3-kinase-Akt/protein kinase C/histone deacetylase pathway. J Biol Chem 2009;
       284(48): 33185-94.
       [http://dx.doi.org/10.1074/jbc.M109.054221] [PMID: 19801684]

[33]   Du J, Xu R, Hu Z, et al. PI3K and ERK-induced Rac1 activation mediates hypoxia-induced HIF-1α
       expression in MCF-7 breast cancer cells. PLoS One 2011; 6(9): e25213.
       [http://dx.doi.org/10.1371/journal.pone.0025213] [PMID: 21980400]

[34]   Podkowińska A, Formanowicz D. Chronic Kidney Disease as Oxidative Stress- and Inflammatory-
       Mediated Cardiovascular Disease. Antioxidants 2020; 9(8): 752. Epub ahead of print
       [http://dx.doi.org/10.3390/antiox9080752] [PMID: 32823917]

[35]   Snoeijs MGJ, van Heurn LWE, Buurman WA. Biological modulation of renal ischemia–reperfusion injury. Curr Opin Organ Transplant 2010; 15(2): 190-9.
       [http://dx.doi.org/10.1097/MOT.0b013e32833593eb] [PMID: 20009928]

[36]   Duni A, Liakopoulos V, Roumeliotis S, Peschos D, Dounousi E. Oxidative Stress in the Pathogenesis and Evolution of Chronic Kidney Disease: Untangling Ariadne's Thread. Int J Mol Sci 2019; 20(15): 3711. Epub ahead of print
       [http://dx.doi.org/10.3390/ijms20153711] [PMID: 31362427]

[37]   Granger DN, Kvietys PR. Reperfusion injury and reactive oxygen species: The evolution of a concept. Redox Biol 2015; 6: 524-51.
       [http://dx.doi.org/10.1016/j.redox.2015.08.020] [PMID: 26484802]

[38]   Soares ROS, Losada DM, Jordani MC, Évora P, Castro-e-Silva O. Ischemia/Reperfusion Injury Revisited: An Overview of the Latest Pharmacological Strategies. Int J Mol Sci 2019; 20(20): 5034. Epub ahead of print
       [http://dx.doi.org/10.3390/ijms20205034] [PMID: 31614478]

[39]   Sangeetha Lakshmi B, Harini Devi N, Suchitra MM, Srinivasa Rao PVLN, Siva Kumar V. Changes in the inflammatory and oxidative stress markers during a single hemodialysis session in patients with chronic kidney disease. Ren Fail 2018; 40(1): 534-40.
       [http://dx.doi.org/10.1080/0886022X.2018.1487857] [PMID: 30277113]

[40]   Sasaki K, Shoji T, Kabata D, *et al.* Oxidative Stress and Inflammation as Predictors of Mortality and Cardiovascular Events in Hemodialysis Patients: The DREAM Cohort. J Atheroscler Thromb 2021; 28(3): 249-60.
       [http://dx.doi.org/10.5551/jat.56069] [PMID: 32741893]

[41]   Yari Z, Tabibi H, Najafi I, Hedayati M, Movahedian M. Effects of soy isoflavones on serum systemic and vascular inflammation markers and oxidative stress in peritoneal dialysis patients: A randomized controlled trial. Phytother Res 2020; 34(11): 3011-8.
       [http://dx.doi.org/10.1002/ptr.6729] [PMID: 32419281]

[42]   Russa DL, Pellegrino D, Montesanto A, *et al.* Oxidative Balance and Inflammation in Hemodialysis Patients: Biomarkers of Cardiovascular Risk? Oxid Med Cell Longev 2019; 2019: 1-7.
       [http://dx.doi.org/10.1155/2019/8567275] [PMID: 30886674]

[43]   Stevens PE, O'Donoghue DJ, de Lusignan S, *et al.* Chronic kidney disease management in the United Kingdom: NEOERICA project results. Kidney Int 2007; 72(1): 92-9.
       [http://dx.doi.org/10.1038/sj.ki.5002273] [PMID: 17440495]

[44]   Katz SD, Hryniewicz K, Hriljac I, *et al.* Vascular endothelial dysfunction and mortality risk in patients with chronic heart failure. Circulation 2005; 111(3): 310-4.
       [http://dx.doi.org/10.1161/01.CIR.0000153349.77489.CF] [PMID: 15655134]

[45]   Soppert J, Lehrke M, Marx N, Jankowski J, Noels H. Lipoproteins and lipids in cardiovascular disease: from mechanistic insights to therapeutic targeting. Adv Drug Deliv Rev 2020; 159: 4-33.
       [http://dx.doi.org/10.1016/j.addr.2020.07.019] [PMID: 32730849]

[46]   Weber C, Noels H. Atherosclerosis: current pathogenesis and therapeutic options. Nat Med 2011; 17(11): 1410-22.
       [http://dx.doi.org/10.1038/nm.2538] [PMID: 22064431]

[47]   Cai H, Harrison DG. Endothelial dysfunction in cardiovascular diseases: the role of oxidant stress. Circ Res 2000; 87(10): 840-4.
       [http://dx.doi.org/10.1161/01.RES.87.10.840] [PMID: 11073878]

[48]   Nowak KL, Jovanovich A, Farmer-Bailey H, *et al.* Vascular Dysfunction, Oxidative Stress, and Inflammation in Chronic Kidney Disease. Kidney360 2020; 1(6): 501-9.
       [http://dx.doi.org/10.34067/KID.0000962019] [PMID: 33305290]

[49]   Oberg BP, McMenamin E, Lucas FL, *et al.* Increased prevalence of oxidant stress and inflammation in

patients with moderate to severe chronic kidney disease. Kidney Int 2004; 65(3): 1009-16.
[http://dx.doi.org/10.1111/j.1523-1755.2004.00465.x] [PMID: 14871421]

[50]   Cachofeiro V, Goicochea M, de Vinuesa SG, Oubiña P, Lahera V, Luño J. Oxidative stress and inflammation, a link between chronic kidney disease and cardiovascular disease. Kidney Int 2008; 74(111): S4-9.
[http://dx.doi.org/10.1038/ki.2008.516] [PMID: 19034325]

[51]   Yang K, Nie L, Huang Y, *et al.* Amelioration of uremic toxin indoxyl sulfate-induced endothelial cell dysfunction by Klotho protein. Toxicol Lett 2012; 215(2): 77-83.
[http://dx.doi.org/10.1016/j.toxlet.2012.10.004] [PMID: 23085347]

[52]   El-Gamal D, Rao SP, Holzer M, *et al.* The urea decomposition product cyanate promotes endothelial dysfunction. Kidney Int 2014; 86(5): 923-31.
[http://dx.doi.org/10.1038/ki.2014.218] [PMID: 24940796]

[53]   Wang CC, Lee AS, Liu SH, Chang KC, Shen MY, Chang CT. Spironolactone ameliorates endothelial dysfunction through inhibition of the AGE/RAGE axis in a chronic renal failure rat model. BMC Nephrol 2019; 20(1): 351.
[http://dx.doi.org/10.1186/s12882-019-1534-4] [PMID: 31492107]

[54]   Peng A, Wu T, Zeng C, *et al.* Adverse effects of simulated hyper- and hypo-phosphatemia on endothelial cell function and viability. PLoS One 2011; 6(8): e23268.
[http://dx.doi.org/10.1371/journal.pone.0023268] [PMID: 21858050]

[55]   Li P, Zhang L, Zhang M, Zhou C, Lin N. Uric acid enhances PKC-dependent eNOS phosphorylation and mediates cellular ER stress: A mechanism for uric acid-induced endothelial dysfunction. Int J Mol Med 2016; 37(4): 989-97.
[http://dx.doi.org/10.3892/ijmm.2016.2491] [PMID: 26935704]

[56]   Hao Y, Zhao L, Zhao JY, *et al.* Unveiling the potential of mitochondrial dynamics as a therapeutic strategy for acute kidney injury. Front Cell Dev Biol; 11.
[http://dx.doi.org/10.3389/fcell.2023.1244313]

[57]   Emma F, Montini G, Parikh SM, Salviati L. Mitochondrial dysfunction in inherited renal disease and acute kidney injury. Nat Rev Nephrol 2016; 12(5): 267-80.
[http://dx.doi.org/10.1038/nrneph.2015.214] [PMID: 26804019]

[58]   Tran M, Tam D, Bardia A, *et al.* PGC-1α promotes recovery after acute kidney injury during systemic inflammation in mice. J Clin Invest 2011; 121(10): 4003-14.
[http://dx.doi.org/10.1172/JCI58662] [PMID: 21881206]

[59]   Sweeney TE, Suliman HB, Hollingsworth JW, Welty-Wolf KE, Piantadosi CA. A toll-like receptor 2 pathway regulates the Ppargc1a/b metabolic co-activators in mice with Staphylococcal aureus sepsis. PLoS One 2011; 6(9): e25249.
[http://dx.doi.org/10.1371/journal.pone.0025249] [PMID: 21966468]

[60]   Fontecha-Barriuso M, Martin-Sanchez D, Martinez-Moreno J, *et al.* The role of PGC-1α and mitochondrial biogenesis in kidney diseases. Biomolecules 2020; 10(2): 347.
[http://dx.doi.org/10.3390/biom10020347] [PMID: 32102312]

[61]   Tran MT, Zsengeller ZK, Berg AH, *et al.* PGC1α drives NAD biosynthesis linking oxidative metabolism to renal protection. Nature 2016; 531(7595): 528-32.
[http://dx.doi.org/10.1038/nature17184] [PMID: 26982719]

[62]   Idrovo JP, Yang WL, Nicastro J, Coppa GF, Wang P. Stimulation of carnitine palmitoyltransferase 1 improves renal function and attenuates tissue damage after ischemia/reperfusion. J Surg Res 2012; 177(1): 157-64.
[http://dx.doi.org/10.1016/j.jss.2012.05.053] [PMID: 22698429]

[63]   Ugarte-Uribe B, Müller HM, Otsuki M, Nickel W, García-Sáez AJ. Dynamin-related protein 1 (Drp1) promotes structural intermediates of membrane division. J Biol Chem 2014; 289(44): 30645-56.

[http://dx.doi.org/10.1074/jbc.M114.575779] [PMID: 25237193]

[64] Mukhopadhyay P, Horváth B, Zsengellér Z, *et al.* Mitochondrial-targeted antioxidants represent a promising approach for prevention of cisplatin-induced nephropathy. Free Radic Biol Med 2012; 52(2): 497-506.
[http://dx.doi.org/10.1016/j.freeradbiomed.2011.11.001] [PMID: 22120494]

[65] Perry HM, Huang L, Wilson RJ, *et al.* Dynamin-related protein 1 deficiency promotes recovery from AKI. J Am Soc Nephrol 2018; 29(1): 194-206.
[http://dx.doi.org/10.1681/ASN.2017060659] [PMID: 29084809]

[66] Morigi M, Perico L, Rota C, *et al.* Sirtuin 3–dependent mitochondrial dynamic improvements protect against acute kidney injury. J Clin Invest 2015; 125(2): 715-26.
[http://dx.doi.org/10.1172/JCI77632] [PMID: 25607838]

[67] Gottlieb RA, Carreira RS. Autophagy in health and disease. 5. Mitophagy as a way of life. Am J Physiol Cell Physiol 2010; 299(2): C203-10. Epub ahead of print
[http://dx.doi.org/10.1152/ajpcell.00097.2010] [PMID: 20357180]

[68] Sansanwal P, Yen B, Gahl WA, *et al.* Mitochondrial autophagy promotes cellular injury in nephropathic cystinosis. J Am Soc Nephrol 2010; 21(2): 272-83.
[http://dx.doi.org/10.1681/ASN.2009040383] [PMID: 19959713]

[69] Lee J, Giordano S, Zhang J. Autophagy, mitochondria and oxidative stress: cross-talk and redox signalling. Biochem J 2012; 441(2): 523-40.
[http://dx.doi.org/10.1042/BJ20111451] [PMID: 22187934]

[70] Ishihara M, Urushido M, Hamada K, *et al.* Sestrin-2 and BNIP3 regulate autophagy and mitophagy in renal tubular cells in acute kidney injury. Am J Physiol Renal Physiol 2013; 305(4): F495-509.
[http://dx.doi.org/10.1152/ajprenal.00642.2012] [PMID: 23698117]

[71] Jiang M, Wei Q, Dong G, Komatsu M, Su Y, Dong Z. Autophagy in proximal tubules protects against acute kidney injury. Kidney Int 2012; 82(12): 1271-83.
[http://dx.doi.org/10.1038/ki.2012.261] [PMID: 22854643]

[72] Peasley K, Chiba T, Goetzman E, Sims-Lucas S. Sirtuins play critical and diverse roles in acute kidney injury. Pediatr Nephrol 2021; 36(11): 3539-46. Epub ahead of print
[http://dx.doi.org/10.1007/s00467-020-04866-z] [PMID: 33411071]

[73] Chiba T, Peasley KD, Cargill KR, *et al.* Sirtuin 5 regulates proximal tubule fatty acid oxidation to protect against AKI. J Am Soc Nephrol 2019; 30(12): 2384-98.
[http://dx.doi.org/10.1681/ASN.2019020163] [PMID: 31575700]

[74] Faivre A, Katsyuba E, Verissimo T, *et al.* Differential role of nicotinamide adenine dinucleotide deficiency in acute and chronic kidney disease. Nephrol Dial Transplant 2021; 36(1): 60-8.
[http://dx.doi.org/10.1093/ndt/gfaa124] [PMID: 33099633]

[75] Morigi M, Perico L, Benigni A. Sirtuins in Renal Health and Disease. J Am Soc Nephrol 2018; 29(7): 1799-809.
[http://dx.doi.org/10.1681/ASN.2017111218] [PMID: 29712732]

[76] Jung YJ, Lee AS, Nguyen-Thanh T, *et al.* SIRT2 regulates LPS-induced renal tubular CXCL2 and CCL2 expression. J Am Soc Nephrol 2015; 26(7): 1549-60.
[http://dx.doi.org/10.1681/ASN.2014030226] [PMID: 25349202]

[77] Jung YJ, Park W, Kang KP, Kim W. SIRT2 is involved in cisplatin-induced acute kidney injury through regulation of mitogen-activated protein kinase phosphatase-1. Nephrol Dial Transplant 2020; 35(7): 1145-56.
[http://dx.doi.org/10.1093/ndt/gfaa042] [PMID: 32240312]

[78] Zhao W, Zhang L, Chen R, *et al.* SIRT3 protects against acute kidney injury *via* AMPK/mTOR-regulated autophagy. Front Physiol 2018; 9: 1526.
[http://dx.doi.org/10.3389/fphys.2018.01526] [PMID: 30487750]

[79]   Tennen RI, Chua KF. Chromatin regulation and genome maintenance by mammalian SIRT6. Trends Biochem Sci 2011; 36(1): 39-46.
[http://dx.doi.org/10.1016/j.tibs.2010.07.009] [PMID: 20729089]

[80]   Mao Z, Hine C, Tian X, *et al.* SIRT6 promotes DNA repair under stress by activating PARP1. Science 2011; 332(6036): 1443-6.
[http://dx.doi.org/10.1126/science.1202723] [PMID: 21680843]

[81]   Huang W, Liu H, Zhu S, *et al.* Sirt6 deficiency results in progression of glomerular injury in the kidney. Aging (Albany NY) 2017; 9(3): 1069-83.
[http://dx.doi.org/10.18632/aging.101214] [PMID: 28351995]

[82]   Zhang Y, Wang L, Meng L, Cao G, Wu Y. Sirtuin 6 overexpression relieves sepsis-induced acute kidney injury by promoting autophagy. Cell Cycle 2019; 18(4): 425-36.
[http://dx.doi.org/10.1080/15384101.2019.1568746] [PMID: 30700227]

[83]   Grob A, Roussel P, Wright JE, McStay B, Hernandez-Verdun D, Sirri V. Involvement of SIRT7 in resumption of rDNA transcription at the exit from mitosis. J Cell Sci 2009; 122(4): 489-98.
[http://dx.doi.org/10.1242/jcs.042382] [PMID: 19174463]

[84]   Chen S, Seiler J, Santiago-Reichelt M, Felbel K, Grummt I, Voit R. Repression of RNA polymerase I upon stress is caused by inhibition of RNA-dependent deacetylation of PAF53 by SIRT7. Mol Cell 2013; 52(3): 303-13.
[http://dx.doi.org/10.1016/j.molcel.2013.10.010] [PMID: 24207024]

[85]   Miyasato Y, Yoshizawa T, Sato Y, *et al.* Sirtuin 7 Deficiency Ameliorates Cisplatin-induced Acute Kidney Injury Through Regulation of the Inflammatory Response. Sci Rep 2018; 8(1): 5927.
[http://dx.doi.org/10.1038/s41598-018-24257-7] [PMID: 29651144]

[86]   Zhang H, Sun SC. NF-κB in inflammation and renal diseases. Cell Biosci 2015; 5(1): 63.
[http://dx.doi.org/10.1186/s13578-015-0056-4] [PMID: 26579219]

[87]   Sato Y, Yanagita M. Immune cells and inflammation in AKI to CKD progression. Am J Physiol Renal Physiol 2018; 315(6): F1501-12.
[http://dx.doi.org/10.1152/ajprenal.00195.2018] [PMID: 30156114]

[88]   Patel N, Johnson MA, Vapniarsky N, *et al.* Elamipretide mitigates ischemia-reperfusion injury in a swine model of hemorrhagic shock. Sci Rep 2023; 13(1): 4496.
[http://dx.doi.org/10.1038/s41598-023-31374-5] [PMID: 36934127]

[89]   Alavian KN, Dworetzky SI, Bonanni L, *et al.* The mitochondrial complex V-associated large-conductance inner membrane current is regulated by cyclosporine and dexpramipexole. Mol Pharmacol 2015; 87(1): 1-8.
[http://dx.doi.org/10.1124/mol.114.095661] [PMID: 25332381]

[90]   Song Z, Xia Y, Shi L, *et al.* Inhibition of Drp1- Fis1 interaction alleviates aberrant mitochondrial fragmentation and acute kidney injury. Cell Mol Biol Lett 2024; 29(1): 31.
[http://dx.doi.org/10.1186/s11658-024-00553-1] [PMID: 38439028]

[91]   Aranda-Rivera AK, Cruz-Gregorio A, Amador-Martínez I, Hernández-Cruz EY, Tapia E, Pedraza-Chaverri J. Antioxidants targeting mitochondria function in kidney diseases. Mitochondrial Communications 2024; 2: 21-37.
[http://dx.doi.org/10.1016/j.mitoco.2024.03.002]

[92]   Morevati M, Fang EF, Mace ML, *et al.* Roles of NAD$^+$ in Acute and Chronic Kidney Diseases. Int J Mol Sci 2022; 24(1): 137. Epub ahead of print
[http://dx.doi.org/10.3390/ijms24010137] [PMID: 36613582]

[93]   Cui L, Zhou Q, Zheng X, Sun B, Zhao S. Mitoquinone attenuates vascular calcification by suppressing oxidative stress and reducing apoptosis of vascular smooth muscle cells *via* the Keap1/Nrf2 pathway. Free Radic Biol Med 2020; 161: 23-31.
[http://dx.doi.org/10.1016/j.freeradbiomed.2020.09.028] [PMID: 33011276]

[94]   Zhu Z, Liang W, Chen Z, *et al.* Mitoquinone Protects Podocytes from Angiotensin II□Induced Mitochondrial Dysfunction and Injury *via* the Keap1□Nrf2 Signaling Pathway. Oxid Med Cell Longev 2021; 2021(1): 1394486.
[http://dx.doi.org/10.1155/2021/1394486] [PMID: 34426758]

[95]   Hernández-Cruz EY, Aparicio-Trejo OE, Hammami FA, *et al.* N-acetylcysteine in Kidney Disease: Molecular Mechanisms, Pharmacokinetics, and Clinical Effectiveness. Kidney Int Rep 2024; 9(10): 2883-903.
[http://dx.doi.org/10.1016/j.ekir.2024.07.020] [PMID: 39430194]

[96]   Kobroob A, Kongkaew A, Wongmekiat O. Melatonin Reduces Aggravation of Renal Ischemia–Reperfusion Injury in Obese Rats by Maintaining Mitochondrial Homeostasis and Integrity through AMPK/PGC-1α/SIRT3/SOD2 Activation. Curr Issues Mol Biol 2023; 45(10): 8239-54.
[http://dx.doi.org/10.3390/cimb45100520] [PMID: 37886963]

[97]   Bai XZ, He T, Gao JX, *et al.* Melatonin prevents acute kidney injury in severely burned rats *via* the activation of SIRT1. Sci Rep 2016; 6(1): 32199.
[http://dx.doi.org/10.1038/srep32199] [PMID: 27599451]

[98]   Zhao H, Ning J, Lemaire A, *et al.* Necroptosis and parthanatos are involved in remote lung injury after receiving ischemic renal allografts in rats. Kidney Int 2015; 87(4): 738-48.
[http://dx.doi.org/10.1038/ki.2014.388] [PMID: 25517913]

CHAPTER 3

Inflammation in Kidney Diseases

Azalia Ávila-Nava[1], Nayeli Goreti Nieto-Velázquez[2] and Isabel Medina-Vera[3,*]

[1] *Research Division, Hospital Regional de Alta Especialidad de la Península de Yucatán IMSS-Bienestar, Mérida, Yucatán, Mexico*

[2] *Research Division, Hospital Juárez de México, Mexico City, Mexico*

[3] *Methodology of Investigation, Instituto Nacional de Pediatría, Mexico City, Mexico*

Abstract: Inflammation is a complex network of interactions between renal parenchymal cells and resident immune cells, such as macrophages and dendritic cells, in conjunction with the recruitment of circulating monocytes, lymphocytes, and neutrophils. Inflammation is an important defense mechanism intended primarily to detect and fight pathogens; resident and circulating immune cells can interact with renal parenchymal cells to trigger the inflammatory response when subjected to stress, leading to irreversible tissue damage and organ failure. Although more evidence of the impact of exercise and omega-3 supplementation on the inflammatory status of these patients has yet to be generated, current evidence suggests that these types of interventions could have a beneficial impact on reducing inflammatory reactions in this population.

Keywords: Adaptative immune system, Dendritic cells, Immune cells, Innate immune system, Interleukins.

INTRODUCTION

The immune system plays an important role in renal homeostasis throughout life. Aging leads to immunosenescence, which is associated with a decrease in the capacity for tissue regeneration and increased susceptibility to kidney disease due to defective immune responses and increased systemic inflammation [1]. Changes in the availability of nutrients and biomolecules, such as cytokines, growth factors, and hormones, initiate cell signaling events involving energy-sensitive molecules and other metabolism-related proteins to coordinate the differentiation, activation, and function of immune cells. The homeostasis alteration causes the metabolic reorganization of immune cells and kidney cells, promoting inflammation and tissue damage [2].

* **Corresponding author Isabel Medina Vera:** Methodology of Investigation, Instituto Nacional de Pediatría, Coyoacán 04530, Mexico City, Mexico; E-mail: isabelj.medinav@gmail.com

Rafael Valdez-Ortiz, Katy Sánchez-Pozos, Ana Carolina Ariza & Enzo C. Vásquez-Jiménez (Eds.)

The inflammation is defined as a complex network of interactions between renal parenchymal cells and resident immune cells, such as macrophages and dendritic cells, in conjunction with the recruitment of circulating monocytes, lymphocytes, and neutrophils [3]. The stimulation of these cells, in turn, can activate other specialized structures, and upon detection of danger-associated molecules, receptors activate the main pathways of innate immunity. An example of this is the activation of Nuclear Factor Kappa-B (NF-κB), Nuclear Factor of Activated T cells (NFAT), or Activator Protein 1 (AP-1). This process causes metabolic reprogramming and phenotypic changes of immune and parenchymal cells, triggering the secretion of inflammatory mediators that are signaled as inflammatory biomarkers: cytokines, Tumor Necrosis Factor-α (TNF-α), Interleukins 1, 6 and 8 (IL-1, IL-6, IL-8), Monocyte Chemotactic Protein 1; or other enzymes and proteins, such as Cyclooxygenase-2 (COX-2), 5-Lipoxygenase (5-LOX), C-Reactive Proteins, Vascular Endothelial Growth Factor (VEGF). Activation of these pathways promoted irreversible tissue damage and functional loss [4]. Kidney inflammation can cause kidney tissue injury and progressive fibrosis, which contributes to the development of glomerulonephritis, acute or chronic kidney disease, and finally end-stage renal disease (ESRD). Kidney inflammation can be caused by several factors, including infection, ischemia/reperfusion, tissue damage, and prolonged exposure to toxic agents [5].

Inflammation: Acute Kidney Injury to Chronic Kidney Disease Progression

The underlying mechanisms in acute kidney injury (AKI) and chronic kidney disease (CKD) are different, but both conditions are interconnected by inflammation. Inflammation is an important defense mechanism intended primarily to detect and fight pathogens; resident and circulating immune cells can interact with renal parenchymal cells to trigger the inflammatory response when subjected to stress, leading to irreversible tissue damage and organ failure [6].

The pathophysiology of AKI is generally characterized by a common pathway, including a cascade of cell death and inflammation induced by injury. The first progression approach from AKI to CKD has been reported as a function of tubule injury, an important source of proinflammatory cytokines. Renal tubular cells recruit immune cells to the tissue. Some of the immune cell populations that are recruited to kidney tissue are mucosal-associated invariant T cells (MAIT), neutrophils, monocytes/macrophages, NK cells, dendritic cells, and T and B lymphocytes, essential components of the innate and adaptive immune response, which play a crucial role in the pathophysiology of kidney disease [4, 7 - 9].

MAIT cells are a subpopulation of unconventional T lymphocytes because they express a minimal repertoire of T cell receptors (TCR) defined by the invariant

TCR Va7.2 (iTCR) alpha chain. They can be activated for their iTCR, which mainly recognizes metabolites derived from vitamin B through the protein related to the major histocompatibility complex class I (MR1). Once activated, they can secrete cytokines of the Th1 type, such as interferon-gamma (IFN-γ), or the Th17 type, such as interleukin 17 (IL-17), in addition to cytotoxic proteins such as granzymes and perforins so that they can protect the host from invasive pathogens and the growth of malignant cells [10].

Although discovered in the mucosa, MAIT cells are distributed in various tissues. Its protective function is limited to barrier tissues; when MAIT cells migrate from peripheral blood to these tissues, their function is tissue repair, the proliferation of other cell types, and the regulation of their activation. In the kidney, a population of MAIT cells that produce IL-17 (MAIT17) with anti-inflammatory properties resides. Such MAIT cells are activated when an inflammatory process such as glomerulonephritis begins. MAIT17 cells can interact with proinflammatory myeloid cells of the kidney, neutrophils, and macrophages, through the CXCR6/ CXCL16 axis, suppressing their destructive capacity. However, the persistence of MAIT17 cells in other tissues can drive the development of chronic and metabolic diseases, which is why they are still being studied since their plasticity is of particular interest [4, 9].

Renal infiltration by neutrophils can be detected in the first hours after ischemia-reperfusion injury. Upon reaching the renal parenchyma, neutrophils are exposed to damage-associated molecular patterns (DAMPs) and/or pathogen-associated molecular patterns (PAMPs), leading to the activation of pattern recognition Toll-like receptors (TLRs) and Nod-like receptors (NLRs), as well as to the secretion of inflammatory factors such as proteases, reactive oxygen species (ROS) and lytic enzymes that alter the homeostasis of the vascular endothelium. DAMPs and PAMPs also induce one of the defense mechanisms against pathogens of neutrophils, which is the formation of extracellular traps (NETs). These network-shaped chromatin structures trap pathogens and eliminate them. However, although NETosis is efficient if not adequately regulated, it can cause damage to the surrounding tissue by itself or by increasing the proinflammatory response; this could be one of the mechanisms by which neutrophils cause tissue damage during the AKI. In removing NETs, macrophages play a leading role [11].

Macrophages are monocyte-derived phagocytic cells that act as important mediators of inflammation and immune modulation. Usually, once they are activated, they can have two phenotypes: proinflammatory macrophages or M1 and anti-inflammatory macrophages or M2. Interestingly, it is known that the phenotype of macrophages can change depending on the microenvironment; in such a way they can contribute to both the pathophysiology and the maintenance of the physiological function of the tissue in which they are found [12]. The subpopulation associated with kidney disease is the proinflammatory M1 macrophages, which are differentiated and activated by inflammatory cytokines such as IFN-γ or TNF-α. However, they can also be activated by advanced glycation end products (AGEs). Once activated, M1 macrophages produce cytokines such as transforming growth factor beta (TGF-β), TNF-α, IL-1β, IL-6, and IL-23, which, together with the generation of reactive oxygen/nitrogen species, promote inflammation and tissue damage. Although macrophages play an important role in the elimination of cellular waste, an increase in the macrophage's infiltration into the tissue has been reported in both, AKI and CKD, so it has been suggested that their activation can promote kidney injury, tubulointerstitial fibrosis, and renal failure through the release of cytokines derived from macrophages and by endorsing the deposition of extracellular matrix [12, 13].

NK cells produce IFN-γ and promote the polarization of macrophages to the M1 phenotype. NK cell function is regulated by inhibitory and activating receptors that detect abnormal or decreased expression of major histocompatibility complex class I (MHC-I) molecules on the cell surface. They can also be activated directly by cytokine signaling or recognizing bacterial components such as lipopolysaccharide (LPS), superantigens of Gram-positive bacteria, or streptococcal derivatives. Once the target cell is identified, NK cells, without the cooperation of other immune cells, exert their cytotoxic action by releasing perforin and granzyme, thus eliminating infected cells, cancer cells, or autoreactive cells. In the kidney, the recruitment of NK cells and their overactivation promote tubular epithelial cell death and AKI, leading to the progression of kidney disease [14].

On the other hand, antigen-presenting dendritic cells (DCs), a key step in the activation of adaptive immunity, are located between the tubules and peritubular capillaries, which allows them to interact with both epithelial and endothelial cells. When the stimulus is tissue damage, DCs are activated by recognizing DAMPs, while in infectious processes, they are activated by PAMPs. Once activated, they migrate to the lymph nodes, activating T lymphocytes through antigen recognition. The activated T lymphocytes differentiate into CD4+ T helper lymphocytes (CD4+ T) or CD8+ cytotoxic T lymphocytes (CD8+ T). The latter infiltrate the kidney and release IFN-γ and TNF-α that finally induce glomerulonephritis, chronic inflammation, and fibrosis. Furthermore, its exacerbated activity can induce cell death of tubular cells, contributing to tubulointerstitial fibrosis. T cells also mount an antibody-dependent response that requires activation of B cells by CD4+ T cells. These antibodies that mediate the effector functions of the humoral immune system are produced and secreted from a population of differentiated B lymphocyte cells called plasma cells [14, 15].

Antibodies function by opsonizing target cells and promoting their elimination by activating complement proteins. The complement system amplifies the innate and adaptive immune response because, in addition to opsonization, the complement system mediates functions such as cell lysis, chemotaxis, inflammation, cellular activation, removal of antigen/antibody complexes, and elimination of autoreactive B cells [15]. However, some autoreactive B cells occur to produce autoantibodies. In that case, antigen-autoantibody complexes can be deposited in the glomerulus promoting the activation of complement proteins, which induces glomerulonephritis and AKI. Activated B cells also produce proinflammatory cytokines that contribute to infiltrating more inflammatory cells into the kidney [16].

The inflammatory response must be regulated and ultimately suppressed To prevent the progression from acute to persistent chronic inflammation. The resolution of inflammation is a well-managed process that recovers tissue homeostasis, reducing the production of inflammatory mediators, decreasing tissue infiltration by immune cells, and modifying the profile of M1 macrophages to an M2 phenotype, whose anti-inflammatory effect facilitates the repair of kidney tissue. To promote this process of recovery of homeostasis, DCs produce IL-10, an anti-inflammatory cytokine that promotes the differentiation of regulatory T lymphocytes (Treg) with $CD^{4+}CD2^{5+}$ phenotype, whose function is to counteract the inflammatory response promoted by lymphocytes. T CD4+ and T CD^{8+}. Treg cells participate in both development and tissue repair after AKI. However, deregulation of this process can cause uncontrolled chronic inflammation; it has been proven that there is altered Treg activity in AKI due to cellular exhaustion [16 - 19].

In response to severe tubule injury, the cells enter the cell cycle and arrest in the G2/M phase in which proinflammatory cytokines are released. Additionally, connective tissue growth factor (CTGF) and transforming growth factor beta (TGF-β), which are profibrotic factors involved in fibrosis development, are upregulated, leading to kidney fibrosis [20]. It has been documented that after an episode of AKI, some of the signaling pathways during normal kidney development are activated; one of these pathways is Wnt/B-catenin, stimulated in the acute phase of AKI. This process has been observed to increase apoptosis, which is a programmed cell death that eliminates the tubular cells' inflammation to protect them from renal injury. However, if this pathway remains permanently active, signaling can activate myofibroblasts and promote fibrosis until progression to CKD [21]. Moreover, one of the signaling pathways activated in AKI progression to CKD is that of TGF-β, consequently inducing renal cells to produce fibrotic extracellular matrix proteins, leading to glomerulosclerosis and tubulointerstitial fibrosis. Although activation of this pathway in AKI is implicated in the regeneration of functional renal tubules, if it is continuously active and upregulated, this could lead to CKD progression [22]. The canonical function of fibroblasts is a mechanism that has been implicated in the progression of AKI to CKD and has recently been recognized as a driver of inflammation as they have been shown to respond after injury to damage-associated molecular patterns through Toll-like receptors (TLRs) more sensitively than other cell types, producing higher amounts of proinflammatory cytokines [23].

Etiology and Outcomes of Inflammation in CKD

The kidney is a very vulnerable tissue due to its limited mechanisms of antioxidant, detoxifying, and anti-inflammatory defense mechanisms compared with other intensively vascularized organs [24]. Furthermore, inflammation is one of the major contributors to the uremic phenotype in CKD. Indeed, the role of inflammation in the pathogenesis and progression of CKD has been recognized since the 1990s. A study showed that IL-1 release was the starting point of the main complications and the increasing mortality rate in patients undergoing chronic dialysis. Inflammatory status in CKD is a multifactorial process, which includes deregulation of the microvascular response, acidosis, and chronic and recurrent infections. Another major underlying cause of systemic inflammation is uremic immune dysfunction, affecting the innate and adaptive immune systems [25]. During CKD, renal dysfunction inevitably results in alterations in the retention of fluid and small and large solutes, many of which may act as proinflammatory uremic toxins. Among these toxins are indoxyl sulfate (IS), p-cresol (PC), and p-cresol sulfate (PCS) involved in the inflammatory state of CKD [26]. Uremic toxins have also been shown to contribute to many uremia-associated dysfunctions, including an altered immune response [27]. These can activate immune cells such as neutrophils, monocytes, and lymphocytes, resulting in high oxidative stress and the production of proinflammatory cytokines, creating a persistent inflammatory state [28 - 30]. In addition, inflammation contributes to the deregulation of the microvascular response and, consequently, the sustained production of an array of tubular toxins, including reactive oxygen species (ROS). These alterations modify or interfere with the intrarenal microcirculatory regulation and perfusion distribution and can induce tubular injury and nephron dropout, causing renal damage and thus accelerating CKD progression [31]. Clinical studies have demonstrated that inflammatory markers are associated with many complications during CKD, such as malnutrition, coronary artery calcification, atherosclerosis, atrial fibrillation, left ventricular hypertrophy, heart failure and enhanced CKD mortality [32 - 34]. Moreover, inflammation contributes to the progression of CKD by favoring insulin resistance, oxidative stress, endothelial dysfunction, mineral and bone diseases, anemia, and erythropoietin [35 - 38].

One of the key pathways involved in the development of CKD is the activation of the NLRP3 inflammasome and the subsequent production of proinflammatory cytokines, such as IL-1β and IL-18 [39]. Inflammasomes are a multiprotein complex that mediates the activation of caspase 1, which promotes the secretion of cytokines (IL-1β and IL-18) and cell death by pyroptosis of renal tubular cells. Pyroptosis of renal cells can exacerbate tissue injury and contribute to loss of renal function [40, 41]. Depending on the receptors that make up the inflammasome, they are classified into NLRP1, NLRP3, and NLRC4. In various studies, an increase in the expression and activation of NLRP3 has been observed in tubular epithelial cells, glomerular cells, and immune system cells infiltrating the kidney of patients with CKD. The activation of the NLRP3 inflammasome, as a mechanism of the innate immune response, is induced by the presence of DAMPs and PAMPs in the kidney tissue. In the renal microenvironment, the production of large amounts of IL-1β and IL-18 by the inflammasome and the consequent activation of the NF-κB transcription factor and MAPK signaling, amplifying the proinflammatory response and perpetuating it, contribute to the pathogenesis and progression of AKI-CKD. IL-1β and IL-18 also promote immune cell recruitment, exacerbate tissue damage, and stimulate fibrotic responses in the kidney [42, 43].

Role of Proinflammatory Biomarkers in Renal Injury

The inflammasomes have recently become the subject of intensive research since they play a significant role in the pathogenic mechanisms of renal diseases. The inflammasomes are large, multiprotein complexes that could be induced by lipopolysaccharide (LPS) [44]. Increased inflammatory markers by innate immune signaling pathways characterize inflammation. This signal involved activation of NF-κB, which regulates the expression of proinflammatory markers. Among these markers are cytokines, acute phase proteins, and adhesion molecules, which are stimulated by the cells of the innate immune response system [24, 45]. Proinflammatory markers in CKD are CRP, IL-6, IL-1, TNF-α, monocyte chemoattractant peptide protein 1 (MCP-1), adipokines, adhesion molecules, and the CD40 ligand. Circulating proinflammatory cytokines generally activate intrarenal microvessels, promoting modifications that affect cell-surface adhesion molecules. These alterations disrupt endothelial barrier function, activation of the coagulation system, and receptor-mediated vasoreactivity; together, they can promote irreversible tubular injury and nephron failure [31]. Specifically, IL-1 and IL-6 have been shown to suppress the secretion of parathyroid hormone (PTH). Low PTH levels in hemodialysis patients have been associated with malnutrition, cachexia syndrome, as well as low bone turnover disease [46]. In addition, TNF-α, CRP, and MCP-1 have been linked to lower levels of glomerular filtration rate, malnutrition, vascular injury, atherosclerosis, erythropoietin resistance, and cardiovascular morbidity and mortality [45, 47, 48]. Also, high levels of these cytokines increased the activity of pro-inflammatory enzymes such as COX-2 and inducible nitric oxide synthase (iNOS), which is also associated with the activation of NF-κB in patients with CKD. Uremic toxins also activate NF-κB, exhibiting positive correlations with CRP levels, iNOS, and COX-2 expression [45].

Furthermore, other specific inflammatory molecules, such as pentraxin-3 (PTX3) and TNF-Related weak inducer of apoptosis (TWEAK), have gained increasing interest. PTX3 and TWEAK promote kidney infiltration of inflammatory cells, stimulate the proliferation of kidney cells, and the development of glomerulonephritis [49].

Anti-inflammatory Therapies in CKD: Diet Bioactive Compounds, Prebiotics, Probiotics Use, and Intradialytic Exercise

Various interventions have been proposed to counteract the inflammation produced in CKD, among which are the consumption of bioactive compounds in the diet, prebiotics and probiotics, and intradialytic exercise programs. One of the bioactive compounds studied to mitigate inflammation in these patients has been omega-3 supplementation, a polyunsaturated fatty acid reported to be therapeutically helpful in patients at high inflammatory risk. It was reported that after supplementation of 2.4 g of omega-3 for 12 weeks in CKD patients on hemodialysis, the authors observed a decrease in CRP (-26.1%, $P < 0.001$), IL-6 (-25.1%, $P < 0.001$) and TNF-α concentrations (-13.13%, $P< 0.009$) when compared to the control group [50]. One of the proposed mechanisms by which omega-3 has anti-inflammatory effects is that these fatty acids act on adhesion molecules, thereby inhibiting the NF-κB pathway's activation. Since NF-κB activation requires the presence of ROS, such as hydrogen peroxide, a plausible mechanism would involve a decrease in the production of ROS by n-3 fatty acids [51].

Monitoring and controlling inflammation biomarkers is a promising therapeutic approach. The accumulation of high-molecular polymeric IgA1 stimulates the proliferation of mesangial cells with the release of IL-6. The activation of AT1R is linked to the IL-6 secretion in the mesangial [52]. Therefore, the use of losartan, which is a blocker of AT1R, might result in decreasing levels of IL-6 [53]. Tocilizumab is a monoclonal antibody (mAb) specific for the IL-6 receptor (IL-6R) meaning a therapeutic improvement for patients with renal insufficiency [54].

Finally, intradialytic exercise programs are among the most recent therapeutics that could benefit the inflammatory profile. Sovatzidis *et al.* studied the effect of intradialytic exercise for 6 months on redox status, inflammation, and physical performance in patients with end-stage renal disease. As a result, there was an increase in maximal oxygen consumption (VO_2 peak) (15%, P <0.01). This intervention promoted the reduction of lipoperoxidation products (- 28%) and proinflammatory markers such as PCR (-31%) and hs-CRP (-15%). In addition, it also increased antioxidants such as reduced glutathione (52%) and total antioxidant activity (59%) (P < 0.01). These findings suggest that regular intradialytic cardiovascular exercise reduces inflammation [55]. On the other hand, Min-Tser Liao *et al.* showed the effects of intradialytic aerobic cycling exercise in hemodialysis patients; after 3 months of intervention, the patients showed a significant decrease in concentrations of hs-CRP (1.25 ± 2.021 to 0.78 ± 0.83 mg/dL) and IL-6 (4.23 ± 2.65 to 3.48 ± 2.95 pg/mL) [56].

CONCLUSION

Although more evidence of the impact of exercise and omega-3 supplementation on the inflammatory status of these patients has yet to be generated, current evidence suggests that these types of interventions could have a beneficial impact in reducing inflammatory reactions in this population. Therefore, the effect of some NLRP3 inflammasome inhibitors has been studied in animal models of kidney injury, which have not yet reached treatment phases in humans. In conclusion, modulation of the immune response in kidney disease is a possible therapeutic strategy.

REFERENCES

[1]   Sato Y, Yanagita M. Immunology of the ageing kidney. Nat Rev Nephrol 2019; 15(10): 625-40.
       [http://dx.doi.org/10.1038/s41581-019-0185-9] [PMID: 31477915]

[2]   Basso PJ, Andrade-Oliveira V, Câmara NOS. Targeting immune cell metabolism in kidney diseases.
       Nat Rev Nephrol 2021; 17(7): 465-80.
       [http://dx.doi.org/10.1038/s41581-021-00413-7] [PMID: 33828286]

[3]   Yoshikawa T, Yanagita M. Single-Cell Analysis Provides New Insights into the Roles of Tertiary
       Lymphoid Structures and Immune Cell Infiltration in Kidney Injury and Chronic Kidney Disease. Am
       J Pathol 2024; 195(1): 40-54.
       [http://dx.doi.org/10.1016/j.ajpath.2024.07.008] [PMID: 39097168]

[4]   Andrade-Oliveira V, Foresto-Neto O, Watanabe IKM, Zatz R, Câmara NOS. Inflammation in renal
       diseases: New and old players. Front Pharmacol 2019; 10: 1192.
       [http://dx.doi.org/10.3389/fphar.2019.01192] [PMID: 31649546]

[5]   Chen L, Deng H, Cui H, *et al.* Inflammatory responses and inflammation-associated diseases in
       organs. Oncotarget 2018; 9(6): 7204-18.
       [http://dx.doi.org/10.18632/oncotarget.23208] [PMID: 29467962]

[6]   Singbartl K, Formeck CL, Kellum JA. Kidney-Immune System Crosstalk in AKI. Semin Nephrol
       2019; 39(1): 96-106.
       [http://dx.doi.org/10.1016/j.semnephrol.2018.10.007] [PMID: 30606411]

[7]   Qu L, Jiao B. The Interplay between Immune and Metabolic Pathways in Kidney Disease. Cells 2023;
       12(12): 1584. Epub ahead of print
       [http://dx.doi.org/10.3390/cells12121584] [PMID: 37371054]

[8]   Imig JD, Ryan MJ. Immune and Inflammatory Role in Renal Disease. In: Compr Physiol, pp. 957–976.
         [http://dx.doi.org/10.1002/cphy.c120028]

[9]   Gnirck AC, Philipp MS, Waterhölter A, *et al.* Mucosal-associated invariant T cells contribute to suppression of inflammatory myeloid cells in immune-mediated kidney disease. Nat Commun 2023; 14(1): 7372.
         [http://dx.doi.org/10.1038/s41467-023-43269-0] [PMID: 37968302]

[10]   Xiao X, Cai J. Mucosal-Associated Invariant T Cells: New Insights into Antigen Recognition and Activation. Front Immunol 2017; 8: 1540.
         [http://dx.doi.org/10.3389/fimmu.2017.01540] [PMID: 29176983]

[11]   Mutua V, Gershwin LJ. A Review of Neutrophil Extracellular Traps (NETs) in Disease: Potential Anti-NETs Therapeutics. Clin Rev Allergy Immunol 2021; 61(2): 194-211.
         [http://dx.doi.org/10.1007/s12016-020-08804-7] [PMID: 32740860]

[12]   Papayannopoulos V. Neutrophil extracellular traps in immunity and disease. Nat Rev Immunol 2018; 18(2): 134-47.
         [http://dx.doi.org/10.1038/nri.2017.105] [PMID: 28990587]

[13]   Yunna C, Mengru H, Lei W, Weidong C. Macrophage M1/M2 polarization. Eur J Pharmacol 2020; 877: 173090.
         [http://dx.doi.org/10.1016/j.ejphar.2020.173090] [PMID: 32234529]

[14]   Sun S, Chen R, Dou X, *et al.* Immunoregulatory mechanism of acute kidney injury in sepsis: A Narrative Review. Biomed Pharmacother 2023; 159: 114202.
         [http://dx.doi.org/10.1016/j.biopha.2022.114202] [PMID: 36621143]

[15]   Petr V, Thurman JM. The role of complement in kidney disease. Nat Rev Nephrol 2023; 19(12): 771-87.
         [http://dx.doi.org/10.1038/s41581-023-00766-1] [PMID: 37735215]

[16]   Bavikar P, Dighe T, Wakhare P, Shinde N, Bale C, Sajgure A. Role of T-lymphocytes in Kidney Disease. Cureus 2021; 13(10): e19153.
         [http://dx.doi.org/10.7759/cureus.19153] [PMID: 34868786]

[17]   Kong L, Andrikopoulos S, MacIsaac RJ, *et al.* Role of the adaptive immune system in diabetic kidney disease. J Diabetes Investig 2022; 13(2): 213-26.
         [http://dx.doi.org/10.1111/jdi.13725] [PMID: 34845863]

[18]   Lee SA, Noel S, Sadasivam M, Hamad ARA, Rabb H. Role of Immune Cells in Acute Kidney Injury and Repair. Nephron J 2017; 137(4): 282-6.
         [http://dx.doi.org/10.1159/000477181] [PMID: 28601878]

[19]   Lee K, Jang HR. Role of T cells in ischemic acute kidney injury and repair. Korean J Intern Med (Korean Assoc Intern Med) 2022; 37(3): 534-50.
         [http://dx.doi.org/10.3904/kjim.2021.526] [PMID: 35508946]

[20]   Yang L, Besschetnova TY, Brooks CR, Shah JV, Bonventre JV. Epithelial cell cycle arrest in G2/M mediates kidney fibrosis after injury. Nat Med 2010; 16(5): 535-543, 1p, 143.
         [http://dx.doi.org/10.1038/nm.2144] [PMID: 20436483]

[21]   Xiao L, Zhou D, Tan RJ, *et al.* Sustained activation of Wnt/b-catenin signaling drives AKI to CKD progression. J Am Soc Nephrol 2016; 27(6): 1727-40.
         [http://dx.doi.org/10.1681/ASN.2015040449] [PMID: 26453613]

[22]   He L, Wei Q, Liu J, *et al.* AKI on CKD: heightened injury, suppressed repair, and the underlying mechanisms. Kidney Int 2017; 92(5): 1071-83.
         [http://dx.doi.org/10.1016/j.kint.2017.06.030] [PMID: 28890325]

[23]   Leaf IA, Nakagawa S, Johnson BG, *et al.* Pericyte MyD88 and IRAK4 control inflammatory and

fibrotic responses to tissue injury. J Clin Invest 2016; 127(1): 321-34.
[http://dx.doi.org/10.1172/JCI87532] [PMID: 27869651]

[24]   Mihai S, Codrici E, Popescu ID, *et al.* Inflammation-related mechanisms in chronic kidney disease prediction, progression, and outcome. J Immunol Res; 2018. Epub ahead of print 2018.
[http://dx.doi.org/10.1155/2018/2180373]

[25]   Machowska A, Carrero JJ, Lindholm B, Stenvinkel P. Therapeutics targeting persistent inflammation in chronic kidney disease. Transl Res 2016; 167(1): 204-13.
[http://dx.doi.org/10.1016/j.trsl.2015.06.012] [PMID: 26173187]

[26]   Huang SY, Chen YA, Chen SA, Chen YJ, Lin YK. Uremic toxins-novel arrhythmogenic factor in chronic kidney disease-related atrial fibrillation. Zhonghua Minguo Xinzangxue Hui Zazhi 2016; 32(3): 259-64.
[http://dx.doi.org/10.6515/acs20151116a] [PMID: 27274165]

[27]   Adesso S, Popolo A, Bianco G, *et al.* The uremic toxin indoxyl sulphate enhances macrophage response to LPS. PLoS One 2013; 8(9): e76778. Epub ahead of print
[http://dx.doi.org/10.1371/journal.pone.0076778] [PMID: 24098806]

[28]   Shimizu H, Bolati D, Adijiang A, *et al.* NF-κB plays an important role in indoxyl sulfate-induced cellular senescence, fibrotic gene expression, and inhibition of proliferation in proximal tubular cells. Am J Physiol Cell Physiol 2011; 301(5): C1201-12.
[http://dx.doi.org/10.1152/ajpcell.00471.2010] [PMID: 21832251]

[29]   Watanabe H, Miyamoto Y, Honda D, *et al.* p -Cresyl sulfate causes renal tubular cell damage by inducing oxidative stress by activation of NADPH oxidase. Kidney Int 2013; 83(4): 582-92.
[http://dx.doi.org/10.1038/ki.2012.448] [PMID: 23325087]

[30]   Hasegawa T, Nakai S, Masakane I, *et al.* Dialysis fluid endotoxin level and mortality in maintenance hemodialysis: a nationwide cohort study. Am J Kidney Dis 2015; 65(6): 899-904.
[http://dx.doi.org/10.1053/j.ajkd.2014.12.009] [PMID: 25641063]

[31]   Qian Q. Inflammation: A key contributor to the genesis and progression of chronic kidney disease. Contrib Nephrol 2017; 191: 72-83.
[http://dx.doi.org/10.1159/000479257] [PMID: 28910792]

[32]   Gupta J, Mitra N, Kanetsky PA, *et al.* Association between albuminuria, kidney function, and inflammatory biomarker profile in CKD in CRIC. Clin J Am Soc Nephrol 2012; 7(12): 1938-46.
[http://dx.doi.org/10.2215/CJN.03500412] [PMID: 23024164]

[33]   Ishigami J, Taliercio J, I Feldman H, *et al.* Inflammatory markers and incidence of hospitalization with infection in chronic kidney disease. Am J Epidemiol 2020; 189(5): 433-44.
[http://dx.doi.org/10.1093/aje/kwz246] [PMID: 31673705]

[34]   Jagadeswaran D, Indhumathi E, Hemamalini AJ, Sivakumar V, Soundararajan P, Jayakumar M. Inflammation and nutritional status assessment by malnutrition inflammation score and its outcome in pre-dialysis chronic kidney disease patients. Clin Nutr 2019; 38(1): 341-7.
[http://dx.doi.org/10.1016/j.clnu.2018.01.001] [PMID: 29398341]

[35]   Akchurin OM, Kaskel F. Update on inflammation in chronic kidney disease. Blood Purif 2015; 39(1-3): 84-92.
[http://dx.doi.org/10.1159/000368940] [PMID: 25662331]

[36]   Kosmas CE, Silverio D, Tsomidou C, *et al.* The impact of insulin resistance and chronic kidney disease on inflammation and cardiovascular disease. Clin Med Insights Endocrinol Diabetes 2018; 11: 0–5.
[http://dx.doi.org/10.1177/1179551418792257]

[37]   Ravarotto V, Simioni F, Pagnin E, Davis PA, Calò LA. Oxidative stress – chronic kidney disease – cardiovascular disease: A vicious circle. Life Sci 2018; 210: 125-31.
[http://dx.doi.org/10.1016/j.lfs.2018.08.067] [PMID: 30172705]

[38] Lunyera J, Scialla JJ. Update on chronic kidney disease mineral and bone disorder in cardiovascular disease. Semin Nephrol 2018; 38(6): 542-58.
[http://dx.doi.org/10.1016/j.semnephrol.2018.08.001] [PMID: 30413250]

[39] Hickey FB, Martin F. Role of the immune system in diabetic kidney disease. Curr Diab Rep 2018; 18(4): 20.
[http://dx.doi.org/10.1007/s11892-018-0984-6] [PMID: 29532281]

[40] Kadatane SP, Satariano M, Massey M, Mongan K, Raina R. The role of inflammation in CKD. Cells 2023; 12(12): 1581. Epub ahead of print
[http://dx.doi.org/10.3390/cells12121581] [PMID: 37371050]

[41] Chen Q, Zhang X, Yang H, *et al.* CD8 + CD103 + iTregs protect against ischemia-reperfusion-induced acute kidney Injury by inhibiting pyroptosis. Apoptosis 2024; 29(9-10): 1709-22.
[http://dx.doi.org/10.1007/s10495-024-02001-z] [PMID: 39068624]

[42] Tan YF, Wang M, Chen ZY, Wang L, Liu XH. Inhibition of BRD4 prevents proliferation and epithelial–mesenchymal transition in renal cell carcinoma *via* NLRP3 inflammasome-induced pyroptosis. Cell Death Dis 2020; 11(4): 239.
[http://dx.doi.org/10.1038/s41419-020-2431-2] [PMID: 32303673]

[43] Chi H-H, Hua K-F, Lin Y-C, *et al.* IL-36 signaling facilitates activation of the NLRP3 inflammasome and IL-23/IL-17 axis in renal inflammation and fibrosis. J Am Soc Nephrol; 28.
[http://dx.doi.org/10.1681/ASN.2016080840]

[44] Martinon F, Burns K, Tschopp J. The Inflammasome. Mol Cell 2002; 10(2): 417-26.
[http://dx.doi.org/10.1016/S1097-2765(02)00599-3] [PMID: 12191486]

[45] Rapa SF, Di Iorio BR, Campiglia P, Heidland A, Marzocco S. Inflammation and oxidative stress in chronic kidney disease—potential therapeutic role of minerals, vitamins and plant-derived metabolites. Int J Mol Sci 2019; 21(1): 263. Epub ahead of print
[http://dx.doi.org/10.3390/ijms21010263] [PMID: 31906008]

[46] Feroze U, Molnar MZ, Dukkipati R, Kovesdy CP, Kalantar-Zadeh K. Insights into nutritional and inflammatory aspects of low parathyroid hormone in dialysis patients. J Ren Nutr 2011; 21(1): 100-4.
[http://dx.doi.org/10.1053/j.jrn.2010.10.006] [PMID: 21195929]

[47] Bazeley J, Bieber B, Li Y, *et al.* C-reactive protein and prediction of 1-year mortality in prevalent hemodialysis patients. Clin J Am Soc Nephrol 2011; 6(10): 2452-61.
[http://dx.doi.org/10.2215/CJN.00710111] [PMID: 21868617]

[48] Grabulosa CC, Manfredi SR, Canziani ME, *et al.* Chronic kidney disease induces inflammation by increasing Toll-like receptor-4, cytokine and cathelicidin expression in neutrophils and monocytes. Exp Cell Res 2018; 365(2): 157-62.
[http://dx.doi.org/10.1016/j.yexcr.2018.02.022] [PMID: 29481790]

[49] Gao HX, Campbell SR, Burkly LC, *et al.* TNF-like weak inducer of apoptosis (TWEAK) induces inflammatory and proliferative effects in human kidney cells. Cytokine 2009; 46(1): 24-35.
[http://dx.doi.org/10.1016/j.cyto.2008.12.001] [PMID: 19233685]

[50] Valle Flores JA, Fariño Cortéz JE, Mayner Tresol GA, Perozo Romero J, Blasco Carlos M, Nestares T. Oral supplementation with omega-3 fatty acids and inflammation markers in patients with chronic kidney disease in hemodialysis. Appl Physiol Nutr Metab 2020; 45(8): 805-11.
[http://dx.doi.org/10.1139/apnm-2019-0729] [PMID: 31935118]

[51] Mori TA, Beilin LJ. Omega-3 fatty acids and inflammation. Curr Atheroscler Rep 2004; 6(6): 461-7.
[http://dx.doi.org/10.1007/s11883-004-0087-5] [PMID: 15485592]

[52] Su H, Lei CT, Zhang C. Interleukin-6 Signaling Pathway and Its Role in Kidney Disease: An Update. Front Immunol 2017; 8: 405.
[http://dx.doi.org/10.3389/fimmu.2017.00405] [PMID: 28484449]

[53]   Tamouza H, Chemouny JM, Raskova Kafkova L, *et al.* The IgA1 immune complex–mediated activation of the MAPK/ERK kinase pathway in mesangial cells is associated with glomerular damage in IgA nephropathy. Kidney Int 2012; 82(12): 1284-96.
[http://dx.doi.org/10.1038/ki.2012.192] [PMID: 22951891]

[54]   Mori S, Yoshitama T, Hidaka T, Hirakata N, Ueki Y. Effectiveness and safety of tocilizumab therapy for patients with rheumatoid arthritis and renal insufficiency: a real-life registry study in Japan (the ACTRA-RI study). Ann Rheum Dis 2015; 74(3): 627-30.
[http://dx.doi.org/10.1136/annrheumdis-2014-206695] [PMID: 25561361]

[55]   Sovatzidis A, Chatzinikolaou A, Fatouros IG, *et al.* Intradialytic cardiovascular exercise training alters redox status, reduces inflammation, and improves physical performance in patients with chronic kidney disease. Antioxidants 2020; 9(9): 868.
[http://dx.doi.org/10.3390/antiox9090868] [PMID: 32942555]

[56]   Liao MT, Liu WC, Lin FH, *et al.* Intradialytic aerobic cycling exercise alleviates inflammation and improves endothelial progenitor cell count and bone density in hemodialysis patients. Medicine (Baltimore) 2016; 95(27): e4134. Epub ahead of print
[http://dx.doi.org/10.1097/MD.0000000000004134] [PMID: 27399127]

CHAPTER 4

Metabolic Syndrome as a Risk Factor for Chronic Kidney Disease

Ana Ligia Gutiérrez-Solís[1,2,*] and **Nina Mendez-Domínguez**[1]

[1] *Research Division, Hospital Regional de Alta Especialidad de la Península de Yucatán IMSS-Bienestar, Mérida, Yucatán, Mexico*

[2] *Centro de Investigación y de Estudios Avanzados del IPN (CINVESTAV-IPN) Mérida, Yucatán, Mexico*

Abstract: Recent evidence suggests that MetS significantly increases individuals' risk of developing CKD. Among individuals with CKD, the MetS incidence can reach 70%. Epidemiological studies have reported an independent and positive association between MetS and CKD; accordingly, patients with MetS have up to a 2.6-fold greater risk of CKD than individuals without MetS. On the other hand, the presence of microalbuminuria is also more frequent among patients with MetS. This chapter aims to explore the association between MetS and precursor factors of kidney disease, including prevalence, pathophysiology, and clinical and laboratory diagnosis, including progression monitoring. The factors contributing to kidney injury onset in MetS patients may include oxidative stress and systemic inflammation, endothelial dysfunction, altered renal hemodynamics, excessive renal sodium reabsorption, activation of the RAAS and sympathetic nervous system, an atherogenic lipid profile, and even physical compression of the kidneys by adipose tissue. In conclusion, measures for broadly addressing the impact of CKD and MetS may not be understood as separate approaches but may be complementary. The need to ensure effective primary prevention based on nutritional and lifestyle approaches is fundamental.

Keywords: Chronic kidney disease, Inflammation, Metabolic syndrome, Microalbuminuria, Renin-angiotensin system.

INTRODUCTION

Chronic kidney disease (CKD) is defined as an alteration in renal function characterized by the excretion of urinary albumin between 30-300 mg/dL and/or a decrease in the estimated glomerular filtration rate (eGFR) ≤ 60 mL/min/1.73 m2 that persists for at least three months, independent of its origin, whether structural

---

* **First and Corresponding author Ana Ligia Gutiérrez Solís:** Research Division, Hospital Regional de Alta Especialidad de la Península de Yucatán IMSS-Bienestar, Altabrisa, 97130 Mérida, Yucatán, Mexico; E-mail: ganaligia@gmail.com

Rafael Valdez-Ortiz, Katy Sánchez-Pozos, Ana Carolina Ariza & Enzo C. Vásquez-Jiménez (Eds.)

or functional. CKD is a widespread health problem worldwide and is associated with increased morbidity and mortality. CKD decreases the quality of life by generating disability and loss of independence and involves social and psychological burdens for caregivers. These factors, taken together, result in a high economic impact on families and institutions [1].

The worldwide prevalence of CKD is estimated to be close to 10.6%, including patients in 3-5 stages, with CKD being greatest among females (12.1%) [2]. The prevalence varies with geographic region: in China, a prevalence of 1.7% has been reported [3]; with 3.1% in Canada [4]; 5.8% in Australia [5]; and 6.7% in the United States [6], while in Europe, the prevalence varies from 2.3% to 5.2% [7, 8]. Moreover, in America, the prevalence from 2015 to 2016 was 15.3% [9]. According to the Renal Data System of the United States, Taiwan, Mexico (Jalisco), and the United States contributed the most significant number of patients with terminal CKD in 2015 (CKDT, glomerular filtration rate < 15 mL/min/1.73 m^2), with 378-476 patients per million of the general population [10].

The disturbances in CKD correlate with several clinical manifestations, such as insulin resistance (IR), hypertension, central obesity, and/or dyslipidemia, which are the main manifestations of metabolic syndrome (MetS). Overall, the main risk factors for CKD are T2D (57.6%) and systemic arterial hypertension (SAH) (3.2%). An increase in body mass index (BMI) (26.6%), a diet rich in sodium (9.5%), and an unintentional consumption of lead (3.6%) can increase the risk of CKD [11, 12]. Additionally, MetS is linked to aging and unhealthy lifestyles, such as a lack of physical activity and smoking, and it has been well established that MetS is a good predictive factor for T2D and cardiovascular disease (CVD) [13].

MetS is defined as a combination of risk factors, including abdominal obesity based on waist circumference (WC), increased blood pressure (BP), low levels of high-density lipoprotein-cholesterol (HDL-C), and elevated glucose and triglyceride levels. MetS occurs when three or more risk factors are met [13]. Although global data regarding the prevalence of MetS are unavailable for each country, several studies have reported high variation among populations due to differences in demographic characteristics such as ethnic backgrounds, locations, and clinical conditions. The estimated prevalence of MetS in 2011-2016 in the United States was 34.7% in adults [14]. In African populations, the MetS incidence is as high as 50% [15]. Furthermore, in Mexico, a recent meta-analysis reported a MetS prevalence of 41% among adults [16].

Recent evidence suggests that MetS significantly increases individuals' chances of developing CKD. The MetS incidence among individuals with CKD can reach

70% [17]. Several studies have reported an independent and positive association between MetS and CKD; accordingly, patients with MetS have up to a 2.6-fold greater risk of CKD than individuals without MetS [18, 19]. On the other hand, the presence of microalbuminuria is also more frequent among patients with MetS [20]. Furthermore, individuals with advanced CKD have higher prevalence rates of MetS components than individuals without CKD [21].

The increase in CKD incidence has emerged simultaneously with the rise of the obesity epidemic and obesity-related diseases, including MetS. Thus, it is unsurprising that CKD may be more prevalent in regions where MetS has a high incidence. In addition, both conditions share physiopathological pathways; therefore, CKD and MetS may also have common approaches to decrease their burden. Among the reliable strategies may be those that help to prevent and control obesity and its related diseases, promoting multilevel approaches to healthier lifestyles [22]. In this context, favorable outcomes in patients with CKD can be achieved with dietetic and lifestyle changes [23]. However, adopting these changes toward healthier nutrition and active lifestyles depends not only on patients' commitment but also on societal, economic, and political factors. Food insecurity, social violence, production chains, and costs of healthy food and medication are thus limiting factors related to MetS and renal failure progression worldwide [24].

There is an incipient impairment in renal function in patients with MetS long before clinical diagnosis, as microvascular changes are found to be present before metabolic components are integrated as a syndrome. Tubular atrophy, along with increased microvascular disease, interstitial fibrosis, and global and segmental arterial sclerosis occur gradually, and all of these processes, in combination with the presence of inflammatory cytokines (interleukin 6, IL-6; tumor necrosis factor-alpha, TNF-α; and other cytokines), potentiate kidney damage, leading to renal fibrosis [20].

Patients at early stages of CKD can be asymptomatic until the illness is advanced, and renal function deteriorates by more than 50%. This latter favors the accumulation of uremic toxins, alterations in the production of erythrocytes, calcium and phosphorus metabolism, metabolic acidosis, hydro electrolyte alterations, and immune system dysfunction. Together, these factors can contribute to the occurrence of comorbidities and gradual worsening of general conditions, leading to patient death without adequate management [25].

Several studies from different populations have linked MetS to CKD progression. A cohort study of 15,605 patients with stage 3 and 4 CKD (eGFR=15–59 mL/min/1.73 m^2) revealed that MetS was associated with end-stage renal disease

(ESRD), with a hazard ratio of 1.33 (95% CI: 1.08–1.64) and a mean follow-up period of 2.3 years. Among MetS components, impaired glucose metabolism, elevated triglyceride levels, and hypertension have been shown to increase the risk of ESRD [26]. In a large cross-sectional study of 12,335 participants, MetS, but not obesity, was associated with kidney damage [27]. Among the 37,537 elderly Chinese population, it was concluded that aging, prehypertension, hypertension, elevated triglyceride concentrations, and fasting blood glucose were associated with the risk of CKD [28]. Altogether, conditions underlying MetS deserve special attention regarding the incidence and progression of CKD. Thus, this chapter explores the association between MetS as a precursor of kidney disease, including its prevalence, pathophysiology, clinical, laboratory diagnosis, and progression monitoring.

PATHOPHYSIOLOGY OF METS COMPONENTS IN CKD

Although microalbuminuria was associated with insulin resistance and MetS more than two decades ago [29, 30], the pathophysiological mechanisms and pathways by which MetS induces kidney disease are still under study. Before MetS was associated with the risk of CKD, earlier studies established that individual components of MetS, such as hypertension and hyperglycemia, confer themselves with a risk of CKD [18].

Hypertension, a MetS component, is the most common condition associated with CKD onset. The mechanisms leading to CKD have been well established, including salt retention, inappropriate renin-angiotensin system activity, sympathetic overactivity, and impaired endothelial cell-mediated vasodilatation [31]. Metabolic visceral adipocytes secrete angiotensinogen, stimulating the renin-angiotensin-aldosterone system (RAAS), which comprises the key blood pressure (BP) regulators. Hence, alterations in the RAAS in obese individuals eventually result in a systematic increase in BP and ultimately generate hyperfiltration and kidney damage [32, 33].

Another component of MetS is dyslipidemia, which may alter renal function through the excessive hepatic production of triglycerides, resulting in an increase in free fatty acid flux into the liver and nonadipose organs, stimulating the recruitment of inflammatory cells and resulting in tissue damage [34]. Excess lipids can accumulate ectopically in the kidney, contributing to damage through lipotoxicity. Lipid accumulation tends to occur in proximal tubular cells, and in more severe metabolic states, lipid droplets frequently accumulate in both glomeruli and proximal tubules [35, 36]. Lipid accumulation is also enhanced by albumin, which acts as a passive carrier of lipids, bringing nonesterified free fatty acids into the proximal tubule [37]. Consequently, lipid accumulation results in lipotoxicity caused by IR, the generation of reactive oxygen species, endoplasmic reticulum stress, alterations in cell signaling pathways, and the release of proinflammatory and profibrotic factors [35, 38 - 40]. All these alterations lead to renal fat accumulation, mesangial expansion, and the development of glomerulosclerosis, manifestations of CKD [34].

Although obesity is one of the main components of MetS, the exact mechanisms linked to renal damage are still unclear. Obesity, especially visceral obesity, is closely related to kidney dysfunction [41]. Investigations in humans and animal models have suggested that overweight and obesity result in hemodynamic changes in kidney function characterized by an increase in the eGFR [42]. In one study on healthy men, an independent association was found between BMI and CKD risk [43]. However, contradictory results have been observed. Other studies that adjusted for cardiovascular risk factors reported that the association between BMI and CKD stage 3 was not significant. Another study on CKD patients in stages 3–5 showed no association between BMI and eGFR reduction [44]. Ciardullo *et al.* reported that obesity was not associated with kidney damage. Subjects who were obese but did not have MetS did not present an increased risk of kidney disease, although it is important to note that MetS as an entity was associated with kidney damage [27].

Insulin resistance (IR) causes hyperinsulinemia and hyperglycemia, the latter of which are components of MetS, which are fundamental factors in the development of atherosclerosis, one of the major contributors to kidney damage [45]. Dysfunctional secretion of adiponectin, leptin, and inflammatory mediators interferes with the insulin receptor pathway, causing IR [46, 47]. Finally, IR impairs renal hemodynamics through sodium retention, increased sympathetic activity, and endothelial dysfunction. Furthermore, angiotensin II, a component of the RAAS, may play a role in the development of IR by inducing oxidative stress and developing salt-sensitive hypertension by promoting sodium reabsorption [48].

Thus, contributing factors for kidney injury development in individuals affected by MetS may include oxidative stress and systemic inflammation, endothelial dysfunction, altered renal hemodynamics, excessive renal sodium reabsorption, activation of the RAAS and sympathetic nervous system, atherogenic dyslipidemia, and even physical compression of the kidneys by adipose tissue. Complex interactions between these factors lead to glomerular hyperfiltration, glomerular cell proliferation, matrix accumulation, and glomerulosclerosis with nephron loss (Fig. **1**) [49]. Research to improve understanding of MetS pathophysiology as a marker or precursor for CKD is ongoing. However, there is less evidence for causation.

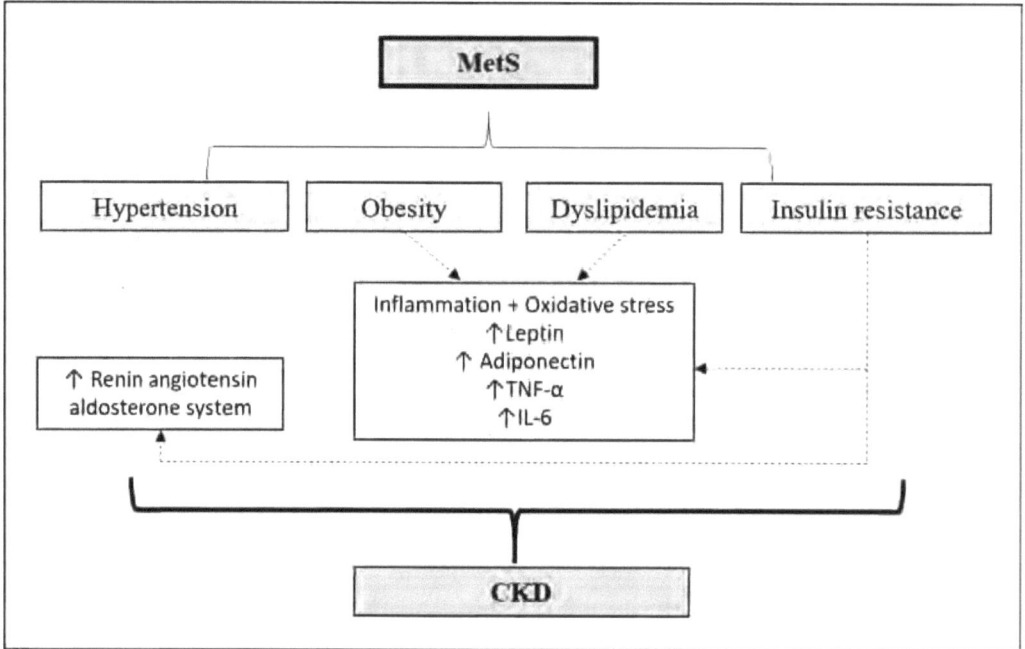

Fig. (1). Potential mechanisms of metabolic syndrome and its components in chronic kidney disease.

In summary, regarding the role of MetS components in CKD, some studies have reported that hypertension is a decisive, independent risk factor for renal injury, followed by hyperglycemia. However, MetS was found to be an independent risk factor for CKD after adjustment for hypertension and diabetes [50]. Dyslipidemia, characterized by elevated levels of triglycerides and low levels of HDL-C, is also associated with an increased risk of CKD and poor kidney function [51, 52]. Finally, visceral obesity might result in changes in the hemodynamics of kidney function [53, 54].

DIAGNOSIS OF METS IN PATIENTS WITH CKD

Reports have highlighted the impact of MetS on the progression of CKD. Therefore, it is important to address MetS and its components to prevent progression to CKD. The clinical manifestations of kidney disease are proteinuria and a reduced glomerular filtration rate; however, at this point, kidney damage has already started; thus, early screenings are always preferred.

As a risk factor for CVD, MetS remains the leading cause of CKD-related morbidity and mortality in patients with kidney failure [55]. Consequently, targeting MetS to predict the risk of developing CKD is reasonable. Hence, long-term studies on identifying and treating MetS that consider markers of kidney function tests are urgently needed.

Several criteria are used to define MetS, which complicates its diagnosis. Currently, there are two most commonly used definitions: the one proposed by the Adult Treatment Panel III (ATP III) and the one defined by the American Heart Association/National Heart, Lung, and Blood Institute (AHA/NHLBI) [13, 56]. Table **1** shows the most practical and used criteria.

Table 1. Current concepts to define MetS.

MetS Components	NCEP/ATP III	AHA/NHLBI
Obesity (WC)	>102 cm in males and >80 cm in females	Population- and country-specific cutoff values.
Triglycerides	≥150 mg/dL or with treatment	≥150 mg/dL or with treatment
HDL	Males HDL <40 mg/dL, females <50 mg/dL or with treatment.	Males HDL <40 mg/dL, females <50 mg/dL or with treatment.
Blood pressure	≥130/85 mm Hg or with treatment.	≥130/85 mm Hg or with treatment.
Glycemia	Fasting plasma glucose >100 mg/dL or with treatment	Fasting plasma glucose >100 mg/dL or with treatment

Abbreviations: WC, waist circumference; NCEP, National Cholesterol Education Program; ATP III, Adult Treatment Panel III; AHA, American Heart Association; NHLBI, National Heart, Lung and Blood Institute.

Recently, different scores have been proposed to avoid biases in selecting cutoff values for MetS components in diverse populations (Table **2**) [57]. The scores' goal was to determine MetS progression to T2D or CDV; however, their clinical utility must be demonstrated considering cohorts of populations with different ethnic backgrounds. Today, these scores could be an alternative to identify more precisely and with more precision those individuals at risk of developing diabetes and cardiometabolic outcomes [58 - 64].

The reported data indicate that some lipid ratios performed better than traditional parameters. Given the similar pathogenic mechanisms involved in atherosclerosis and glomerulosclerosis, elevated lipid ratios may also indicate the development and progression of CKD. Lipid ratios such as the Castelli risk indices I and II (CRI-I and CRI-II, respectively), atherogenic index of plasma (AIP), lipid accumulation product (LAP), and cardiometabolic index (CMI) have been extensively studied in the context of MetS and CKD, while other authors have proposed that LAP is the optimal predictor of MetS in CKD patients [65]. In a series of 11,578 middle-aged adults, the study suggested that a greater CMI was independently associated with a reduced eGFR; these findings from CKD patients on hemodialysis confirmed that the use of the CRI-I and CRI-II can facilitate the early diagnosis of hypertension and related CVD [66]. The early screening of these lipid parameters could lead to timely interventions that, together with diet and lifestyle changes, will effectively prevent CKD progression.

Table 2. Proposed scores to identify individuals with MetS.

Score	Population	Sample Size	References
MetS-Z	Caucasian African American	8,273	DeBoer *et al.* 2018 [58, 59]
cMetS	Caucasian	1,453	Magnussen *et al.* 2016 [60]
cMetS	Caucasian	1,869	Janghorbani and Amini 2016 [61]
MetS risk score	Asian	3,598	Kang *et al.* 2012 [62]
Percentiles of NCEP criteria	Hispanic	2,158	Aguilar-Salinas *et al.* 2006 [63]
cMsy	Caucasian	1,020	Wijndaele *et al.* 2006 [64]

Abbreviations: NCEP, National Cholesterol Education Program.

Among the different organizations that define MetS, the 1998 WHO defined the presence of microalbuminuria, as this condition is critical for CKD [67]. A recent study revealed that albuminuria increased the hazard ratio for worsening renal function. Moreover, MetS and albuminuria could provide a better stratification model for diabetic kidney disease (DKD) progression than albuminuria alone [68].

TREATMENT OF METS IN PATIENTS WITH COEXISTING CKD

MetS, CVD, and CKD share common traditional risk factors, namely, diabetes, hypertension, aging, a sedentary lifestyle, a hypercaloric diet, and a genetic predisposition. However, some risk factors only occur in CKD patients, such as toxic metabolites that are produced and accumulated during uremia, aggravating the health status of individuals with other comorbidities. Therefore, another treatment alternative might be novel metabolite markers for uremic toxins in CKD patients. Some studies have reported the benefit of resveratrol (RSV), a polyphenol found in red wine and grapes. RSV has been found to improve MetS components, resulting in the prevention of CVD. In addition, RSV can also reduce the levels of uremic toxins [69].

Currently, high frequencies of obesity are found among populations worldwide [70], and early detection, monitoring, and/or modulation of the effects of MetS are significant challenges for health professionals. A better understanding of the harmful effects of MetS on CKD patients is required to design strategies for earlier diagnosis, intervention, and treatment. Therefore, interventions should focus on treating the multiple risk factors for MetS. In a cohort study using nationally representative data from the Korean National Health Insurance System, 13,310,924 subjects were followed for at least 4 years or more, and it was found that improvements in MetS components had an impact on the incidence of ESRD [71]. Therefore, modulating MetS in the general population is a good strategy for preventing the development of ESRD.

Although the lack of well-designed studies is an issue, some studies that evaluated interventions for MetS treatment in CKD patients have revealed a clear association between lifestyle modifications, such as dietary weight loss and physical activity, and MetS components. In a cohort study of more than 3,000 individuals with mild-to-moderate CKD, the associations of adherence to healthy lifestyle factors (smoking habits, BMI, physical activity, and diet) with mortality were evaluated, and the results showed that abstinence from smoking was the most significant lifestyle factor linked to survival improvement [72]. Another meta-analysis reported that active smoking is associated with the development of MetS; however, stopping smoking seems to decrease the risk of MetS [73]. Regarding obesity, moderate weight loss, together with exercise cointervention in obese MetS patients, was associated with a reduction in albuminuria and an improvement in the eGFR [74]. Therefore, the use of medication or bariatric surgery for weight loss could be a helpful alternative; however, only a few studies have explored these approaches, and the results are inconclusive. A meta-analysis including 15 studies that reported surgery-related changes in the urinary albumin-to-creatinine ratio (UACR) in patients with obesity and T2D concluded that neither weight loss nor glycemic improvement correlated with albuminuria reduction [75].

Hypertension is a risk factor for CKD and has been increasingly studied. In one systematic review that pooled nine randomized clinical trials with a median follow-up of 3.3 years in patients with CKD without diabetes, the authors concluded that targeting BP did not provide additional benefit for renal outcomes compared with standard treatment [76].

Lipid reduction may preserve the glomerular filtration rate and decrease proteinuria in patients with renal disease [77]. Statins can decrease proteinuria in patients with renal disease [78]. Although statin therapy is recommended for the treatment of dyslipidemia in CKD patients, the results obtained are controversial. Most studies converge on reducing CDV events but not mortality [79 - 81]. Regarding kidney disease progression, in the study by Rahman et al., statin therapy did not reduce the risk of ESRD progression [82]. Nonetheless, post hoc analysis of randomized controlled trials revealed variable effects on ESRD progression [79].

On the other hand, metformin is widely used as an option to decrease glucose concentrations and improve insulin sensitivity in patients with T2D. In one systemic review, the authors suggest a potential benefit of metformin on macrovascular outcomes, conclusions derived from observational studies. However, there are some concerns regarding the occurrence of lactic acidosis in individuals with impaired kidney function [83]. A more recent meta-analysis and systemic review that included 19 randomized controlled trials revealed no effect on renal parameters such as the urinary albumin–creatinine ratio, serum creatinine, or ESRD. Thus, the authors comment that there is no clinically significant beneficial effect of metformin therapy compared to other glucose-lowering medications or placebo on microvascular complications [84].

Currently, high frequencies of obesity are found among populations worldwide [70], and early detection, monitoring, and/or modulation of the effects of MetS are significant challenges for health professionals. A better understanding of the harmful effects of MetS on CKD patients is required to design strategies for earlier diagnosis, intervention, and treatment. Therefore, interventions should focus on treating multiple risk factors for MetS. In a cohort study using nationally representative data from the Korean National Health Insurance System, 13,310,924 subjects were followed for at least 4 years or more, and it was found that improvements in MetS components had an impact on the incidence of ESRD [71]. Therefore, modulating MetS in the general population is a good strategy for preventing the development of ESRD.

Although the lack of well-designed studies is an issue, some studies that evaluated interventions for MetS treatment in CKD patients have revealed a clear association between lifestyle modifications, such as dietary weight loss and physical activity, and MetS components. In a cohort study of more than 3,000 individuals with mild-to-moderate CKD, the associations of adherence to healthy lifestyle factors (smoking habits, BMI, physical activity, and diet) with mortality were evaluated, and the results showed that abstinence from smoking was the most significant lifestyle factor linked to survival improvement [72]. Another meta-analysis reported that active smoking is associated with the development of MetS; however, stopping smoking seems to decrease the risk of MetS [73]. Regarding obesity, moderate weight loss, together with exercise cointervention in obese MetS patients, was associated with a reduction in albuminuria and an improvement in the eGFR [74]. Therefore, using medication or bariatric surgery for weight loss could be a helpful alternative; however, only a few studies have explored these approaches, and the results are inconclusive. A meta-analysis that included 15 studies reported surgery-related changes in the urinary albumin-to-creatinine ratio (UACR) in patients with obesity and T2D concluded that neither weight loss nor glycemic improvement correlated with albuminuria reduction [75].

Hypertension is a risk factor for CKD and has been increasingly studied. In one systematic review that pooled nine randomized clinical trials with a median follow-up of 3.3 years in patients with CKD without diabetes, the authors concluded that targeting BP did not provide additional benefit for renal outcomes compared with standard treatment [76].

Lipid reduction may preserve the glomerular filtration rate and decrease proteinuria in patients with renal disease [77]. Statins can decrease proteinuria in patients with renal disease [78]. Although statin therapy is recommended for the treatment of dyslipidemia in CKD patients, the results obtained are controversial. Most studies converge on reducing CDV events but not mortality [79 - 81]. Regarding kidney disease progression, in the study by Rahman et al., statin therapy did not reduce the risk of ESRD progression [82]. Nonetheless, post hoc analysis of randomized controlled trials revealed variable effects on ESRD progression [79].

On the other hand, metformin is widely used as an option to decrease glucose concentrations and improve insulin sensitivity in patients with T2D. In one systemic review, the authors suggest a potential benefit of metformin on macrovascular outcomes, conclusions derived from observational studies. However, there are some concerns regarding the occurrence of lactic acidosis in individuals with impaired kidney function [83]. A more recent meta-analysis and systemic review that included 19 randomized controlled trials revealed no effect on renal parameters such as the urinary albumin–creatinine ratio, serum creatinine, or ESRD. Thus, the authors comment that there is no clinically significant beneficial effect of metformin therapy compared to other glucose-lowering medications or placebo on microvascular complications [84].

CONCLUSION

In conclusion, measures for broadly addressing the impact of CKD and MetS may not be understood as separate approaches but may be complementary. The need to ensure effective primary prevention based on nutritional and lifestyle approaches is fundamental, particularly in LMICs where the burdens of CKD and MetS are still rising. Health promotion, access to and availability of health resources, and food safety are basic needs to effectively reduce MetS at the population level while screening and timely diagnosis are needed for surveillance to maintain and monitor renal disease progression even before any clinical manifestations appear.

REFERENCES

[1]   Levey AS, Eckardt K-U, Dorman NM, *et al.* Nomenclature for kidney function and disease: report of a Kidney Disease: Improving Global Outcomes (KDIGO) Consensus Conference. Kidney Int 2020; 97(6): 1117-29.
[http://dx.doi.org/10.1016/j.kint.2020.02.010] [PMID: 32409237]

[2]   Hill NR, Fatoba ST, Oke JL, *et al.* Global Prevalence of Chronic Kidney Disease – A Systematic Review and Meta-Analysis. PLoS One 2016; 11(7): e0158765.
[http://dx.doi.org/10.1371/journal.pone.0158765] [PMID: 27383068]

[3]   Zhang L, Wang F, Wang L, *et al.* Prevalence of chronic kidney disease in China: a cross-sectional survey. Lancet 2012; 379(9818): 815-22.
[http://dx.doi.org/10.1016/S0140-6736(12)60033-6] [PMID: 22386035]

[4]   Arora P, Vasa P, Brenner D, *et al.* Prevalence estimates of chronic kidney disease in Canada: results of a nationally representative survey. CMAJ 2013; 185(9): E417-23.
[http://dx.doi.org/10.1503/cmaj.120833] [PMID: 23649413]

[5]   White SL, Polkinghorne KR, Atkins RC, Chadban SJ. Comparison of the Prevalence and Mortality Risk of CKD in Australia Using the CKD Epidemiology Collaboration (CKD-EPI) and Modification of Diet in Renal Disease (MDRD) Study GFR Estimating Equations: The AusDiab (Australian Diabetes, Obesity and Lifestyle) Study. Am J Kidney Dis 2010; 55(4): 660-70.
[http://dx.doi.org/10.1053/j.ajkd.2009.12.011] [PMID: 20138414]

[6]   Levey AS, Coresh J. Chronic kidney disease. Lancet 2012; 379(9811): 165-80.
[http://dx.doi.org/10.1016/S0140-6736(11)60178-5] [PMID: 21840587]

[7]   Girndt M, Trocchi P, Scheidt-Nave C, Markau S, Stang A. The Prevalence of Renal Failure. Dtsch Arztebl Int 2016; 113(6): 85-91.
[http://dx.doi.org/10.3238/arztebl.2016.0085] [PMID: 26931624]

[8]   Brück K, Stel VS, Gambaro G, *et al.* CKD Prevalence Varies across the European General Population. J Am Soc Nephrol 2016; 27(7): 2135-47.
[http://dx.doi.org/10.1681/ASN.2015050542] [PMID: 26701975]

[9]   Kovesdy CP. Epidemiology of chronic kidney disease: an update 2022. Kidney Int Suppl 2022; 12(1): 7-11.
[http://dx.doi.org/10.1016/j.kisu.2021.11.003] [PMID: 35529086]

[10]   Fraser SDS, Aitken G, Taal MW, *et al.* Exploration of chronic kidney disease prevalence estimates using new measures of kidney function in the health survey for England. PLoS One 2015; 10(2): e0118676.
[http://dx.doi.org/10.1371/journal.pone.0118676] [PMID: 25700182]

[11]   Singh AK, Kari JA. Metabolic syndrome and chronic kidney disease. Curr Opin Nephrol Hypertens 2013; 22(2): 198-203.
[http://dx.doi.org/10.1097/MNH.0b013e32835dda78] [PMID: 23340215]

[12]   Bikbov B, Purcell CA, Levey AS, *et al.* Global, regional, and national burden of chronic kidney disease, 1990–2017: a systematic analysis for the Global Burden of Disease Study 2017. Lancet 2020; 395(10225): 709-33.
[http://dx.doi.org/10.1016/S0140-6736(20)30045-3] [PMID: 32061315]

[13]   Alberti KGMM, Eckel RH, Grundy SM, *et al.* Harmonizing the Metabolic Syndrome. Circulation 2009; 120(16): 1640-5.
[http://dx.doi.org/10.1161/CIRCULATIONAHA.109.192644] [PMID: 19805654]

[14]   Hirode G, Wong RJ. Trends in the Prevalence of Metabolic Syndrome in the United States, 2011-2016. JAMA 2020; 323(24): 2526-8.
[http://dx.doi.org/10.1001/jama.2020.4501] [PMID: 32573660]

[15]   Okafor C. The metabolic syndrome in Africa: Current trends. Indian J Endocrinol Metab 2012; 16(1): 56-66.
[http://dx.doi.org/10.4103/2230-8210.91191] [PMID: 22276253]

[16]   Gutiérrez-Solis AL, Datta Banik S, Méndez-González RM. Prevalence of Metabolic Syndrome in Mexico: A Systematic Review and Meta-Analysis. Metab Syndr Relat Disord 2018; 16(8): 395-405.
[http://dx.doi.org/10.1089/met.2017.0157] [PMID: 30063173]

[17]   Faenza A, Fuga G, Nardo B, *et al.* Metabolic syndrome after kidney transplantation. Transplant Proc 2007; 39(6): 1843-6.
[http://dx.doi.org/10.1016/j.transproceed.2007.07.019] [PMID: 17692629]

[18]   Chen J, Muntner P, Hamm LL, *et al.* The metabolic syndrome and chronic kidney disease in U.S. adults. Ann Intern Med 2004; 140(3): 167-74.
[http://dx.doi.org/10.7326/0003-4819-140-3-200402030-00007] [PMID: 14757614]

[19]   Nashar K, Egan B. Relationship between chronic kidney disease and metabolic syndrome: current perspectives. Diabetes Metab Syndr Obes 2014; 7: 421-35.
[http://dx.doi.org/10.2147/DMSO.S45183] [PMID: 25258547]

[20]   Li XH, Lin HY, Wang SH, Guan LY, Wang YB. Association of Microalbuminuria with Metabolic Syndrome among Aged Population. BioMed Res Int 2016; 2016: 1-7.
[http://dx.doi.org/10.1155/2016/9241278] [PMID: 27200378]

[21]   Raikou V, Gavriil S. Metabolic Syndrome and Chronic Renal Disease. Diseases 2018; 6(1): 12. Epub ahead of print
[http://dx.doi.org/10.3390/diseases6010012] [PMID: 29364162]

[22]   Crews DC, Bello AK, Saadi G. Burden, Access, and Disparities in Kidney Disease. Nephron J 2019; 141(4): 219-26.
[http://dx.doi.org/10.1159/000495557] [PMID: 30783033]

[23]   Rysz J, Franczyk B, Ciałkowska-Rysz A, Gluba-Brzózka A. The effect of diet on the survival of patients with chronic kidney disease. Nutrients 2017; 9(5): 495. Epub ahead of print
[http://dx.doi.org/10.3390/nu9050495] [PMID: 28505087]

[24]   Rosas-Cortez N, Hernández-Ibarra LE, Zillmer JGV, *et al.* Structural barriers in care nutrition for people with chronic kidney disease in Mexico. Saude Soc 2020; 29: e190476.
[http://dx.doi.org/10.1590/s0104-12902020190476]

[25]   Romagnani P, Remuzzi G, Glassock R, *et al.* Chronic kidney disease. Nat Rev Dis Primers 2017; 3(1): 17088.
[http://dx.doi.org/10.1038/nrdp.2017.88] [PMID: 29168475]

[26]   Navaneethan SD, Schold JD, Kirwan JP, *et al.* Metabolic syndrome, ESRD, and death in CKD. Clin J Am Soc Nephrol 2013; 8(6): 945-52.
[http://dx.doi.org/10.2215/CJN.09870912] [PMID: 23411425]

[27]   Ciardullo S, Ballabeni C, Trevisan R, Perseghin G. Metabolic Syndrome, and Not Obesity, Is Associated with Chronic Kidney Disease. Am J Nephrol 2021; 52(8): 666-72.
[http://dx.doi.org/10.1159/000518111] [PMID: 34569517]

[28]   Xu L, Liu J, Li D, Yang H, Zhou Y, Yang J. Association between metabolic syndrome components and chronic kidney disease among 37,533 old Chinese individuals. Int Urol Nephrol 2022; 54(6): 1445-54.
[http://dx.doi.org/10.1007/s11255-021-03013-3] [PMID: 34671893]

[29]   Hoehner CM, Greenlund KJ, Rith-Najarian S, Casper ML, McClellan WM. Association of the insulin resistance syndrome and microalbuminuria among nondiabetic native Americans. The Inter-Tribal Heart Project. J Am Soc Nephrol 2002; 13(6): 1626-34.
[http://dx.doi.org/10.1097/01.ASN.0000015762.92814.85] [PMID: 12039992]

[30]   Schelling JR, Sedor JR. The metabolic syndrome as a risk factor for chronic kidney disease: more than a fat chance? J Am Soc Nephrol 2004; 15(11): 2773-4.
[http://dx.doi.org/10.1097/01.ASN.0000141964.68839.BB] [PMID: 15504930]

[31]   Adamczak M, Zeier M, Dikow R, Ritz E. Kidney and hypertension. Kidney Int 2002; 61: S62-7.
[http://dx.doi.org/10.1046/j.1523-1755.61.s80.28.x]

[32]   Kawarazaki W, Fujita T. The Role of Aldosterone in Obesity-Related Hypertension. Am J Hypertens 2016; 29(4): 415-23.
[http://dx.doi.org/10.1093/ajh/hpw003] [PMID: 26927805]

[33]   Lea J, Cheek D, Thornley-Brown D, *et al.* Metabolic syndrome, proteinuria, and the risk of progressive CKD in hypertensive African Americans. Am J Kidney Dis 2008; 51(5): 732-40.
[http://dx.doi.org/10.1053/j.ajkd.2008.01.013] [PMID: 18436083]

[34]   Gai Z, Wang T, Visentin M, Kullak-Ublick G, Fu X, Wang Z. Lipid accumulation and chronic kidney disease. Nutrients 2019; 11(4): 722.
[http://dx.doi.org/10.3390/nu11040722] [PMID: 30925738]

[35]   Martínez-García C, Izquierdo A, Velagapudi V, *et al.* Accelerated renal disease is associated with the development of metabolic syndrome in a glucolipotoxic mouse model. Dis Model Mech 2012; 5(5): dmm.009266.
[http://dx.doi.org/10.1242/dmm.009266] [PMID: 22773754]

[36]   Izquierdo-Lahuerta A, Martínez-García C, Medina-Gómez G. Lipotoxicity as a trigger factor of renal disease. J Nephrol 2016; 29(5): 603-10.
[http://dx.doi.org/10.1007/s40620-016-0278-5] [PMID: 26956132]

[37]   Iglesias J, Levine JS. Albuminuria and renal injury—beware of proteins bearing gifts. Nephrol Dial Transplant 2001; 16(2): 215-8.
[http://dx.doi.org/10.1093/ndt/16.2.215] [PMID: 11158389]

[38]   Katsoulieris E, Mabley JG, Samai M, Sharpe MA, Green IC, Chatterjee PK. Lipotoxicity in renal proximal tubular cells: Relationship between endoplasmic reticulum stress and oxidative stress pathways. Free Radic Biol Med 2010; 48(12): 1654-62.
[http://dx.doi.org/10.1016/j.freeradbiomed.2010.03.021] [PMID: 20363316]

[39]   Lennon R, Pons D, Sabin MA, *et al.* Saturated fatty acids induce insulin resistance in human podocytes: implications for diabetic nephropathy. Nephrol Dial Transplant 2009; 24(11): 3288-96.
[http://dx.doi.org/10.1093/ndt/gfp302] [PMID: 19556298]

[40]   Sieber J, Lindenmeyer MT, Kampe K, *et al.* Regulation of podocyte survival and endoplasmic reticulum stress by fatty acids. Am J Physiol Renal Physiol 2010; 299(4): F821-9.
[http://dx.doi.org/10.1152/ajprenal.00196.2010] [PMID: 20668104]

[41]   Hall JE, do Carmo JM, da Silva AA, Wang Z, Hall ME. Obesity-Induced Hypertension. Circ Res 2015; 116(6): 991-1006.
[http://dx.doi.org/10.1161/CIRCRESAHA.116.305697] [PMID: 25767285]

[42]   Henegar JR, Bigler SA, Henegar LK, Tyagi SC, Hall J. Functional and structural changes in the kidney in the early stages of obesity. J Am Soc Nephrol 2001; 12(6): 1211-7.
[http://dx.doi.org/10.1681/ASN.V1261211] [PMID: 11373344]

[43]   Gelber RP, Kurth T, Kausz AT, *et al.* Association between body mass index and CKD in apparently healthy men. Am J Kidney Dis 2005; 46(5): 871-80.
[http://dx.doi.org/10.1053/j.ajkd.2005.08.015] [PMID: 16253727]

[44]   Foster MC, Hwang SJ, Larson MG, *et al.* Overweight, obesity, and the development of stage 3 CKD: the Framingham Heart Study. Am J Kidney Dis 2008; 52(1): 39-48.
[http://dx.doi.org/10.1053/j.ajkd.2008.03.003] [PMID: 18440684]

[45]   Abate N, Chandalia M, Cabo-Chan AV Jr, Moe OW, Sakhaee K. The metabolic syndrome and uric

acid nephrolithiasis: Novel features of renal manifestation of insulin resistance. Kidney Int 2004; 65(2): 386-92.
[http://dx.doi.org/10.1111/j.1523-1755.2004.00386.x] [PMID: 14717908]

[46]   Fernández-Real JM, Castro A, Vázquez G, *et al*. Adiponectin is associated with vascular function independent of insulin sensitivity. Diabetes Care 2004; 27(3): 739-45.
[http://dx.doi.org/10.2337/diacare.27.3.739] [PMID: 14988295]

[47]   Cheng HT, Huang JW, Chiang CK, Yen CJ, Hung KY, Wu KD. Metabolic syndrome and insulin resistance as risk factors for development of chronic kidney disease and rapid decline in renal function in elderly. J Clin Endocrinol Metab 2012; 97(4): 1268-76.
[http://dx.doi.org/10.1210/jc.2011-2658] [PMID: 22337909]

[48]   Fujita T. Spotlight on renin. The renin system, salt-sensitivity and metabolic syndrome. J Renin Angiotensin Aldosterone Syst 2006; 7(3): 181-3.
[http://dx.doi.org/10.3317/jraas.2006.029] [PMID: 17094057]

[49]   Raimundo M, Lopes JA. Metabolic syndrome, chronic kidney disease, and cardiovascular disease: a dynamic and life-threatening triad. Cardiol Res Pract 2011; 2011: 1-16.
[http://dx.doi.org/10.4061/2011/747861] [PMID: 21403897]

[50]   Gluba A, Mikhailidis DP, Lip GYH, Hannam S, Rysz J, Banach M. Metabolic syndrome and renal disease. Int J Cardiol 2013; 164(2): 141-50.
[http://dx.doi.org/10.1016/j.ijcard.2012.01.013] [PMID: 22305775]

[51]   McMahon GM, Preis SR, Hwang SJ, Fox CS. Mid-adulthood risk factor profiles for CKD. J Am Soc Nephrol 2014; 25(11): 2633-41.
[http://dx.doi.org/10.1681/ASN.2013070750] [PMID: 24970884]

[52]   Bowe B, Xie Y, Xian H, Balasubramanian S, Al-Aly Z. Low levels of high-density lipoprotein cholesterol increase the risk of incident kidney disease and its progression. Kidney Int 2016; 89(4): 886-96.
[http://dx.doi.org/10.1016/j.kint.2015.12.034] [PMID: 26924057]

[53]   Thomas G, Sehgal AR, Kashyap SR, Srinivas TR, Kirwan JP, Navaneethan SD. Metabolic syndrome and kidney disease: a systematic review and meta-analysis. Clin J Am Soc Nephrol 2011; 6(10): 2364-73.
[http://dx.doi.org/10.2215/CJN.02180311] [PMID: 21852664]

[54]   Eknoyan G. Obesity and chronic kidney disease. Nefrología 2011; 31(4): 397-403.
[http://dx.doi.org/10.3265/Nefrologia.pre2011.May.10963] [PMID: 21623393]

[55]   Cardiovascular disease, chronic kidney disease, and diabetes mortality burden of cardiometabolic risk factors from 1980 to 2010: a comparative risk assessment. Lancet Diabetes Endocrinol 2014; 2(8): 634-47.
[http://dx.doi.org/10.1016/S2213-8587(14)70102-0] [PMID: 24842598]

[56]   Grundy SM, Cleeman JI, Daniels SR, *et al*. Diagnosis and Management of the Metabolic Syndrome. Circulation 2005; 112(17): 2735-52.
[http://dx.doi.org/10.1161/CIRCULATIONAHA.105.169404] [PMID: 16157765]

[57]   Aguilar-Salinas CA, Viveros-Ruiz T. Recent advances in managing/understanding the metabolic syndrome. F1000Res; 8. Epub ahead of print 2019.
[http://dx.doi.org/10.12688/f1000research.17122.1]

[58]   DeBoer MD, Filipp SL, Gurka MJ. Use of a Metabolic Syndrome Severity Z Score to Track Risk During Treatment of Prediabetes: An Analysis of the Diabetes Prevention Program. Diabetes Care 2018; 41(11): 2421-30.
[http://dx.doi.org/10.2337/dc18-1079] [PMID: 30275282]

[59]   Gurka MJ, Filipp SL, Pearson TA, DeBoer MD. Assessing Baseline and Temporal Changes in Cardiometabolic Risk Using Metabolic Syndrome Severity and Common Risk Scores. J Am Heart

Assoc 2018; 7(16): e009754.
[http://dx.doi.org/10.1161/JAHA.118.009754] [PMID: 30369320]

[60]   Magnussen CG, Cheriyan S, Sabin MA, *et al.* Continuous and Dichotomous Metabolic Syndrome Definitions in Youth Predict Adult Type 2 Diabetes and Carotid Artery Intima Media Thickness: The Cardiovascular Risk in Young Finns Study. J Pediatr 2016; 171: 97-103.e3, 3.
[http://dx.doi.org/10.1016/j.jpeds.2015.10.093] [PMID: 26681473]

[61]   Janghorbani M, Amini M. Utility of Continuous Metabolic Syndrome Score in Assessing Risk of Type 2 Diabetes: The Isfahan Diabetes Prevention Study. Ann Nutr Metab 2016; 68(1): 19-25.
[http://dx.doi.org/10.1159/000441851] [PMID: 26559166]

[62]   Kang G-D, Guo L, Guo Z-R, Hu XS, Wu M, Yang HT. Continuous metabolic syndrome risk score for predicting cardiovascular disease in the Chinese population. Asia Pac J Clin Nutr 2012; 21(1): 88-96.
[http://dx.doi.org/10.6133/apjcn.2012.21.1.12] [PMID: 22374565]

[63]   Aguilar-Salinas CA, Rojas R, Gonzalez-Villalpando C, *et al.* Design and validation of a population-based definition of the metabolic syndrome. Diabetes Care 2006; 29(11): 2420-6.
[http://dx.doi.org/10.2337/dc06-0611] [PMID: 17065678]

[64]   Wijndaele K, Beunen G, Duvigneaud N, *et al.* A continuous metabolic syndrome risk score: utility for epidemiological analyses. Diabetes Care 2006; 29(10): 2329.
[http://dx.doi.org/10.2337/dc06-1341] [PMID: 17003322]

[65]   Olamoyegun M, Oluyombo R, Asaolu S. Evaluation of dyslipidemia, lipid ratios, and atherogenic index as cardiovascular risk factors among semi-urban dwellers in Nigeria. Ann Afr Med 2016; 15(4): 194-9.
[http://dx.doi.org/10.4103/1596-3519.194280] [PMID: 27853034]

[66]   Onat A, Can G, Kaya H, Hergenç G. "Atherogenic index of plasma" (log10 triglyceride/high-density lipoprotein−cholesterol) predicts high blood pressure, diabetes, and vascular events. J Clin Lipidol 2010; 4(2): 89-98.
[http://dx.doi.org/10.1016/j.jacl.2010.02.005] [PMID: 21122635]

[67]   Palaniappan L, Carnethon M, Fortmann SP. Association between microalbuminuria and the metabolic syndrome: NHANES III. Am J Hypertens 2003; 16(11): 952-8.
[http://dx.doi.org/10.1016/S0895-7061(03)01009-4] [PMID: 14573334]

[68]   Shih HM, Chuang SM, Lee CC, Liu SC, Tsai MC. Addition of Metabolic Syndrome to Albuminuria Provides a New Risk Stratification Model for Diabetic Kidney Disease Progression in Elderly Patients. Sci Rep 2020; 10(1): 6788.
[http://dx.doi.org/10.1038/s41598-020-63967-9] [PMID: 32321994]

[69]   Song JY, Shen TC, Hou YC, *et al.* Influence of Resveratrol on the Cardiovascular Health Effects of Chronic Kidney Disease. Int J Mol Sci 2020; 21(17): 6294.
[http://dx.doi.org/10.3390/ijms21176294] [PMID: 32878067]

[70]   Ogden CL, Fryar CD, Martin CB, *et al.* Trends in Obesity Prevalence by Race and Hispanic Origin—1999-2000 to 2017-2018. JAMA 2020; 324(12): 1208-10.
[http://dx.doi.org/10.1001/jama.2020.14590] [PMID: 32857101]

[71]   Koh ES, Do Han K, Kim MK, *et al.* Changes in metabolic syndrome status affect the incidence of end-stage renal disease in the general population: a nationwide cohort study. Sci Rep 2021; 11(1): 1957.
[http://dx.doi.org/10.1038/s41598-021-81396-0] [PMID: 33479302]

[72]   Hu EA, Coresh J, Anderson CAM, *et al.* Adherence to Healthy Dietary Patterns and Risk of CKD Progression and All-Cause Mortality: Findings From the CRIC (Chronic Renal Insufficiency Cohort) Study. Am J Kidney Dis 2021; 77(2): 235-44.
[http://dx.doi.org/10.1053/j.ajkd.2020.04.019] [PMID: 32768632]

[73]   Sun K, Liu J, Ning G. Active smoking and risk of metabolic syndrome: a meta-analysis of prospective

studies. PLoS One 2012; 7(10): e47791.
[http://dx.doi.org/10.1371/journal.pone.0047791] [PMID: 23082217]

[74]   Straznicky NE, Grima MT, Lambert EA, *et al.* Exercise augments weight loss induced improvement in renal function in obese metabolic syndrome individuals. J Hypertens 2011; 29(3): 553-64.
[http://dx.doi.org/10.1097/HJH.0b013e3283418875] [PMID: 21119532]

[75]   Docherty NG, le Roux CW. Bariatric surgery for the treatment of chronic kidney disease in obesity and type 2 diabetes mellitus. Nat Rev Nephrol 2020; 16(12): 709-20.
[http://dx.doi.org/10.1038/s41581-020-0323-4] [PMID: 32778788]

[76]   Tsai WC, Wu HY, Peng YS, *et al.* Association of Intensive Blood Pressure Control and Kidney Disease Progression in Nondiabetic Patients With Chronic Kidney Disease. JAMA Intern Med 2017; 177(6): 792-9.
[http://dx.doi.org/10.1001/jamainternmed.2017.0197] [PMID: 28288249]

[77]   Fried LF, Orchard TJ, Kasiske BL. Effect of lipid reduction on the progression of renal disease: A meta-analysis. Kidney Int 2001; 59(1): 260-9.
[http://dx.doi.org/10.1046/j.1523-1755.2001.00487.x] [PMID: 11135079]

[78]   Tonelli M, Wanner C. Lipid management in chronic kidney disease: synopsis of the Kidney Disease: Improving Global Outcomes 2013 clinical practice guideline. Ann Intern Med 2014; 160(3): 182-9.
[http://dx.doi.org/10.7326/M13-2453] [PMID: 24323134]

[79]   Tonelli M, Isles C, Craven T, *et al.* Effect of pravastatin on rate of kidney function loss in people with or at risk for coronary disease. Circulation 2005; 112(2): 171-8.
[http://dx.doi.org/10.1161/CIRCULATIONAHA.104.517565] [PMID: 15998677]

[80]   Soohoo M, Moradi H, Obi Y, *et al.* Statin Therapy Before Transition to End☐Stage Renal Disease With Posttransition Outcomes. J Am Heart Assoc 2019; 8(6): e011869.
[http://dx.doi.org/10.1161/JAHA.118.011869] [PMID: 30885048]

[81]   Tunnicliffe DJ, Palmer SC, Cashmore BA, *et al.* HMG CoA reductase inhibitors (statins) for people with chronic kidney disease not requiring dialysis. Cochrane Libr 2023; 2023(12): CD007784.
[http://dx.doi.org/10.1002/14651858.CD007784.pub3] [PMID: 24880031]

[82]   Rahman M, Baimbridge C, Davis BR, *et al.* Progression of kidney disease in moderately hypercholesterolemic, hypertensive patients randomized to pravastatin versus usual care: a report from the Antihypertensive and Lipid-Lowering Treatment to Prevent Heart Attack Trial (ALLHAT). Am J Kidney Dis 2008; 52(3): 412-24.
[http://dx.doi.org/10.1053/j.ajkd.2008.05.027] [PMID: 18676075]

[83]   Inzucchi SE, Lipska KJ, Mayo H, Bailey CJ, McGuire DK. Metformin in patients with type 2 diabetes and kidney disease: a systematic review. JAMA 2014; 312(24): 2668-75.
[http://dx.doi.org/10.1001/jama.2014.15298] [PMID: 25536258]

[84]   Gerardo González-González J, Cesar Solis R, Díaz González-Colmenero A, *et al.* Effect of metformin on microvascular outcomes in patients with type 2 diabetes: A systematic review and meta-analysis. Diabetes Res Clin Pract 2022; 186: 109821.
[http://dx.doi.org/10.1016/j.diabres.2022.109821] [PMID: 35247521]

CHAPTER 5

Current Definitions, Biomarkers, and Treatments for Acute Kidney Injury

Juan Carlos Diaz Núñez[1] and **Rafael Valdez Ortiz**[1,*]

[1] *Department of Nephrology, Hospital General de México Dr. Eduardo Liceaga, Mexico City, Mexico*

Abstract: An unexpected reduction in renal function during the first seven days after a triggering event is known as acute kidney injury (AKI). AKI is diagnosed when serum creatinine increases by 0.3 mg/dL in 48 h, or an increase $\geq 50\%$ in the first seven days of follow-up or a urinary volume < 0.5 mL/kg/h for six hours. AKI affects between 7% and 20% of hospitalized patients, and the incidence in the community is estimated to be between 20 and 200 per million inhabitants. Among critically ill patients, the incidence of AKI varies between 30% and 70%. AKI is multifactorial and can develop in a heterogeneous population in terms of genetics, age, previous renal function, and different comorbidities. The limitations in classifying and diagnosing AKI lie in the scarce variable specificity since serum creatinine and urine output do not always represent the severity of damage and are only markers of excretory function. Hence, owing to a lack of evidence of kidney damage in some cases (patients who did not present increased creatinine or decreased urine volume at the time of evaluation) and despite patients meeting the criteria for AKI, timely detection of functional changes with more precise and effective biomarkers is urgently needed.

Keywords: ADQI, Acid-base balance, Glomerular filtration rate, KDIGO, Metabolic acidosis.

INTRODUCTION

Acute kidney injury (AKI) is characterized by a sudden reduction in renal function during the first seven days after a triggering event [1]. AKI causes the accumulation of waste products derived from protein metabolism (urea, urea nitrogen, and creatinine) in conjunction with an alteration in acid-base balance (metabolic acidosis) and fluid and electrolyte homeostasis [2, 3]. AKI spectrum is broad, fluctuating from minor changes in biochemical markers of renal function to a total impaired kidney function, which demands the beginning of life-supporting treatments that involve renal replacement therapy (RRT) [4].

---

[*] **Corresponding author Rafael Valdez Ortiz:** Department of Nephrology, Hospital General de México Dr. Eduardo Liceaga, Mexico City, Mexico; E-mail: rafavaldez@gmail.com.

Rafael Valdez-Ortiz, Katy Sánchez-Pozos, Ana Carolina Ariza & Enzo C. Vásquez-Jiménez (Eds.)

The name of this abrupt decrease in renal function has transformed over time from "insufficiency" to "failure" to "injury." Hence, to obtain better outcomes for patients with AKI, in 2007, the report of the Acute Kidney Injury Network (AKIN) group recommended the word "injury," except for other terms that dichotomously suggest either normal kidney function or organ failure [2]. Later, the International Consensus of the Kidney Disease Improving Global Outcomes (KDIGO) group used the AKIN initiative and published the operational concept of AKI in 2012. Therefore, AKI is defined as a rise in serum creatinine (>0.3 mg/dL in 48 h), an increase oφ ≥50% in the first 7 days of follow-up, or a urinary volume < 0.5 mL/Kg/h for six hours [5]. Table 1 shows the categorization of AKI based on the serum creatinine level and urine volume.

Table 1. KDIGO severity classification of AKI.

Stage	Serum Creatinine Concentration	Urine Volume Output
1	sCr basal value increase ≥ 1.5 to 1.9 times in 7 days or baseline increase ≥ 0.3 mg/dL in 48 h	<0.5 mL/Kg/h for 6 h
2	Baseline sCr rise > 2 to 2.9 times the baseline value	<0.5 mL/Kg/h for 12 h
3	sCr ≥4 mg/dL or baseline sCr increase ≥ 3 times the baseline value or need for RRT	<0.3 mL/Kg/h for 24 h or anuria for 12 h

Abbreviations: AKI, Acute Kidney Injury; KDIGO, Kidney Disease: Improving Global Outcomes; RRT, Renal Replacement Therapy; sCr, serum creatinine.

The importance of classifying the spectrum from AKI to chronic kidney disease (CKD) was advertised in the Working Group of the Acute Disease Quality Initiative (ADQI) report [1, 6]. The acute kidney disease (AKD) concept was first proposed to delineate the course of the disease after patients were affected with AKI and progressed to advanced stages. Moreover, regardless of the severity of AKI, the complete and continuous reversal of an episode within 48 hours of its onset is known as "transient AKI" [5, 7]. Other methods to classify AKI have used the concepts of community-acquired AKI and hospital-acquired AKI. The last proposed classification system considers the origin of AKI and the prognosis and survival of patients [8]. Table 2 shows the definitions proposed by the latest ADQI consensus for AKI, AKD, and CKD.

EPIDEMIOLOGY

The importance of AKI lies in its consistent association with increased mortality, elevated progression risk to chronic kidney disease (CKD), and increased healthcare spending [9].

Table 2. AKI classification according to the Acute Disease Quality Initiative (ADQI).

-	AKI	AKD	CKD	Without kidney disease
Duration	≤ 7 days	< 3 months	> 3 months	Not applicable
Functional criteria	Oliguria for ≥ 6 h or sCr increased by ≥ 50% in 7 days, or sCr increased by ≥ 0.3 mg/dL in 2 days	GFR reduction ≥ 35% over baseline or sCr increase > 50% over baseline or AKI or GFR < 60 mL/min/1.73 m²	GFR < 60 mL/min/1.73m²	Unchanging sCr (no 50% rise in 3 months nor 0.3 mg/dL increase in 2 days), GFR ≥ 60 mL/min/1.73m², constant GFR (no 35% reduction in 3 months), no oliguria for ≥ 6 h
Either	Either	Either	Either	Either
Structural criteria	Not Defined	Increased albuminuria, hematuria, or pyuria, which are the most common biomarkers of kidney injury	Commonly elevated albuminuria	No marker of kidney damage

Abbreviations: AKI, Acute Kidney Injury; AKD, Acute Kidney Disease; CKD, Chronic Kidney Disease; sCr, serum creatinine; GFR, glomerular filtration rate.

The changes in the operational definitions of AKI have increased the incidence and reports of the disease to the extent that long-term economic and clinical impacts on health are recognized. Publications from upper-income countries have provided data for comparisons of incidence, course, and clinical settings. Nonetheless, this information is scarce in low- and middle-income countries, which has led to a deficient and restricted perspective of AKI as a pathology that affects only hospitalized and critically ill patients [10, 11]. In this context, the incidence and prevalence of AKI worldwide are very heterogeneous, not only among ethnic groups but also among different studies in the same population, mainly depending on the hospital and community setting. AKI affects between 7% and 20% of hospitalized patients, and the incidence in the community is estimated to be between 20 and 200 per million inhabitants [10, 12].

In the hospitalization setting, AKI affects mainly older adult patients, whereas outpatients with AKI tend to be younger and healthier. AKI incidence varies between 30% and 70% in critical care patients; moreover, it is estimated that around 5% of patients admitted to the intensive care unit (ICU) will need RRT [4, 5, 12].

In high-income countries, AKI is more prevalent in ICUs, where it occurs mainly in older patients with multiple organ failure. In this sense, the costs related to AKI are high, and prevention is difficult due to its unexpected appearance [8]. In general, the mortality associated with AKI is 25%, which is close to 40% in those with stage 3 AKI, according to KDIGO [8, 13]. In a cohort of more than 19,000 hospitalizations, AKI was independently associated with hospital mortality [OR = 4.43 (95% CI, 3.68–5.35)], even after adjusting for admission creatinine concentration, age, sex, race, and disease severity index [14]. Worldwide, the estimated mean age of AKI presentation is around 60 years old, but the mean age decreases to 50 years in low-income countries regardless of socioeconomic class. Furthermore, 60% of patients affected with AKI are men, with minimal ethnic variation [8, 14, 15].

ETIOLOGY

AKI is classified as "prerenal" when the injury is due to intravascular volume deficiency or impaired perfusion renal function. The term "intrarenal" AKI refers to AKI caused by acute tubular necrosis, drug nephrotoxicity, or interstitial or glomerular nephritis, and "postrenal" AKI is associated with urinary tract acute obstruction (Table **3**) [5, 16]. These categories are helpful because they provide an overview of the usual clinical course and management; however, the causes frequently overlap since the events precipitating AKI are multifactorial and develop in a heterogeneous population regarding genetics, age, previous renal function, and different comorbidities. In the last decade, acute kidney injury has been grouped as a syndrome in which the pathophysiological processes converge as a central problem, for example, AKI associated with sepsis, AKI due to cardiorenal syndrome, AKI associated with malignant neoplasms, *etc.* The initial approach for an AKI patient is based on an exhaustive medical history and physical examination complemented with laboratory assessments, urinary sediment, and even renal biopsy when the etiology is unclear after 7 days of general treatment [16 - 18].

Table 3. Etiology of acute kidney injury.

Prerenal	Renal	Postrenal
♦ Shock (hypovolemic, hemorrhagic, and septic) ♦ Cardiorenal syndrome ♦ Right heart failure ♦ Abdominal compartment syndrome ♦ Medications, including ECA inhibitors and angiotensin receptor blockers	♦ Systemic immunological causes (lupus, rheumatoid arthritis) ♦ Vasculitis ♦ Acute interstitial nephritis ♦ Atheroembolic disease ♦ Renal artery or vein thrombosis ♦ Thrombotic microangiopathy	♦ Urethral obstruction ♦ Bilateral ureteral obstruction ♦ Bladder dysfunction

Abbreviations: ECA, angiotensin converting enzyme.

DIAGNOSIS

The limitations in classifying AKI lie in the lack of specificity of the variables since serum creatinine and urine output do not always represent the same severity of damage and do not provide any information on metabolic, endocrine, or immunological functions. In some cases, they are considered only markers of excretory function. Creatinine is a constantly produced biomarker of hepatic, renal, and muscular origin that is altered even by nonpathological situations, and given that its half-life increases if the GFR decreases, its concentration in plasma increases up to 36 hours after renal injury. However, an actual decrease in the GFR may not be reflected in a timely manner in affected subjects with sepsis, liver disease, or severe malnutrition [4, 6, 8]. Because some patients meet the criteria for AKI but do not have kidney damage (for example, at the start of treatment with iSGLT2) or clear evidence of kidney damage (they do not have increased creatinine or decreased urine volume) at the time of evaluation, timely detection of functional changes with more precise and effective biomarkers are needed.

The novel biomarkers differ in their anatomical origin, physiology, excretion time from the onset of kidney injury, kinetics, and distribution. These biomarkers can be measured in blood and, more usefully, in urine. They can predict the subsequent development of traditionally defined AKI. Furthermore, they can offer information about the causal etiology and reveal different disease stages implicated in AKI, from injury to recovery. Interleukin 6 (IL-6), interleukin 18 (IL-18), and neutrophil gelatinase-associated lipocalin (NGAL) are markers of inflammation. Other molecules, such as the liver fatty acid binding protein (L-FABP) and the kidney injury molecule (KIM-1), have been proposed to define cell injury. On the other hand, tissue inhibitors of metalloproteinases type 2 (TIMP-2) and insulin-like growth factor-binding protein type-7 (IGFBP-7), cell cycle stress markers, have been revealed as potential diagnostic tools and prognostic markers. Perhaps in the future, new clinical studies can help define therapeutic interventions (Table **4**) [19, 20].

Table 4. Characteristics of common biomarkers used in AKI.

Biomarker	Function	Sample	Role in clinical practice in AKI assessment	References
Cystatin C	Cystatin C is found in all nucleated cells. It is a potent inhibitor of cysteine proteases that have a pleiotropic role in vascular pathophysiology and is freely filtered.	Plasma	- Diagnosis - Severity	[19, 21 - 23]

(Table 4) cont.....

Biomarker	Function	Sample	Role in clinical practice in AKI assessment	References
TIMP-2	Inhibitors of matrix metalloproteinases and TIMP family members can suppress the proliferation of endothelial cells.	Urine	- Prediction - Diagnosis - Severity	[24 - 26]
IGFBP-7	Protein that inhibits cell proliferation during cell cycle arrest.			
IL-18	Pro-inflammatory cytokine produced by monocytes, macrophages, and proximal tubular epithelial cells; detected in urine.		- Prediction - Diagnosis	[19 - 21]
KIM-1	Kidney Injury Molecule-1 is a transmembrane protein upregulated in the proximal tubule following tubular damage.		- Prediction - Diagnosis - Severity	[19, 21, 27]
L-FABP	A protein located at the cytoplasm of proximal renal tubular cells, its expression is upregulated after tubular cell damage.	Urine and plasma	- Diagnosis	[21]
NGAL	This protein is a member of the lipocalin family. It is synthesized and secreted by tubular epithelial cells and freely filtered by the glomerulus.		- Diagnosis - Severity	[19, 21, 28]
PENK	Proenkephalin A 119-159 is a novel biomarker; enkephalins are endogenous opioids; it has been suggested that they possibly regulate cardiac function and have roles in diverse physiologic and pathophysiological conditions; freely filtered.	Plasma	- Diagnosis - Severity - Kidney Recovery	[29]

On the other hand, the 23rd ADQI Consensus Meeting recommends identifying populations that can benefit from preventive interventions through validated biomarkers to obtain improved outcomes. In this consensus statement, the use of clinical data together with functional biomarkers was suggested in order to get more specific AKI definitions. In this proposal, the Consensus Statement recommends a modification of KDIGO stage 1 AKI into three substages (1S, 1A, and 1B) as well as to subclassify stages 2 and 3 (2A and 2B, 3A, and 3B) (Table 5). Therefore, it was proposed at the same meeting to include these functionally validated biomarkers in the severity classification. The functional biomarkers included were serum creatinine and urine output. However, the Consensus Statement did not rule out the inclusion of novel biomarkers. For example, stage 1S includes an early phase with a positive biomarker without compelling proof of kidney injury, but it does not meet the serum and urine creatinine diagnostic criteria. Similarly, it was proposed to subdivide with letter A if the biomarker is negative and B if the biomarker is positive [19, 30].

Table 5. Classification of acute kidney injury based on functional criteria and biomarkers.

Functional Criterion	Stage	Damage Criterion Based on some Biomarkers
No changes in sCr or increase <0.3 mg/dl and no criteria in urine output.	1S	Positive
Increase in sCr from baseline value ≥ 1.5 to 1.9 times in 7 days, basal increase ≥ 0.3 mg/dL in 48 h or and/or < 0.5 mL/Kg/h for 6 h.	1A	Negative
	1B	Positive
sCr ≥ 4 mg/dL with the need for RRT, baseline sCr increase ≥ 3 times the baseline value and/or < 0.3 mL/Kg/h for 24 h or anuria for 12 h	2A	Negative
	2B	Positive
sCr increase >2 to 2.9 times the baseline value and/or < 0.5 mL/Kg/h for 12 h.	3A	Negative
	3B	Positive

Abbreviations: sCr, serum creatinine.

TREATMENT

The therapeutic approach for treating AKI depends on the clinical syndrome's etiology and the patients' risk stratification. Risk models based on demographic, clinical, and environmental characteristics, such as persistent elevation of creatinine, the need for RRT, or mortality, are used to predict complex clinical outcomes. The models for contrast-associated AKI [31], perioperative AKI [32 - 34], and AKI in critically ill patients [35, 36] stand out.

One of the traditional interventions for the management of patients at high risk for or with established AKI frequently involves the administration of fluids for fear of untreated hypovolemia. This strategy is only valid when the AKI is of hypovolemic origin. The administration of intravenous fluids should focus on crystalloid solutions, preferably balanced. It should cover particular objectives based on clinical and imaging findings (POCUS: cardiac, VEXUs) since indiscriminate use can worsen the mechanism of kidney damage or stop kidney recovery, given the knowledge that we currently have about fluid overload and kidney congestion [37, 38].

When AKI is severe, RRT should be considered. Classically, there are absolute indications for the initiation of RRT, such as severe refractory hyperkalemia, volume overload with pulmonary edema, pericarditis, and uremic encephalopathy. Notably, RRT has a minimal capacity for eliminating endogenous waste products, including electrolytes, and does not replace other functions, such as metabolic and endocrine [39]. In the absence of indications for urgent dialysis, choosing when to start RRT in AKI patients is a challenge. Despite the evidence collected in the past decade, the indication remains unclear. Some trials, such as the ELAIN trial, recommended early RRT initiation to facilitate a better balance of fluids, electrolytes, and acid-base homeostasis in a timely manner. However, other trials, such as the AKIKI and AKIKI 2 trials, have shown that initiation before emergency surgery carries an increased risk of dialysis-related complications and vascular access placement, together with higher healthcare costs. It is important to note that no improvement in mortality has been demonstrated in patients who are likely to recover renal function without substitution therapy [39, 40]. Algorithms have been proposed that standardize the management of AKI according to risks and clinical characteristics to improve decision-making. Therefore, treatment ordering of patients with AKI can improve hospital mortality [41]. The evidence continues to build, and treatment decisions are likely to be modified with the advent of new technologies in biomarkers and volume status assessment.

CONCLUSION

AKI is a common complication in the hospitalization setting, affecting up to 7% of hospitalized patients, whereas in the ICU, the prevalence of AKI is much higher, ranging from 20% to 50%. It is linked with augmented mortality, morbidity, and long-term renal disease. AKI identification is conventionally ground on variations in serum creatinine and urine output. However, these measures are often delayed, reflecting changes in kidney function that have already occurred. Several biomarkers are helpful for the diagnosis and prognosis of AKI. These include NGAL, which can be detected in the urine as early as 2 hours after injury; KIM-1 and IL18, which can be detected in the urine and serum; and L-FABP, which can be detected in the urine. These biomarkers can be used to diagnose AKI earlier than traditional measures of kidney function. Also, they can be used to assess AKI severity and the risk of progression and follow the response to treatment. The use of biomarkers in diagnosing and managing AKI is still an area of active research.

Nevertheless, biomarkers can improve patient outcomes by allowing for earlier diagnosis and more effective treatment. Despite these advantages, there are challenges in using new classifications and biomarkers, such as the fact that some biomarkers can be expensive to measure, not all biomarkers are available in all hospitals, and the interpretation of biomarker results can be complex. The new classification and biomarkers for AKI could improve patient outcomes. However, some challenges must be addressed before they can be widely adopted.

REFERENCES

[1]   Chawla LS, Bellomo R, Bihorac A, *et al.* Acute kidney disease and renal recovery: consensus report of the Acute Disease Quality Initiative (ADQI) 16 Workgroup. Nat Rev Nephrol 2017; 13(4): 241-57. [http://dx.doi.org/10.1038/nrneph.2017.2] [PMID: 28239173]

[2]   Mehta RL, Kellum JA, Shah SV, *et al.* Acute Kidney Injury Network: report of an initiative to

improve outcomes in acute kidney injury. Crit Care 2007; 11(2): R31.
[http://dx.doi.org/10.1186/cc5713] [PMID: 17331245]

[3]   Stevens PE, Levin A. Evaluation and management of chronic kidney disease: synopsis of the kidney disease: improving global outcomes 2012 clinical practice guideline. Ann Intern Med 2013; 158(11): 825-30.
[http://dx.doi.org/10.7326/0003-4819-158-11-201306040-00007] [PMID: 23732715]

[4]   Ronco C, Bellomo R, Kellum JA. Acute kidney injury. Lancet 2019; 394(10212): 1949-64.
[http://dx.doi.org/10.1016/S0140-6736(19)32563-2] [PMID: 31777389]

[5]   Ostermann M, Joannidis M. Acute kidney injury 2016: diagnosis and diagnostic workup. Crit Care 2016; 20(1): 299.
[http://dx.doi.org/10.1186/s13054-016-1478-z] [PMID: 27670788]

[6]   Thomas ME, Blaine C, Dawnay A, *et al.* The definition of acute kidney injury and its use in practice. Kidney Int 2015; 87(1): 62-73.
[http://dx.doi.org/10.1038/ki.2014.328] [PMID: 25317932]

[7]   Nagata K, Horino T, Hatakeyama Y, Matsumoto T, Terada Y, Okuhara Y. Effects of transient acute kidney injury, persistent acute kidney injury and acute kidney disease on the long□term renal prognosis after an initial acute kidney injury event. Nephrology (Carlton) 2021; 26(4): 312-8.
[http://dx.doi.org/10.1111/nep.13831] [PMID: 33207040]

[8]   Kellum JA, Romagnani P, Ashuntantang G, Ronco C, Zarbock A, Anders HJ. Acute kidney injury. Nat Rev Dis Primers 2021; 7(1): 52.
[http://dx.doi.org/10.1038/s41572-021-00284-z] [PMID: 34267223]

[9]   Lameire NH, Bagga A, Cruz D, *et al.* Acute kidney injury: an increasing global concern. Lancet 2013; 382(9887): 170-9.
[http://dx.doi.org/10.1016/S0140-6736(13)60647-9] [PMID: 23727171]

[10] Rewa O, Bagshaw SM. Acute kidney injury—epidemiology, outcomes and economics. Nat Rev Nephrol 2014; 10(4): 193-207.
[http://dx.doi.org/10.1038/nrneph.2013.282] [PMID: 24445744]

[11] Li PKT, Burdmann EA, Mehta RL. Acute kidney injury: global health alert. Kidney Int 2013; 83(3): 372-6.
[http://dx.doi.org/10.1038/ki.2012.427] [PMID: 23302721]

[12] Hoste EAJ, Kellum JA, Selby NM, *et al.* Global epidemiology and outcomes of acute kidney injury. Nat Rev Nephrol 2018; 14(10): 607-25.
[http://dx.doi.org/10.1038/s41581-018-0052-0] [PMID: 30135570]

[13] Abebe A, Kumela K, Belay M, Kebede B, Wobie Y. Mortality and predictors of acute kidney injury in adults: a hospital-based prospective observational study. Sci Rep 2021; 11(1): 15672.
[http://dx.doi.org/10.1038/s41598-021-94946-3] [PMID: 34341369]

[14] Wang HE, Muntner P, Chertow GM, Warnock DG. Acute kidney injury and mortality in hospitalized patients. Am J Nephrol 2012; 35(4): 349-55.
[http://dx.doi.org/10.1159/000337487] [PMID: 22473149]

[15] Mehta RL, Burdmann EA, Cerdá J, *et al.* Recognition and management of acute kidney injury in the International Society of Nephrology 0by25 Global Snapshot: a multinational cross-sectional study. Lancet 2016; 387(10032): 2017-25.
[http://dx.doi.org/10.1016/S0140-6736(16)30240-9] [PMID: 27086173]

[16] Barasch J, Zager R, Bonventre JV. Acute kidney injury: a problem of definition. Lancet 2017; 389(10071): 779-81.
[http://dx.doi.org/10.1016/S0140-6736(17)30543-3] [PMID: 28248160]

[17] Moore PK, Hsu RK, Liu KD. Management of Acute Kidney Injury: Core Curriculum 2018. Am J Kidney Dis 2018; 72(1): 136-48.

[http://dx.doi.org/10.1053/j.ajkd.2017.11.021] [PMID: 29478864]

[18] Rosner MH, Perazella MA. Acute Kidney Injury in Patients with Cancer. N Engl J Med 2017; 376(18): 1770-81.
[http://dx.doi.org/10.1056/NEJMra1613984] [PMID: 28467867]

[19] Ostermann M, Zarbock A, Goldstein S, *et al.* Recommendations on Acute Kidney Injury Biomarkers From the Acute Disease Quality Initiative Consensus Conference. JAMA Netw Open 2020; 3(10): e2019209.
[http://dx.doi.org/10.1001/jamanetworkopen.2020.19209] [PMID: 33021646]

[20] Kane-Gill SL, Meersch M, Bell M. Biomarker-guided management of acute kidney injury. Curr Opin Crit Care 2020; 26(6): 556-62.
[http://dx.doi.org/10.1097/MCC.0000000000000777] [PMID: 33027146]

[21] Ho J, Tangri N, Komenda P, *et al.* Urinary, Plasma, and Serum Biomarkers' Utility for Predicting Acute Kidney Injury Associated With Cardiac Surgery in Adults: A Meta-analysis. Am J Kidney Dis 2015; 66(6): 993-1005.
[http://dx.doi.org/10.1053/j.ajkd.2015.06.018] [PMID: 26253993]

[22] Lin LC, Chuan MH, Liu JH, *et al.* Proenkephalin as a biomarker correlates with acute kidney injury: a systematic review with meta-analysis and trial sequential analysis. Crit Care 2023; 27(1): 481.
[http://dx.doi.org/10.1186/s13054-023-04747-5] [PMID: 38057904]

[23] Ravn B, Rimes-Stigare C, Bell M, *et al.* Creatinine versus cystatin C based glomerular filtration rate in critically ill patients. J Crit Care 2019; 52: 136-40.
[http://dx.doi.org/10.1016/j.jcrc.2019.04.007] [PMID: 31039451]

[24] Kashani K, Al-Khafaji A, Ardiles T, *et al.* Discovery and validation of cell cycle arrest biomarkers in human acute kidney injury. Crit Care 2013; 17(1): R25.
[http://dx.doi.org/10.1186/cc12503] [PMID: 23388612]

[25] Ostermann M, McCullough PA, Forni LG, *et al.* Kinetics of urinary cell cycle arrest markers for acute kidney injury following exposure to potential renal insults. Crit Care Med 2018; 46(3): 375-83.
[http://dx.doi.org/10.1097/CCM.0000000000002847] [PMID: 29189343]

[26] Joannidis M, Forni LG, Haase M, *et al.* Use of Cell Cycle Arrest Biomarkers in Conjunction With Classical Markers of Acute Kidney Injury. Crit Care Med 2019; 47(10): e820-6.
[http://dx.doi.org/10.1097/CCM.0000000000003907] [PMID: 31343478]

[27] Koyner JL, Vaidya VS, Bennett MR, *et al.* Urinary biomarkers in the clinical prognosis and early detection of acute kidney injury. Clin J Am Soc Nephrol 2010; 5(12): 2154-65.
[http://dx.doi.org/10.2215/CJN.00740110] [PMID: 20798258]

[28] Charlton JR, Portilla D, Okusa MD. A basic science view of acute kidney injury biomarkers. Nephrol Dial Transplant 2014; 29(7): 1301-11.
[http://dx.doi.org/10.1093/ndt/gft510] [PMID: 24385545]

[29] Legrand M, Hollinger A, Vieillard-Baron A, *et al.* One-Year Prognosis of Kidney Injury at Discharge From the ICU: A Multicenter Observational Study. Crit Care Med 2019; 47(12): e953-61.
[http://dx.doi.org/10.1097/CCM.0000000000004010] [PMID: 31567524]

[30] Murray PT, Mehta RL, Shaw A, *et al.* Potential use of biomarkers in acute kidney injury: report and summary of recommendations from the 10th Acute Dialysis Quality Initiative consensus conference. Kidney Int 2014; 85(3): 513-21.
[http://dx.doi.org/10.1038/ki.2013.374] [PMID: 24107851]

[31] Mehran R, Aymong ED, Nikolsky E, *et al.* A simple risk score for prediction of contrast-induced nephropathy after percutaneous coronary intervention. J Am Coll Cardiol 2004; 44(7): 1393-9.
[http://dx.doi.org/10.1016/j.jacc.2004.06.068] [PMID: 15464318]

[32] Woo SH, Zavodnick J, Ackermann L, Maarouf OH, Zhang J, Cowan SW. Development and Validation of a Web-Based Prediction Model for AKI after Surgery. Kidney360 2021; 2(2): 215-23.

[http://dx.doi.org/10.34067/KID.0004732020] [PMID: 35373024]

[33]   Gharaibeh KA, Hamadah AM, Sierra RJ, Leung N, Kremers WK, El-Zoghby ZM. The Rate of Acute Kidney Injury After Total Hip Arthroplasty Is Low but Increases Significantly in Patients with Specific Comorbidities. J Bone Joint Surg Am 2017; 99(21): 1819-26.
[http://dx.doi.org/10.2106/JBJS.16.01027] [PMID: 29088036]

[34]   Mehta RH, Grab JD, O'Brien SM, *et al.* Bedside tool for predicting the risk of postoperative dialysis in patients undergoing cardiac surgery. Circulation 2006; 114(21): 2208-16.
[http://dx.doi.org/10.1161/CIRCULATIONAHA.106.635573] [PMID: 17088458]

[35]   Basu RK, Zappitelli M, Brunner L, *et al.* Derivation and validation of the renal angina index to improve the prediction of acute kidney injury in critically ill children. Kidney Int 2014; 85(3): 659-67.
[http://dx.doi.org/10.1038/ki.2013.349] [PMID: 24048379]

[36]   Matsuura R, Srisawat N, Claure-Del Granado R, *et al.* Use of the Renal Angina Index in Determining Acute Kidney Injury. Kidney Int Rep 2018; 3(3): 677-83.
[http://dx.doi.org/10.1016/j.ekir.2018.01.013] [PMID: 29854976]

[37]   Ostermann M, Liu K, Kashani K. Fluid Management in Acute Kidney Injury. Chest 2019; 156(3): 594-603.
[http://dx.doi.org/10.1016/j.chest.2019.04.004] [PMID: 31002784]

[38]   Ostermann M, Bellomo R, Burdmann EA, *et al.* Controversies in acute kidney injury: conclusions from a Kidney Disease: Improving Global Outcomes (KDIGO) Conference. Kidney Int 2020; 98(2): 294-309.
[http://dx.doi.org/10.1016/j.kint.2020.04.020] [PMID: 32709292]

[39]   Ostermann M, Bagshaw SM, Lumlertgul N, Wald R. Indications for and Timing of Initiation of KRT. Clin J Am Soc Nephrol 2023; 18(1): 113-20.
[http://dx.doi.org/10.2215/CJN.05450522] [PMID: 36100262]

[40]   Zarbock A, Mehta RL. Timing of Kidney Replacement Therapy in Acute Kidney Injury. Clin J Am Soc Nephrol 2019; 14(1): 147-9.
[http://dx.doi.org/10.2215/CJN.08810718] [PMID: 30504248]

[41]   Mendu ML, Ciociolo GR Jr, McLaughlin SR, *et al.* A Decision-Making Algorithm for Initiation and Discontinuation of RRT in Severe AKI. Clin J Am Soc Nephrol 2017; 12(2): 228-36.
[http://dx.doi.org/10.2215/CJN.07170716] [PMID: 28119408]

CHAPTER 6

Non-Anion Gap Metabolic Acidosis: Renal Tubular Acidosis

Juan Reyna-Blanco[1,*]

[1] *Department of Nephrology, Hospital General de México Dr. Eduardo Liceaga, Mexico City, Mexico*

Abstract: Renal tubular acidosis (RTA) is a condition in which there is a defect in the reabsorption of bicarbonate, the excretion of hydrogen ions, or both, generating a clinical syndrome characterized by normal anion gap metabolic acidosis, hyperchloremia, and impaired urinary acidification.

Keywords: Ammoniagenesis, Hyperchloremic acidosis, Metabolic acidosis, Reabsorption of bicarbonate.

INTRODUCTION

Renal tubular acidosis (RTA) is a condition in which there is a defect in the reabsorption of bicarbonate, the excretion of hydrogen ions, or both, generating a clinical syndrome characterized by normal anion gap metabolic acidosis, hyperchloremia, and impaired urinary acidification [1]. According to the site of tubular involvement, RTA is classified as RTA type 1 (distal), RTA type 2 (proximal), or RTA type 4 (aldosterone deficiency). Rarely, due to carbonic anhydrase II (CAII) deficiency, a mixed or type 3 RTA can be generated. However, some authors have removed it from the classification because most of these patients progress to a distal RTA. In these patients, bicarbonate reabsorption is characterized by a reduced renal threshold for bicarbonate reabsorption with developmental immaturity of the proximal tubule, which subsequently normalizes [2].

PHYSIOLOGY OF ACID-BASE BALANCE

The lungs and kidneys are primarily responsible for regulating the acid-base balance of the blood. They do so by independently controlling the two primary components of the body's central buffering system: CO_2 and HCO_3^-. Whereas the

---

[*] **Corresponding author Juan Reyna Blanco:** Department of Nephrology, Hospital General de México Dr. Eduardo Liceaga, Mexico City, Mexico; E-mail: juanrb07@gmail.com.

Rafael Valdez-Ortiz, Katy Sánchez-Pozos, Ana Carolina Ariza & Enzo C. Vásquez-Jiménez (Eds.)

lungs are responsible for excreting a large amount of CO_2 that is produced during the oxidation of carbohydrates, fats, and amino acids, the kidneys are responsible for removing nonvolatile acids such as sulfuric acid, phosphoric acid, oxalic acid, lactic acid, keto acids, and other organic acids. These molecules are generated through the following processes: oxidation of sulfur-containing amino acids, metabolism of phosphorus-containing compounds, oxidation of cationic amino acids, production of nonmetabolizable organic acids, and incomplete oxidation of carbohydrates and fats. In addition, metabolism generates nonvolatile bases, which are converted into HCO_3^-. Subtracting the metabolically generated base from the metabolically generated acid leaves a net endogenous H^+ production of ~40 mmol/day for a person weighing 70 kg. The strong acids in a typical Western diet (20 mmol/day of H^+ gained) and the loss of bases in the stool (10 mmol/day of OH^- lost) represent an additional acid load to the body of 30 mmol/day. Thus, the body faces a total load of nonvolatile acids of ~70 mmol/day (0.75-1.5 mmol/kg body weight) derived from metabolism, diet, and intestinal losses [3]. The kidneys face two problems in addressing this. The first problem is the need to excrete H^+, which implies the need to reabsorb all the HCO_3^- filtered through the glomeruli. Every day, 180 liters of blood are filtered through the kidneys. If each liter of blood contains 23 to 25 mmol of HCO_3^-, then the filtered load of HCO_3^- per day is 180 L x 24 mmol/L = 4,320 mmol of HCO_3^- (4140-4500 mmol) [4]. The kidneys solve this problem by secreting H^+ into the tubular lumen and titrating filtered HCO_3^- to form CO_2 and H_2O. According to the following chemical reaction, for each H^+ consumed, the HCO_3^- is reduced in the same proportion, ultimately generating the same amount of CO_2:

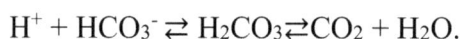

$$H^+ + HCO_3^- \rightleftarrows H_2CO_3 \rightleftarrows CO_2 + H_2O.$$

The carbonic anhydrase enzyme accelerates this process.

Second, 70 mmol of nonvolatile acids were excreted in the form of free H^+ in an "unbuffered" urinary volume of 1,500 mL per day, consequently producing urine with an H^+ concentration of 0.046 M (0.07 mol of H^+/1.5 L of urine). This latter would lead to a urinary pH of ~1.3 (pH = -log $[H^+]$). Physiologically, the lowest urinary pH that can occur is ~4.2, corresponding to an H^+ concentration of 0.000063 M, meaning that H+ is ~1000 times less concentrated than in "unbuffered" urine. The kidneys overcome this problem by binding H^+ with buffers such as phosphates and NH_3^+/NH_4^+ that maintain the urinary pH within a physiological range. Likewise, the H^+ secreted into the lumen has three destinations: the reaction with the filtered HCO_3^- to favor its reabsorption (80-85% is reabsorbed in the proximal convoluted tubule (PCT) and the rest in the thick ascending loop of the Henle and collecting tubules); titration with filtered phosphates ($HPO_4^{2-}/H_2PO_4^-$); and titration with secreted or, to a lesser extent, filtered NH_3^+ to form NH_4^+. The net acid excretion (NAE) is defined with the following equation:

$$NAE= [\text{titratable acid}]u + [NH_4^+]u - [HCO_3^-]u \times \text{urinary volume/day}$$

Titratable acid is obtained as the amount of alkali needed to increase the urinary pH to 7.4. It is the excreted acid load in the form of phosphates ($HPO_4^{2-}/H_2PO_4^-$) or, to a lesser extent, H^+ bound to creatinine or uric acid. Under normal conditions, the amount of excreted HCO_3^- is negligible, and the amount of excreted titratable acid is almost constant. However, NH_4^+ excretion is variable and can increase to more than 300 mmol/day in severe nonrenal metabolic acidosis states. Therefore, an increase in the NAE is due to an increase in the amount of excreted NH_4^+, and conversely, a decrease in the NAE is due to a decrease in the amount of excreted NH_4^+ or an increase in HCO_3^- loss.

Acid-base Balance in Proximal Tubules and Ammonia Genesis

Bicarbonate is freely filtered through the glomerulus, so PCT indirectly reabsorbs most of the filtered HCO_3 load through H^+ secretion. The leading players in this process are the apical Na^+/H^+ exchanger (NHE3), luminal H^+ ATPase, carbonic anhydrase IV located at the brush border (CAIV), cytoplasmic carbonic anhydrase II (CAII), basolateral $Na^+/3HCO_3^-$ cotransporter (NBCe1) and Na-K ATPase, which supply the necessary Na^+ gradient. As shown in Fig. **1**, filtered HCO_3^- reacts with H^+, which is secreted through NHE3 (coupled with Na+ reabsorption) and to a lesser extent through H^+ ATPase, forming H_2CO_3 [5], and in a reaction catalyzed by CAIV, where water and CO_2 are released, which diffuse freely through the cell membrane. Once CO_2 is in the cytoplasm, it reacts with water to reform H+ and HCO_3^- through cytoplasmic ACII. HCO_3^- leaves the basolateral membrane along with Na+, through which the basolateral $Na^+/3HCO_3^-$ cotransporter (NBCe1) reaches the systemic circulation, while H^+ is recycled through NHE3 and H^+ ATPase, repeating the process.

PCT is also responsible for the synthesis and secretion of NH_4^+ through ammonia genesis. Glutamine metabolism leads to the formation of glutamate and, finally, α-ketoglutarate with the help of glutaminase (GS) and glutamate dehydrogenase (GDH). In the synthesis of α-ketoglutarate, 2 NH_4^+ ions are formed. Then, α-ketoglutarate enters gluconeogenesis or the Krebs cycle, forming 2 HCO_3^-, which are reabsorbed through the NBCe1 cotransporter in the basolateral membrane, whereas NH_4^+ can be dissociated intracellularly into H^+ and NH_3^+. Then, H^+ is secreted into the tubular lumen through the apical NHE3 exchanger or H^+ ATPase, and NH_3^+ diffuses across the apical membrane to join free H^+ in the lumen to form NH_4^+. Moreover, intracellular NH_4^+ can be secreted directly into the tubular lumen through NHE3, which functions as a Na^+/NH_4^+ exchanger. Not all the NH_4^+ produced in the PCT is secreted into the tubular lumen, as up to 40% is secreted into the systemic circulation for urea synthesis [6]. The rate-limiting enzymes in proximal tubular ammonia genesis, glutaminase, and phosphoenolpyruvate carboxy kinase are induced by metabolic acidosis, hypokalemia, and glucocorticoids and inhibited by hyperkalemia [7].

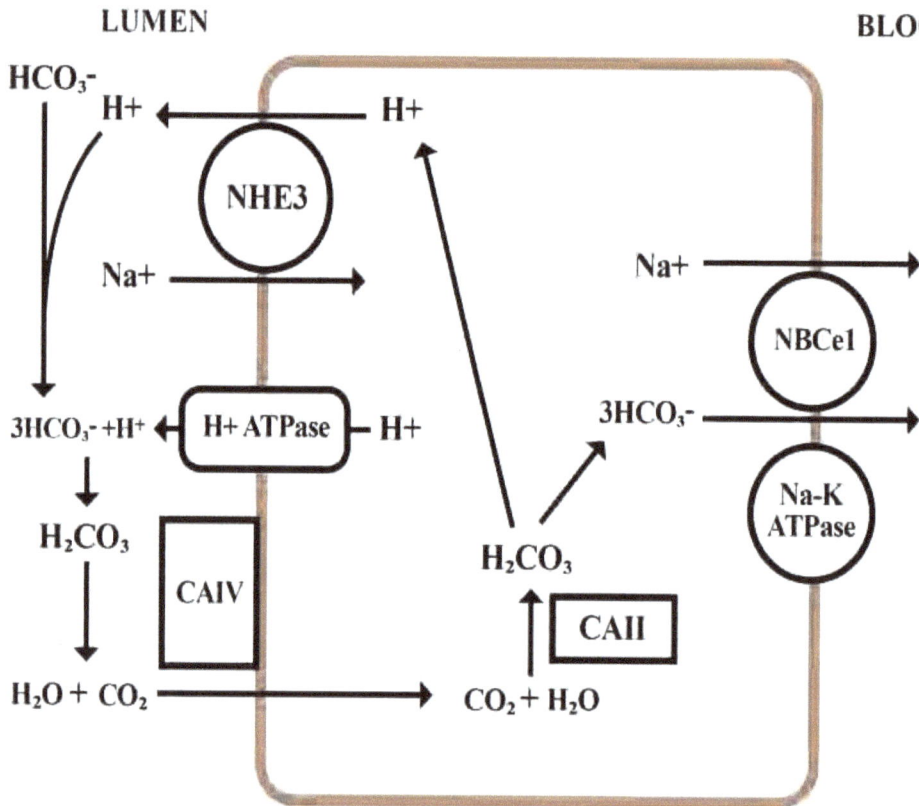

Fig. (1). Proximal tubule cell bicarbonate transport processes.

The thick portion of the ascending loop of Henle (TAL) contributes to the reabsorption of NH_4^+ through the $Na^+/K^+/2Cl^-$ cotransporter (NKCC2), which also functions as a $Na^+/NH_4^+/2Cl^-$ cotransporter. Once in the tubular epithelium, NH_4^+ dissociates into H^+ and NH_3^+, the latter of which passes freely through the basolateral membrane to the medullary interstitium, where it is reabsorbed in the collecting duct to reach the tubular lumen *via* RhCG/RhBG (rhesus proteins), with the remainder delivered to the renal vein. Luminal NH_3^+ buffers secrete H^+ ions from the distal nephron to form NH_4^+, thus contributing to net acid excretion [8].

Acid-base Balance in the Distal Nephron

Approximately 10% of filtered bicarbonate is reabsorbed in the distal nephron *via* H^+ secretion. In the proximal region of the distal convoluted tubule (DCT1), H^+ secretion is carried out through the apical Na^+/H^+ exchanger (NHE2) and by the apical H^+ ATPase, while in the distal region (DCT2), connecting the tubule and collecting duct, there are intercalated cells whose function is the active secretion of H^+ into the tubular lumen through the H^+ ATPase and the H^+/K^+ ATPase that secrete H^+ and reabsorb K^+. At the same time, for each secreted H^+, one molecule of HCO_3^- is reabsorbed through the basolateral exchanger $Cl-/HCO_3^-$ (AE1). In the tubular lumen, the secreted H^+ is buffered by the secreted NH_3^+ in the collecting duct to form NH_4^+ or by filtered HPO_4^{2-} to form $H_2PO_4^-$, contributing to net acid excretion. In addition, principal cells located in the connecting/collecting tubule are responsible for sodium reabsorption through epithelial sodium channels (ENaCs), water reabsorption, and K^+ secretion through apical ROMK transporters (Fig. **2**). Aldosterone positively modulates the ENaC in such a way that the entry of Na^+ into the principal cells promotes the activity of the H^+ ATPase in the intercalated A cells since an electronegative potential is generated in the tubular lumen (- 5 to -30 mV) that favors the secretion of H^+. Furthermore, aldosterone directly modulates the activity of ROMK and H^+ ATPase [9].

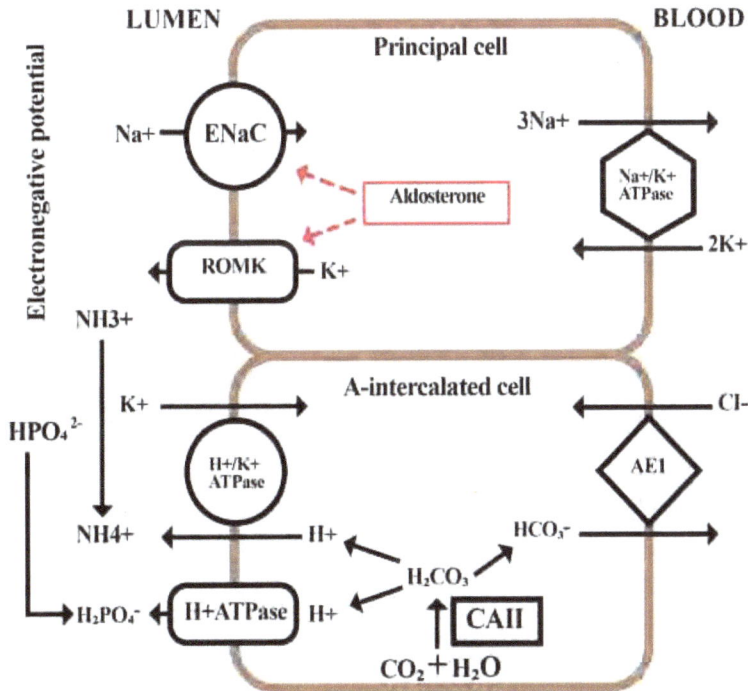

Fig. (2). Distal acidification.

Classification of Renal Tubular Acidosis

Proximal Renal Tubular Acidosis (type 2)

Proximal RTA is characterized by an impairment of bicarbonate reabsorption in the proximal tubule that may theoretically be due to a malfunction of H^+ secretion through the H^+ ATPase or the Na^+/H^+ exchanger (NHE3), altered carbonic anhydrase II/IV (CAII/IV) or an effect on the Na^+/HCO_3^- cotransporter (NBCe1). Proximal RTA (pRTA) can be detected in the context of Fanconi syndrome (genetic or acquired), which is characterized by a generalized effect on the reabsorption of solutes in the proximal tubule manifesting as aminoaciduria, phosphaturia, uricosuria, bicarbonaturia, glucosuria, and other organic acids. pRTA is also characterized by decreased bicarbonate reabsorption threshold, ranging from a normal serum value of 24 mmol/L to <15 mmol/L. Thus, if the patient remains at this new threshold, bicarbonaturia will not be present; however, bicarbonaturia and urinary alkalinization will be observed with a bicarbonate load. Moreover, if ammonium chloride (NH_4Cl) or furosemide/fludrocortisone is administered, adequate urinary acidification will be observed since distal reabsorption of bicarbonate is maintained and secretion of H^+ by the A-intercalated cells is intact. It has been suggested from animal models that there may be other mechanisms that can generate metabolic acidosis in pRTA, such as an impairment in the generation of NH_4^+ in the proximal tubule from glutamine and, consequently, a decrease in the generation of α-ketoglutarate and bicarbonate [10]. Previous studies have shown that in patients with autosomal dominant pRTA, normal urine NH_4^+ excretion occurs in the steady state. However, there is a lack of an appropriate increase in urine NH_4^+ excretion after NH_4Cl loading [11].

Etiology of pRTA

Hereditary: This disorder can manifest as an autosomal recessive, autosomal dominant, sporadic, or X-linked disorder, which occurs in some familial Fanconi syndromes. Patients with autosomal recessive forms are associated with mutations in the gene *SLC4A4*, which encodes the Na^+/HCO_3^- cotransporter (NBCe1) and produces an isolated pRTA accompanied by short stature, glaucoma, cataracts, band keratopathy, dental defects, and basal ganglia calcification [12]. Regarding autosomal dominant forms, only two families with isolated pure autosomal dominant pRTA have been reported, and this was not due to a defect in genes that are known to be involved in proximal bicarbonate reabsorption [13, 14]. No organ system dysfunction or short stature was detected. In animal models, the gene that encodes for NHE3 (*slc9a3*) generates autosomal dominant pRTA [15]; however, this defect has not been demonstrated in humans to date. Sporadic forms that require bicarbonate administration have been reported during childhood; however, they resolve over time without requiring further treatment. The most common forms of familial Fanconi syndrome are cystinosis and Wilson disease; other causes include Dent syndrome, Lowe syndrome, tyrosinemia, and galactosemia.

Acquired: pRTA is the most common cause of pRTA in adults. Its appearance could be due to drugs such as ifosfamide, tenofovir, and carbonic anhydrase inhibitors. Toxins such as cadmium or lead and systemic diseases causing light chain deposition, such as multiple myeloma, amyloidosis, or any monoclonal gammopathy of renal significance with proximal tubule involvement, have been identified (Table **1**).

Table 1. Causes of proximal RTA.

• **Hereditary**
-NBCe1 (AR): short stature, cataracts, glaucoma, band keratopathy and basal ganglia calcification
-CA-II (CA2 gene, AR) on Ch 8q22: cerebral calcification and mental retardation
-Familial Fanconi syndrome: Cystinosis (SLC3A1/SLC7A9 genes) Wilson disease (ATP7B gene) Tyrosinemia (FAH gene) Galactosemia (GALT gene) Fanconi-Bickel syndrome (GLUT-2): pRTA and impaired utilization of glucose and galactose Lowe syndrome (OCRL gene): cataract, mental retardation, and Fanconi-like RTA Dent disease (CLCN5 gene): proteinuria, hypercalciuria, nephrocalcinosis and nephrolithiasis
• **Acquired**
-Multiple myeloma, monoclonal gammopathy of renal significance (MGRS): Light chain proximal tubulopathy (LCPT) Monoclonal immunoglobulin deposition disease (MIDD) Renal amyloidosis
-Toxins: cadmium, mercury, and lead
-Drugs: ifosfamide, valproic acid, carbonic anhydrase inhibitors, aminoglycosides and various antiretrovirals

Clinical Presentation

The cause will depend on the etiology and the age of presentation. If it presents during childhood and is associated with growth retardation, osteomalacia, ocular disorders, and mental retardation, it could be due to a genetic mutation, as previously mentioned. Polyuria, polydipsia, hypovolemia, and hypokalemia are usually observed, and severe conditions can lead to weakness or paralysis. These symptoms generally occur when the bicarbonate reabsorption threshold is exceeded, which causes bicarbonaturia with the consequent excretion of K^+ or Na^+ to maintain electroneutrality, generating, above all, dehydration and exacerbation of hypokalemia [2, 16]. Moreover, increased distal Na^+ increases distal calcium wasting, resulting in hypercalciuria. However, increased citrate excretion increases calcium levels and prevents renal calculi or nephrocalcinosis. In patients with Fanconi syndrome, phosphaturia, tubular proteinuria, aminoaciduria, uricosuria, and glycosuria are also observed. In adults, it could be asymptomatic or present as a finding within a systemic disease, such as in the case of paraproteinemia or with isolated normal anion gap metabolic acidosis with hypokalemia when the cause is drugs or toxins.

Distal Renal Tubular Acidosis (Type 1)

Distal renal tubular acidosis is characterized by a defect in distal tubular acidification, manifested primarily by non-anion gap metabolic acidosis and the inability to acidify the urine during acidaemia.

Etiology of Distal RTA

According to its pathophysiology, this may be due to a secretory defect when the distal secretion of H^+ is compromised or a secondary defect related to the integrity of the secretory mechanism. It can also be classified as hereditary or acquired (Table 2).

Table 2. Causes of distal RTA.

• Hereditary (Familial or sporadic)
-AE1 (SLC4A1 gene, AD/AR): dRTA ±hemolytic anemia without sensorineural deafness -H+ ATPase B1 subunit (ATP6V1B1 gene, AR): dRTA + sensorineural deafness (>90%, early onset) -H+ ATPase A4 subunit (ATP6V0A4 gene, AR): dRTA + sensorineural deafness (35-50%, late onset) -Pseudohypoaldosteronism type 1 and 2 (Gordon syndrome): hyperkalemic dRTA -Other mutations: FOXI1, WDR72
• Acquired
-Autoimmune diseases: Sjogren syndrome, lupus erythematosus, rheumatoid arthritis
-Drugs: ifosfamide (pRTA > dRTA), amphotericin B, lithium, zoledronate, foscarnet, NSAID, amiloride, trimethoprim, pentamidine, cyclosporine
-Toxins: Toluene, Balkan nephropathy
-Nephrocalcinosis: Hyperparathyroidism, milk/alkali, hypervitaminosis D
-Others: Obstructive uropathy, primary biliary cirrhosis, hypergammaglobulinemia

Secretory defect distal RTA (dRTA): also known as classic distal RTA, which occurs due to gene alterations that encode or control the channels involved in urinary acidification in the distal and collecting tubules. Classic dRTA is the most common cause of dRTA in children and presents as an autosomal dominant or recessive pattern. Mutations in the *SLC4A1* gene that encodes the Cl^-/HCO_3^- exchanger (AE1) could be caused by either an autosomal dominant or recessive form. In contrast, mutations in the genes that encode H^+ ATPase (*ATP6V1B1* and *ATP6V0A4*) are presented as an autosomal recessive form. Other genes associated with distal renal tubular acidosis are *FOXI1* (transcription factor) and *WDR72* (involved in intracellular trafficking) [17].

Back leak defect distal RTA (gradient defect): The transport of H^+ and HCO_3^- is intact; however, there is reverse diffusion of secreted H^+ that generates a loss of the H^+ gradient due to either altered membrane permeability or loss of cohesive forces at cell junctions. In this scenario, K^+ is lost instead of H^+. This case is typically generated by the administration of amphotericin [18].

Buffer defect distal RTA: In this category, dRTA is caused by a decrease in the delivery of NH_3^+ to the collecting duct, causing a decreased hydrogen buffering capacity from the intercalated cells. Thus, secreted hydrogen ions saturate the phosphate buffer and cause an early gradient loss. Because there is a decrease in H^+ secretion due to impaired NH3+ secretion, K^+ is lost. This can occur in conditions that lead to chronic tubulointerstitial nephritis or nephrocalcinosis.

Voltage defect distal RTA: Also called hyperkalemic dRTA, aldosterone may be either normal or increased, and there is a tubular defect for H^+ and K^+ secretion generally induced by aldosterone resistance, as occurs in pseudohypoaldosteronism type I (PHA type 1), caused by mutations in either the mineralocorticoid receptor or ENaC; decreased distal Na^+ delivery, such as pseudohypoaldosteronism type II (also known as Gordon syndrome), caused by mutations in *WNKs* that regulate the $Na^+/2Cl^-$ channel (NCC) in the distal tubule. The drugs associated with similar effects are amiloride, triamterene, pentamidine, trimethoprim, and cyclosporine, as well as mixed defects such as obstructive uropathy, lupus, and sickle cell nephropathy. These alterations commonly involve a loss of electronegative potential in the tubular lumen; therefore, the voltage gradient necessary for H^+ secretion by intercalated cells is not created, and the secretion of K^+ is reduced [19].

Combined defects: In many cases, dRTA is generated by the combination of several effects, such as systemic lupus erythematosus, Sjogren's syndrome, rheumatoid arthritis, vasculitis, cryoglobulinemia, hypergammaglobulinemia, paraproteinemia, drugs or toxins.

Clinical presentation

Distal RTA is characterized by hyperchloremic metabolic acidosis with a positive urinary anion gap due to decreased NH_4^+ excretion. It can also present as polyuria, polydipsia, muscle weakness, or paralysis caused by hypokalemia, nephrocalcinosis, or nephrolithiasis. Acidaemia in these patients promotes stone formation by increasing calcium phosphate release from bones (to buffer with hydrogen ions secreted from the distal nephron) and decreasing calcium tubular reabsorption due to distal luminal alkalinization. Moreover, the increase in citrate consumption caused by the intracellular acidosis of proximal tubular cells generates a gradient that favors its reabsorption, thus reducing the urinary concentration of citrate and favoring the formation of stones [20]. In children, it is common to observe failure to thrive, growth retardation, rickets, or osteomalacia in adults. In hereditary forms, other defects may be present in addition to the symptoms caused by dRTA. In patients with mutations in the *ATP6V1B1* and *ATP6V0A4* genes (encoding H^+ ATPases), symptoms usually present at an earlier age, between 6 and 24 months after birth, while patients with mutations in the *SLC4A1* gene exhibit symptoms at a later age, between 4 and 13 years. Sensorineural deafness is a characteristic feature in patients with *ATP6V1B1*, *ATP6V0A4*, and *FOXI1* mutations due to the expression of these genes in the kidney and ear [17]. However, mutations in *ATP6V1B1* are associated with a greater incidence of deafness (90%) than are mutations in *ATP6V0A4* (35-50%) [21]. The clinical manifestations are less severe when *SLC4A1* mutations occur due to the later age of presentation, the latter compared to the recessive forms. In these patients, deafness is not present, although hemolytic anemia has been reported [22]. Genetic diseases that cause hyperkalemic dRTA, such as PHA type 1, are characterized by salt loss and a lack of growth. The spectrum of clinical manifestations varies from severely affected patients who die in childhood to asymptomatic carriers. Infants typically present with weight loss, dehydration, hypotension, growth retardation, high urinary sodium despite volume depletion, hypotension, hyperchloremic metabolic acidosis, and hyperkalemia.

Plasma and urine aldosterone levels are elevated, and plasma renin activity is increased. PHA type 1 is divided into type 1a, which is caused by a defect in the mineralocorticoid receptor and is transmitted in an autosomal dominant pattern, and type 1b, which is caused by a defect in the epithelial sodium channel and is transmitted in an autosomal recessive pattern. PHA type 2, better known as Gordon syndrome, is the mirror image of Gitelman syndrome and is characterized by hyperchloremic metabolic acidosis, hypertension with suppressed renin activity, hyperkalemia, and a normal glomerular filtration rate (GFR) with normal plasma aldosterone levels. In adults, dRTA can be asymptomatic, and it is not uncommon to find patients with nephrolithiasis without systemic metabolic acidosis who are unable to acidify the urine when challenged with an acid-loading test. This entity has been called incomplete dRTA. The development of chronic kidney disease (CKD) is common in patients with dRTA, and the etiology is multifactorial. The duration of the disease, the presence of nephrocalcinosis, the presence of hypokalemia, and the presence of repeated episodes of hypovolemia are considered causal factors [23].

Hyperkalaemic Renal Tubular Acidosis (Type 4)

Type 4 RTA presents with hyperkalemia due to aldosterone deficiency or aldosterone resistance. The pathophysiology is similar to dRTA voltage defects; however, unlike this, the ability to lower urine pH in systemic acidosis is normal, and nephrocalcinosis or urolithiasis is absent. In addition, ammonia genesis is decreased in the proximal tubule due to the presence of hyperkalemia (per se inhibiting the production of NH_4^+) and decreased ammonium absorption through NKCC2, the latter of which is located in the thick ascending loop of Henle. In most cases, interstitial compromise can lead to a decrease in renin production and thereby promote a state of selective chronic hypoaldosteronism.

Etiology of Hyperkalemic RTA

It can be caused by drugs that inhibit the action of aldosterone or its targets, such as spironolactone, eplerenone, amiloride, triamterene, and trimethoprim; glucocorticoid deficiency, such as Addison's disease, desmolase deficiency, or 21-b-hydroxylase deficiency; and hyporeninemic hypoaldosteronism with chronic interstitial nephropathies, such as diabetes, amyloidosis, obstruction and renal transplantation [19]. Some authors consider PHA states in this category [2].

Clinical Presentation

These patients are commonly middle-aged or elderly and asymptomatic. It is usually due to laboratory findings and is present in the context of chronic degenerative diseases (*e.g.*, diabetes). Hyperchloremic metabolic acidosis, chronic kidney disease, and hyperkalemia commonly can occur together. In most cases, hyperkalemia is characterized by being moderate and not producing electrocardiographic changes. Low plasma and urine aldosterone levels are associated with low plasma renin activity and reduced ammonium excretion with a preserved ability to acidify urine. Renal sodium wasting is rare because this condition commonly occurs in patients who already have chronic kidney damage. In children, it can occur in chronic interstitial nephropathies. Unlike a voltage defect, dRTA does not manifest as nephrocalcinosis or nephrolithiasis.

Approach and Diagnosis of Renal Tubular Acidosis

Evaluating patients with hyperchloremic acidosis should begin with a thorough history and physical examination. The age of presentation, family history, associated symptoms, and use of drugs or toxins must be considered. The environment is also a determining factor for developing certain tubulopathies, as is the case for Balkan nephropathy. In adults, renal tubular acidosis is generally a biochemical finding or can occur in systemic disease (*e.g.*, autoimmunity, paraproteinaemia, kidney transplant). Patients who develop stones exhibit incomplete distal renal tubular acidosis [20].

A direct assay for urine NH_4^+ is not often available in clinical settings, and indirect tests are used to estimate the NH_4^+ excretion rate in patients with hyperchloremic metabolic acidosis. Although these tests provide only semiquantitative estimates, they are adequate for clinical use because the information needed is whether the rate of NH_4^+ excretion is low enough that a defect in renal NH_4^+ excretion is the cause of metabolic acidosis or whether it is sufficiently high that another cause of hyperchloremic metabolic acidosis should be considered. Table **3** shows the clinical and biochemical differences between the different types of RTA.

Table 3. Differences in the types of renal tubular acidosis.

Test/Feature	Proximal RTA (type 2)	Distal RTA (type 1)		Type 4 RTA
-	-	Hypokalemic	Hyperkalemic	-
During acidosis (or with acid loading)				
Urine anion gap	Negative	Positive	Positive	Positive
Urine NH4+ excretion	N/↓	↓	↓	↓
Serum K+	N/↓	N/↓	↑	↑
Urine Ca++	N/↑	↑	↑	N/↓
Urine citrate	N/↑	↓	↓	N/↓
With normal blood pH (or with bicarbonate loading)				
FEHCO₃	>10-15%	<5%	<5%	5-10%
Urinary pCO2	>70 mm Hg	~50 mm Hg	>70 mmHg	>70 mmHg
Other features				
Fanconi syndrome	Often present	Absent	Absent	Absent
Nephrolithiasis	Absent	Present	Present	Absent
Bone disease	Often present	Rare	Rare	Absent
Serum Aldo/K	>3	>3	>3	<3

Modified from Gopal Basu *et al.* [2].

Urine Anion Gap (UAG)

The urine anion gap (UAG), calculated as UNa+UK-UCl, has been used to assess the rate of NH_4^+ excretion in patients with hyperchloremic acidosis. Because NH_4^+

excretion is accompanied by Cl$^-$ excretion, then in a state of acidosis of extrarenal origin (*e.g.*, diarrhea), Cl$^-$ excretion will increase (UNa+UK), so the UAG will be negative. However, if there is a decrease in NH$_4^+$ excretion, Cl$^-$ excretion will be low; therefore, UAG will be positive. The NH$_4^+$ excretion rate can be estimated with the following equation (correlation of 0.72):

$$NH_4^+ \text{ excretion} = -0.8 \text{ (UAG)} + 82 \text{ [24]}$$

It is evident that if the UAG is negative, the NH$_4^+$ excretion rate will be > 82. However, if the UAG is positive, the NH$_4^+$ excretion rate will be < 82. The problem is that UAG detects NH$_4^+$ only if it is excreted with Cl. Therefore, if NH$_4^+$ is excreted with another anion (*e.g.*, hippurate, b-hydroxybutyrate, D-lactate), the UAG will not exhibit a high rate of NH$_4^+$ excretion, and these patients may be misdiagnosed with RTA. In type 1 and 4 renal tubular acidosis, the UAG is positive according to the acid loading test. In contrast, the UAG value may be negative in proximal renal tubular acidosis because NH$_4^+$ excretion in the distal tubule is intact.

Urine Osmolality (UOG)

Another indirect alternative for measuring NH$_4^+$ excretion can be obtained through the following formula:

Urinary osmolality was calculated as follows: urinary osmolality (calculated as [(uNa × uK) × 2]) + urinary urea nitrogen/2.8 + urinary glucose/18.

Normal UOG is usually 80-150 mEq/L, and the concentration of NH$_4^+$ in the urine can be estimated by dividing the UOG by 2. The UOG detects NH$_4^+$ in the urine regardless of its accompanying anion but is unreliable for assessing the rate of NH$_4^+$ excretion if other osmoles (*e.g.*, ethanol, methanol, ethylene glycol, mannitol) are present in the urine [25].

Urine pH

The basis for the low excretion rate of NH$_4^+$ can be inferred from the urine pH. A urine pH of ~5 suggests a defect causing a low rate of NH$_4^+$ production or preventing NH$_4^+$ accumulation in the medullary interstitium/transfer of NH$_3^+$ into the lumen of the collecting duct (Type 4 RTA with acid load challenge). A urinary pH > 6 suggests a defect in HCO$_3^-$ reabsorption in the PCT (Type 2 RTA with bicarbonate load challenge) or a defect in H$^+$ secretion in the distal nephron (Type 1 RTA with acid load challenge) [26].

Citrate Excretion

Normal citrate excretion is 1.6 - 4.5 mmol/24 h (adult) and is related to acid-base status. Under conditions of acidaemia, where proximal intratubular cells have a lower pH, citrate reabsorption is stimulated, generating hypocitraturia, as occurs in the dRTA. Conversely, in pRTA, the alkaline pH of intratubular cells decreases their reabsorption due to low consumption. Hypocitraturia is also observed in patients with carbonic anhydrase IV deficiency, whereas this is not the case in patients with carbonic anhydrase II deficiency [25].

Urine PCO$_2$

The urinary PCO$_2$ is used to assess H$^+$ secretion in the distal nephron. The patient is given a load of NaHCO$_3$ to increase the filtered load and its delivery to the distal tubule. In this way, HCO$_3^-$ reacts with H$^+$ secreted by the intercalated cells to form carbonic acid (H$_2$CO$_3$), which slowly dehydrates to release CO$_2$, which is trapped in the renal tubule because there is no luminal carbonic anhydrase in the distal nephron. A urinary PCO$_2$ > 70 mmHg with a urine-to-blood PCO$_2$ gradient (U-B PCO$_2$) greater than 20 mmHg suggests a normal rate of net H$^+$ secretion in the distal nephron. In back leak dRTA, a urinary PCO$_2$ > 70 mmHg can be found because the filtered HCO$_3^-$ reacts with H$^+$ to prevent its back leak. Similar values can be found in patients with hyperkalaemic RTA (voltage defect dRTA and RTA type 4) with integrity in distal H$^+$ secretion (the problem is generating the electronegative potential to stimulate H$^+$ secretion). In the case of classic dRTA, low urinary pCO$_2$ and a U-B pCO$_2$ gradient < 20 mmHg will be observed [2].

Sodium Bicarbonate Loading Test

The patient is given a load of sodium bicarbonate intravenously or orally. With this test, the excreted fraction of bicarbonate (FEHCO$_3$) can be calculated using the following equation:

$$[u(HCO_3^-) \, p(Cr)/p(HCO_3^-)u(Cr)] \times 100$$

Under normal conditions, this percentage is less than 5% since 85-90% of filtered bicarbonate is reabsorbed in the proximal tubule. If there is a defect in proximal HCO$_3^-$ reabsorption, the amount of filtered bicarbonate will exceed the proximal tubule absorption threshold, and the FE of HCO$_3^-$ will exceed 15% (Table **4**).

Acid Loading Test

It can be performed with ammonium chloride or furosemide; however, the former can trigger nausea, vomiting, and gastric irritation, which is why the administration of furosemide has replaced it to cause urinary acidification. This test was performed with prior administration of fludrocortisone. Typically, in a mineralocorticoid-replete state, the administration of furosemide allows the amplification of the voltage gradient usually found in the cortical collecting tubule. This latter occurs because mineralocorticoid activity increases sodium reabsorption *via* ENaC, whereas the administration of furosemide increases sodium delivery to the distal nephron. In patients with dRTA, the urinary pH at the end of the test will be > 5.3, while in those patients with pRTA or type 4 RTA, the urinary pH will be < 5.3 (Table 4) [26].

Table 4. Differences between the bicarbonate and furosemide loading tests.

Bicarbonate Loading Test	Furosemide Loading Test
-First calculate HCO_3- deficit through the following formula: [(desired HCO_3)- (actual HCO_3-)] x body weight x 0.6. This HCO_3- deficit must be administered intravenously or orally. -IV bicarbonate loading (takes 2-4 hours to achieve a serum HCO_3- of 22-25 mEq/L) -8.4% $NaHCO_3$ solution – 100mEq of $NaHCO_3$ in 100 mL -7.5% $NaHCO_3$ solution = 89mEq of $NaHCO_3$ in 100 mL - Administer 2 ml/kg bolus followed by 2 ml/min infusion -Oral bicarbonate loading -1 g $NaHCO_3$ = 12 mEq of $NaHCO_3$ - It can be performed by administering 2 g $NaHCO_3$ q15 min - It could cause gastric distention -End the test when 3 serial urine samples with pH>7.5 are obtained, measured every 30-60 minutes.	- Administer fludrocortisone 1 mg PO at 22:00 h prev. day + overnight fast - Morning baseline urine pH and serum electrolytes - If Urine pH < 5.5, precludes the need for further testing - Give furosemide 40 mg PO - Measure urine pH q30 min for 5 h - Normally, urine pH falls to <5.5. Failure to do so indicates a distal acidification defect - Useful to screen for incomplete distal acidification defects in the presence of urolithiasis

TREATMENT

The main goal of treatment in patients with RTA is to maintain a normal or near-normal serum pH and bicarbonate concentration, especially in children, for proper development and growth and to reduce the incidence of nephrocalcinosis, nephrolithiasis, rickets, hypokalemia, and CKD progression.

Alkali administration in the form of tablets or solutions can be achieved through sodium bicarbonate or an equivalent organic anion such as citrate, which consumes H^+ during metabolism in the liver [27, 28].

Proximal Renal Tubular Acidosis

Bicarbonate is required since its absorption threshold is exceeded, causing bicarbonaturia and a propensity to develop hypokalemia and polyuria. High doses of sodium bicarbonate (or sodium/potassium citrate) of up to 14 mEq/kg/day are recommended. It is commonly associated with thiazides and a low-sodium diet to decrease bicarbonate loss [29].

Distal Renal Tubular Acidosis

Adults require 1-2 mEq/kg/day of sodium bicarbonate or sodium citrate, while children are treated with much higher doses of alkali (4-8 mEq/kg/day). Thiazide can increase bicarbonate absorption in the proximal tubule and decrease hypercalciuria [30, 31].

Hyperkalemic Renal Tubular Acidosis

In this case, the objective is to reduce the serum potassium level to decrease acidosis and promote ammonia genesis. Sometimes, the use of fludrocortisone is helpful; however, care must be taken for patients who have a certain degree of CKD since most of them have systemic arterial hypertension or cardiovascular disease. All drugs predisposing patients to hyperkalemia should be discontinued, potassium consumption should be reduced, and glycemia should be controlled. Loop diuretics or potassium exchange resins could be helpful [27]. In all cases of renal tubular acidosis, the underlying cause should be treated.

CONCLUSION

Renal tubular acidosis encompasses a group of disorders characterized by the kidneys' inability to acidify urine, leading to hyperchloremic metabolic acidosis. It is classified into three main types: distal (Type 1), proximal (Type 2), and hyperkalemic (Type 4), each with distinct pathophysiological mechanisms and clinical features. Diagnosis is based on laboratory tests assessing blood and urine bicarbonate levels, electrolytes, and pH. Management involves correcting metabolic acidosis with bicarbonate or citrate supplementation and specific treatments for each RTA type, such as thiazide diuretics for Type 1 and potassium supplements for Type 2. Early identification and treatment of RTA are critical to prevent serious complications like nephrocalcinosis, kidney stones, and growth retardation in children. Understanding the underlying mechanisms of each RTA type facilitates effective clinical management and significantly improves patient outcomes.

REFERENCES

[1]   Pereira P, Miranda D, Oliveira E, Simoes e Silva A. Molecular pathophysiology of renal tubular acidosis. Curr Genomics 2009; 10(1): 51-9.
       [http://dx.doi.org/10.2174/138920209787581262] [PMID: 19721811]

[2]   Basu G, Sudhakar G, Mohapatra A. Renal tubular acidosis. Clin Queries Nephrol 2013; 2(4): 166-78.
       [http://dx.doi.org/10.1016/j.cqn.2013.11.006]

[3]   Hamm LL, Nakhoul N, Hering-Smith KS. Acid-Base Homeostasis. Clin J Am Soc Nephrol 2015; 10(12): 2232-42.
[http://dx.doi.org/10.2215/CJN.07400715] [PMID: 26597304]

[4]   Curthoys NP, Moe OW. Proximal tubule function and response to acidosis. Clin J Am Soc Nephrol 2014; 9(9): 1627-38.
[http://dx.doi.org/10.2215/CJN.10391012] [PMID: 23908456]

[5]   Preisig PA, Ives HE, Cragoe EJ Jr, Alpern RJ, Rector FC Jr. Role of the Na+/H+ antiporter in rat proximal tubule bicarbonate absorption. J Clin Invest 1987; 80(4): 970-8.
[http://dx.doi.org/10.1172/JCI113190] [PMID: 2888788]

[6]   Kurtz I. Renal Tubular Acidosis: H$^+$/Base and Ammonia Transport Abnormalities and Clinical Syndromes. Adv Chronic Kidney Dis 2018; 25(4): 334-50.
[http://dx.doi.org/10.1053/j.ackd.2018.05.005] [PMID: 30139460]

[7]   Kaiser S, Curthoys NP. Effect of pH and bicarbonate on phosphoenolpyruvate carboxykinase and glutaminase mRNA levels in cultured renal epithelial cells. J Biol Chem 1991; 266(15): 9397-402.
[http://dx.doi.org/10.1016/S0021-9258(18)92832-2] [PMID: 1851745]

[8]   Caner T, Abdulnour-Nakhoul S, Brown K, Islam MT, Hamm LL, Nakhoul NL. Mechanisms of ammonia and ammonium transport by rhesus-associated glycoproteins. Am J Physiol Cell Physiol 2015; 309(11): C747-58.
[http://dx.doi.org/10.1152/ajpcell.00085.2015] [PMID: 26354748]

[9]   Wagner CA. Effect of mineralocorticoids on acid-base balance. Nephron, Physiol 2014; 128(1-2): 26-34.
[http://dx.doi.org/10.1159/000368266] [PMID: 25377117]

[10]   Lee HW, Osis G, Harris AN, *et al.* NBCe1-A Regulates Proximal Tubule Ammonia Metabolism under Basal Conditions and in Response to Metabolic Acidosis. J Am Soc Nephrol 2018; 29(4): 1182-97.
[http://dx.doi.org/10.1681/ASN.2017080935] [PMID: 29483156]

[11]   Brenes LG, Sánchez MI. Impaired urinary ammonium excretion in patients with isolated proximal renal tubular acidosis. J Am Soc Nephrol 1993; 4(4): 1073-8.
[http://dx.doi.org/10.1681/ASN.V441073] [PMID: 8286715]

[12]   Igarashi T, Sekine T, Inatomi J, Seki G. Unraveling the molecular pathogenesis of isolated proximal renal tubular acidosis. J Am Soc Nephrol 2002; 13(8): 2171-7.
[http://dx.doi.org/10.1097/01.ASN.0000025281.70901.30] [PMID: 12138151]

[13]   Brenes LG, Brenes JN, Hernández MM. Familial proximal renal tubular acidosis. Am J Med 1977; 63(2): 244-52.
[http://dx.doi.org/10.1016/0002-9343(77)90238-8] [PMID: 888846]

[14]   Katzir Z, Dinour D, Reznik-Wolf H, Nissenkorn A, Holtzman E. Familial pure proximal renal tubular acidosis--a clinical and genetic study. Nephrol Dial Transplant 2007; 23(4): 1211-5.
[http://dx.doi.org/10.1093/ndt/gfm583] [PMID: 17881426]

[15]   Gross P, Meye C. Proximal RTA: Are all the charts completed yet? Nephrol Dial Transplant 2007; 23(4): 1101-2.
[http://dx.doi.org/10.1093/ndt/gfm933] [PMID: 18223262]

[16]   Soleimani M, Rastegar A. Pathophysiology of Renal Tubular Acidosis: Core Curriculum 2016. Am J Kidney Dis 2016; 68(3): 488-98.
[http://dx.doi.org/10.1053/j.ajkd.2016.03.422] [PMID: 27188519]

[17]   Gómez-Conde S, García-Castaño A, Aguirre M, *et al.* Hereditary distal renal tubular acidosis: Genotypic correlation, evolution to long term, and new therapeutic perspectives. Nefrología (Engl Ed) 2021; 41(4): 383-90.
[http://dx.doi.org/10.1016/j.nefroe.2021.09.004] [PMID: 36165107]

[18]   Steinmetz PR, Lawson LR. Defect in urinary acidification induced in vitro by amphotericin B. J Clin Invest 1970; 49(3): 596-601.
[http://dx.doi.org/10.1172/JCI106270] [PMID: 5415685]

[19]   Batlle D, Arruda J. Hyperkalemic Forms of Renal Tubular Acidosis: Clinical and Pathophysiological Aspects. Adv Chronic Kidney Dis 2018; 25(4): 321-33.
[http://dx.doi.org/10.1053/j.ackd.2018.05.004] [PMID: 30139459]

[20]   Fuster DG, Moe OW. Incomplete distal renal tubular acidosis and kidney stones. Adv Chronic Kidney Dis 2018; 25(4): 366-74.
[http://dx.doi.org/10.1053/j.ackd.2018.05.007] [PMID: 30139463]

[21]   Palazzo V, Provenzano A, Becherucci F, *et al.* The genetic and clinical spectrum of a large cohort of patients with distal renal tubular acidosis. Kidney Int 2017; 91(5): 1243-55.
[http://dx.doi.org/10.1016/j.kint.2016.12.017] [PMID: 28233610]

[22]   Fawaz NA, Beshlawi IO, Al Zadjali S, *et al.* dRTA and hemolytic anemia: first detailed description of *SLC4A1* A858D mutation in homozygous state. Eur J Haematol 2012; 88(4): 350-5.
[http://dx.doi.org/10.1111/j.1600-0609.2011.01739.x] [PMID: 22126643]

[23]   Evan AP, Lingeman J, Coe F, *et al.* Renal histopathology of stone-forming patients with distal renal tubular acidosis. Kidney Int 2007; 71(8): 795-801.
[http://dx.doi.org/10.1038/sj.ki.5002113] [PMID: 17264873]

[24]   Goldstein MB, Bear R, Richardson RMA, Marsden PA, Halperin ML. The urine anion gap: a clinically useful index of ammonium excretion. Am J Med Sci 1986; 292(4): 198-202.
[http://dx.doi.org/10.1097/00000441-198610000-00003] [PMID: 3752165]

[25]   Kamel KS, Halperin ML. Use of urine electrolytes and urine osmolality in the clinical diagnosis of fluid, electrolytes, and acid-base disorders. Kidney Int Rep 2021; 6(5): 1211-24.
[http://dx.doi.org/10.1016/j.ekir.2021.02.003] [PMID: 34013099]

[26]   Yaxley J, Pirrone C. Review of the diagnostic evaluation of renal tubular acidosis. Ochsner J 2016; 16(4): 525-30.https://pmc.ncbi.nlm.nih.gov/articles/PMC5158160/
[PMID: 27999512]

[27]   Palmer BF, Kelepouris E, Clegg DJ. Renal tubular acidosis and management strategies: A narrative review. Adv Ther 2021; 38(2): 949-68.
[http://dx.doi.org/10.1007/s12325-020-01587-5] [PMID: 33367987]

[28]   Trepiccione F, Walsh SB, Ariceta G, *et al.* Distal renal tubular acidosis: ERKNet/ESPN clinical practice points. Nephrol Dial Transplant 2021; 36(9): 1585-96.
[http://dx.doi.org/10.1093/ndt/gfab171] [PMID: 33914889]

[29]   Pelletier J, Gbadegesin R, Staples B. Renal tubular acidosis. Pediatr Rev 2017; 38(11): 537-9.
[http://dx.doi.org/10.1542/pir.2016-0231] [PMID: 29093127]

[30]   Chaudhury A, Duvoor C, Reddy Dendi VS, *et al.* Clinical review of antidiabetic drugs: Implications for type 2 diabetes mellitus management. Front Endocrinol (Lausanne) 2017; 8: 6.
[http://dx.doi.org/10.3389/fendo.2017.00006] [PMID: 28167928]

[31]   Frías Ordoñez JS, Urrego Díaz JA, Lozano Triana CJ, *et al.* Distal renal tubular acidosis: case series report and literature review. Rev Colomb Nefrol 2020; 7(1): 97-112.
[http://dx.doi.org/10.22265/acnef.7.1.355]

CHAPTER 7

The Genetic Structure of Polycystic Kidney Disease (PKD)

Cristino Cruz[1], **Claudia J. Bautista**[2] and **Victoria Ramírez**[3,*]

[1] *Department of Nephrology, Instituto Nacional de Ciencias Médicas y Nutrición" Salvador Zubirán", Mexico City, Mexico*

[2] *Department of Reproduction Biology, Instituto Nacional de Ciencias Médicas y Nutrición" Salvador Zubirán", Mexico City, Mexico*

[3] *Department of Experimental Surgery, Instituto Nacional de Ciencias Médicas y Nutrición" Salvador Zubirán", Mexico City, Mexico*

Abstract: Polycystic kidney disease (PKD) is characterized by uncontrolled cellular proliferation, leading to fluid accumulation, extracellular matrix remodeling, and cyst formation with progressive kidney damage that leads to renal failure and death. Besides the kidney, other organs, such as the liver, the heart, and vasculature, are damaged.

Keywords: ADPKD, Autosomal dominant, Autosomal recessive, Heritage, Monogenic disease.

INTRODUCTION

Polycystic kidney disease (PKD) is a life-threatening disease with no cure or specific treatment. PKD is characterized by uncontrolled cellular proliferation, leading to fluid accumulation, extracellular matrix remodeling, and cyst formation with progressive kidney damage that leads to renal failure and death. However, in addition to the kidney, other organs, such as the liver, heart, and vasculature, are damaged [1 - 3].

PKD is a monogenic disease classified as heterogeneous. There are two known variants; the first is the most common and least severe variant present in adulthood, known as autosomal dominant polycystic disease (ADPKD). ADPKD is caused by mutations in the polycystin 1 (*PKD1* or *PC1*) and polycystin 2 (*PKD2* or *PC2*) genes. The second is autosomal recessive polycystic kidney disease (ARPKD), a rare and severe disease affecting people before birth or

---

[*] **Corresponding author Victoria Ramírez:** Department of Experimental Surgery, Instituto Nacional de Ciencias Médicas y Nutrición, Salvador Zubirán, Tlalpan 14080, Mexico City, Mexico; E-mail: victoria.ramirezg@incmnsz.mx.

Rafael Valdez-Ortiz, Katy Sánchez-Pozos, Ana Carolina Ariza & Enzo C. Vásquez-Jiménez (Eds.)

childhood. It results from mutations in the fibrocystin or polycystic kidney and liver disease (*PKHD1*) gene. Both disease variants will result in progressive renal function loss until the development of end-stage renal disease (ESRD), and some patients will need replacement therapy or transplantation to survive (Fig. **1**) [4 - 7].

Polycystic Kidney Disease (PKD)

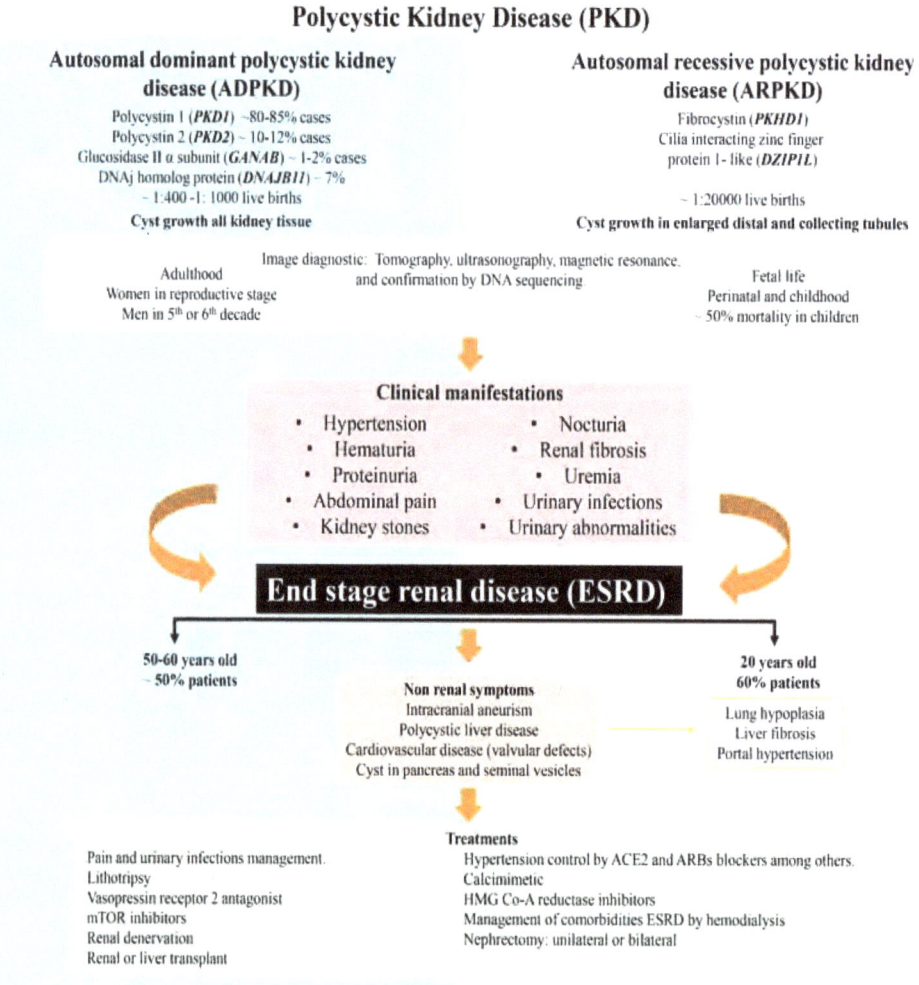

Autosomal dominant polycystic kidney disease (ADPKD)

Polycystin 1 (*PKD1*) ~80-85% cases
Polycystin 2 (*PKD2*) ~ 10-12% cases
Glucosidase II α subunit (*GANAB*) ~ 1-2% cases
DNAj homolog protein (*DNAJB11*) ~ 7%
~ 1:400 -1: 1000 live births
Cyst growth all kidney tissue

Autosomal recessive polycystic kidney disease (ARPKD)

Fibrocystin (*PKHD1*)
Cilia interacting zinc finger protein 1- like (*DZIP1L*)
~ 1:20000 live births
Cyst growth in enlarged distal and collecting tubules

Adulthood
Women in reproductive stage
Men in 5th or 6th decade

Image diagnostic: Tomography, ultrasonography, magnetic resonance. and confirmation by DNA sequencing

Fetal life
Perinatal and childhood
~ 50% mortality in children

Clinical manifestations

- Hypertension
- Hematuria
- Proteinuria
- Abdominal pain
- Kidney stones
- Nocturia
- Renal fibrosis
- Uremia
- Urinary infections
- Urinary abnormalities

End stage renal disease (ESRD)

50-60 years old
~ 50% patients

20 years old
60% patients

Non renal symptoms
Intracranial aneurism
Polycystic liver disease
Cardiovascular disease (valvular defects)
Cyst in pancreas and seminal vesicles

Lung hypoplasia
Liver fibrosis
Portal hypertension

Treatments

Pain and urinary infections management.
Lithotripsy
Vasopressin receptor 2 antagonist
mTOR inhibitors
Renal denervation
Renal or liver transplant

Hypertension control by ACE2 and ARBs blockers among others.
Calcimimetic
HMG Co-A reductase inhibitors
Management of comorbidities ESRD by hemodialysis
Nephrectomy: unilateral or bilateral

Fig. (1). Characteristics of polycystic kidney disease, gene mutations, prevalence, symptoms and treatments. (ACE2) Angiotensin converting enzyme, (ARBs) Angiotensin II receptor blockers, (mTOR) mammalian target of rapamycin.

Frequently, ADPKD patients present germline cell mutations in one allele in any *PKD1* or *PKD2* gene. Consequently, somatic inactivation of the remaining wild-type alleles or loss of heterozygosity can initiate cyst formation. Loss-of-function mutations or truncating mutations determine the phenotypic variability of the disease. Many authors conclude that PKD severity depends directly on the type of mutation present or PKD genes' expression and remaining activity. Patients with truncating *PKD1* mutations develop ESRD faster than those without truncating mutations. Fewer severe cases are diagnosed after 60 years old. Although *PKD2* mutations are related to mild disease progression [8], *PKD1* and *PKD2* inactivating mutations are embryonically lethal. The variety of mutations will generate a different degree of disease or mosaicism, even in the same family members; some of them will have fast cyst growth and loss of renal function, and others will have slow progression with mild or imperceptible symptoms; also, age and hormones may have an essential role in ADPKD disease progression [5, 9, 10].

EPIDEMIOLOGY

The prevalence of PKD is controversial due to the lack of a standard criterion of ascertainment or symptoms; it may vary according to geographical location and ethnicity.

ADPKD

It has been estimated that ADPKD affects 1:400 to 1:1,000 live births [11 - 14]. In 2015, the National Ambulatory Medical Care Survey (NAMCS) in the USA described 170 million registered patients, with a prevalence of 4.3 per 100,000 people. The annual incidence was 0.62 per 10,000 people in the USA. Females were diagnosed early in the reproductive period. Men were diagnosed with comorbidities or complications at 65 years of age [15, 16]. Similar results were found in the European population; a meta-analysis of eight European studies revealed that the prevalence of ADPKD was 2.63:10,000 people; however, in Modena, Italy, the incidence was more than 4.6 per 10,000 people [17]. Comparable results were found in French and Japanese populations [5]. Systematic sequencing of publicly available databases, such as gnomAD and BRAVO, which include all ethnic groups, has shown that the prevalence is greater than the estimated 9.3 cases per 10,000 sequenced individuals; additionally, several new truncate mutations that could be a cyst modifier with clinical importance have been found [12]. In 2020, Suwabe T. *et al.* reported in a retrospective cohort that included data from 1980–2016 that the incidence of ADPKD was 2.2 times greater than that previously reported in the first five decades, which was 3.06 per 100,000 persons per year in Minnesota, USA [18]. As we mentioned before, ADPKD is caused by *PKD1* and *PKD2* mutations; 85% of ADPKD cases are caused by *PKD1* gene truncations (short amino or carboxyl ends), while 15% are caused by *PKD2* mutations [19]. The incidence of ADPKD in children is unknown; however, a Turkish study reported an early diagnosis of ADPKD in children younger than ten years of age. Due to positive family history, the results showed low cyst formation and well-preserved renal function, with close follow-up. Genetic analysis revealed that most cases were due to *PKD1* gene mutations [20].

Patients present with cyst formation in the kidney, liver, spleen, or pancreas; these cysts are more frequently found in adults than children. The majority of ADPKD patients have hypertension, hematuria, proteinuria, cardiovascular diseases, kidney stones, intracranial aneurysms, vascular defects, flank pain, and loss of renal function [17, 21]. It is worth noting that the ADPKD population will progress to ESRD. In 2018, Bergmann C reported that approximately 5-10% of ESRD patients have ADPKD [4, 5, 22]. European epidemiologic data show that the incidence of ESRD in ADPKD patients who need RRT (renal replacement therapy or transplant) increased from 7.6% to 8.3% per million people from 1991–2001 [23]. It is essential to highlight that females are diagnosed earlier than males are, and the number of patients with ESRD increases with age [18]. Approximately 25% of ADPKD patients with ESRD are middle-aged (approximately 45 years old); these figures increase to 40-50% at 60 years of age and even more so in the elderly population, where almost 75% of ADPKD patients are in ESRD [1, 9, 18, 24]. Consequently, ADPKD is the fourth leading cause of ESKD in adult patients [16]. The estimated Medicare cost for the treatment of ESRD in ADPKD patients exceeds $200 million per year, according to a 1994 report [25].

Extrarenal manifestations of ADPKD are hepatic cysts in 90% of patients older than 35 years, and nearly 20% are symptomatic and can cause pain, esophageal reflux, portal hypertension, and, rarely, ascites and pleural effusion. Nearly 12% of these patients develop intracranial aneurysms. The risk of death due to aneurysm rupture is four times greater than that of the average population [10].

ARPKD

The prevalence of ARPKD is even more complex to estimate, and this disease can occur at perinatal age or in childhood. ARPKD is considered the leading cause of morbidity and mortality in neonates and children and has a high mortality rate in young people [26]. It is estimated that it occurs in 1:20,000 to 1:40,000 live births around the globe, with a high frequency of 1:70, affecting all ethnicities [4, 5, 22]. In Finland, the general incidence is 1:8,000 [27, 28], while the prevalence in children is 1:100,000. ARPKD is characterized by early nonobstructive cyst formation in collecting ducts; it can be unilateral or bilateral. The mortality rate is

30-40% due to pulmonary tissue, hyperplasia and oligohydramnios, and hyponatremia, urinary concentration, and Potter facies defects can also be found; it is important to mention that cystic liver disease is always present [29]. Liver complications are more frequently identified in patients first [26]. The survival rate of children after they are ten years old is nearly 82%; however, it has been estimated that nearly 50% of surviving infants with ARPKD will develop ESRD in the second decade of life, and these infants will need RRT earlier than the ADPKD population [22, 29, 30].

Reported Mutations

The ADPKD mutation database revealed at least 2323 mutations in the PKD1 gene, 1273 of which were highly pathogenic; unfortunately, half of these mutations have not been characterized. For the *PKD2* gene, 278 mutations have been described, 202 related to disease development [31, 32]. Finally, *PKHD1* is one of the largest genes and is poorly studied; however, 522 mutations have been reported in the human gene database, among others [33, 34], and almost all of them have a potentially poor prognosis [35].

GENETICS OF PKD DISEASE

As mentioned, ADPKD results from mutations in the *PKD1* and *PKD2* genes.

PKD1

PKD1 or *PC1*, known as polycystin 1, is an 11-transmembrane glycoprotein located primarily in cilia, although there is evidence of lateral membrane, thigh junction, and desmosome mechanosensors. It is located on human chromosome 16p13.3 and is encoded by a 53 kb gene that contains 46 exons, generating a 4303 amino acid protein with a molecular weight of 462 kDa [36, 37]. The presence of at least six pseudogenes with a high homology of 97.7% complicates its study [32]. The protein contains several domains that facilitate interactions for proper trafficking and cell adhesion, such as leucine-rich repeat (LRR), cysteine-rich domain (WSC), lectin type c (C-lectin), low-density lipoprotein receptor class A repeat (LDL-A), PKD, G-coupled receptor (GPCR), and autoproteolysis-inducing domain (GAIN), all of which are essential for PKD1 trafficking. The G protein-binding domain (polycystin, lipoxygenase, and toxin alpha domain, called PLAT) is involved in lipid binding [19, 36 - 38]. PKD1 dimerizes with PKD2 to act as a Ca^{2+} channel, and it has recently been shown that PKD1 could be involved in contractile regulation in cardiomyocytes and is also related to mitochondrial homeostasis [39]. Another function of PKD1 that has been described in recent years is its role as a tumor suppressor in several types of cancer [40].

PKD2

PKD2 or *PC2* is found on the apical and basolateral plasma membrane of the endoplasmic reticulum, Golgi shafts, and cilia of epithelial cells and urinary exosomes [25]. Polycystin 2 is located at chromosome 4q21, is a 15-exon gene with an open reading frame of 2,907 bp, and encodes a 968 amino acid protein. It is significantly smaller than PKD1; the estimated molecular weight is 110 kDa [41, 42]. PKD2 is a six-transmembrane region protein with a long intracellular NH_2 and short COOH termini. The carboxyl end also contains a coil-coil domain for dimerization, with PKD1 functioning as an ion channel. It has been characterized as a Ca^{2+}-responsive cation channel and an indirect regulator of cytoplasmic calcium; this protein is dependent on two intracellular Ca^{2+} channels, the inositol 1,4,5-triphosphate receptor (IP3R) and the ryanodine receptor, and is also considered a mechanosensor [10, 43, 44].

PKHD1

PKHD1, also known as fibrocystin or polyductin, is located mainly in the cilia of epithelial cells and is among the largest human genes. It was mapped to chromosome 6p21.1-p12, with a length of 470 kb and comprising 67 exons. The protein has 4074 amino acids and has a molecular weight of 447 kDa. It is classified as a long-type I transmembrane protein with a single transmembrane region, and it contains a large extracellular NH_2 domain that is highly glycosylated. Additionally, it contains multiple Ig-like, plexin transcription factor (IPT), and IPT-like regions and a short COOH terminal tail that has several potential phosphorylation sites for PKA and a ciliary targeting sequence (CTS) that controls cilia trafficking [42, 45, 46]. Fibrocystin colocalizes with the PKD1 and PKD2 proteins, and its primary function is as a mechanosensor; it also participates in microtubule organization and mediates cell-cell adhesion, proliferation, and differentiation of the renal collecting ducts [22, 42, 46, 47].

New Genes involved in PKD

In recent years, more genes related to PKD disease development have been identified, some of which were included in the two available classifications. In contrast, others describe PKD-like genes that are not described here.

GANAB is a subunit of glucosidase II, a protein belonging to the endoplasmic reticule family and involved in protein processing and folding. Mutations in *GANAB* are associated with poor maturation and localization of PKD1 [5, 10, 48, 49] and have been classified as part of the ADPKD phenotype due to their relationship with cyst formation but less severe disease development. Its prevalence is only 1-2% of ADPKD cases, and the complete pathogenic mechanism is not fully known [50].

DNAJB11 is a glycoprotein of the endoplasmic reticule (ER), which is a cochaperone of Gpr78. *DNAJB11*, as well as *GANAB*, are included in the ADPKD genotype. Both are involved in the processing, folding, and trafficking of proteins in the ER. Mutations in this gene were described in almost 7% of ADPKD patients; they were missense variants that induced microcyst formation, and all patients carrying this mutation had mild symptoms of ADPKD and developed ESRD in the sixth decade with interstitial fibrosis. The mechanism of the disease is related to improper trafficking of PKD1 [48, 49].

Finally, mutations in DAZ interacting zinc finger protein 1-like (*DZIP1L*) have recently been shown to be involved in the development of ARPKD, although the incidence is very low. The clinical manifestation was found prenatally or during early childhood; those patients developed both kidney and liver polycystic disease with moderate symptoms and progression [10, 48]. The described DZIP1L functions to maintain the cilia diffusion barrier and maintain PKD1 stability and trafficking; however, the complete mechanism or interactors are not yet known [22, 27].

PATHOPHYSIOLOGY

The pathophysiology of PKD is described by the development and progressive enlargement of renal cysts, which typically leads to chronic renal failure in middle age [46, 51].

Common clinical and pathological manifestations of ADPKD include abnormal cell proliferation and apoptosis, cell polarity, dedifferentiation disturbance, enhanced transepithelial fluid secretion, extracellular matrix remodeling, and the development of interstitial fibrosis [51, 52]. Progressive loss of kidney function occurs over many decades and frequently leads to ESRD during or after the sixth decade of life; however, it occurs after a stable period due to compensatory hyperfiltration, while other anatomical and molecular changes occur. Once glomerular filtration decreases, progression can occur quickly; total kidney volume (TKV) is considered a potential marker of progression of renal disease unless some patients with large kidney cysts have preserved renal function [53, 54]. The progression of ESRD is faster in the Caucasian population than in the Asian population [55].

Due to cyst formation, pain is frequently reported by ADPKD patients; enlarged kidneys induce organ compression and increase pain, and vomiting can also occur in those patients; in fact, the total kidney volume is considered a risk factor for

PKD progression [49]. One of the most common symptoms of ADPKD and ARPKD is elevated blood pressure. Hypertension develops before renal damage occurs; this will contribute to renal damage and increase the risk of cardiovascular complications, such as cardiovascular hypertrophy and increased albumin excretion. In addition, hypertension in PKD patients is associated with activation of the renin-angiotensin-aldosterone system (RAAS) [53, 56]. Elevated plasma angiotensin II triggers a wide signaling cascade, vascular remodeling, proliferation, hypertrophy, and renal vasoconstriction. Vasoconstriction induces renal ischemia, which induces inflammation, oxidative stress, and apoptosis, damaging renal tissue and accelerating renal failure [57]. Additionally, aldosterone promotes Na^+ conservation through the regulation of $Na^+ K^+$ ATPase, the epithelial sodium channel (ENaC), and the sodium chloride cotransporter (NCC), contributing to fluid accumulation and urinary concentration [53, 57]. RAAS also increases the expression of transcription factors such as endothelial growth factor (EGF), endothelin 1, protein kinase A (PKA), protein kinase C (PKC), and mitogen-activated protein kinases (MAPKs), which participate in proliferation and cyst formation [57, 58].

Another component of PKD physiopathology is repeated genital-urinary infections; these infections are more frequent in this population than in the general population. The proposed mechanism is cyst fluid accumulation, and the most common bacterial strains are *E. coli* and *S. aureus* [58]. Kidney stones are one of the most significant complications in PKD patients; it was estimated that 20-40% of these patients present with pain and hematuria due to kidney stones. Hematuria is caused by a cyst, vascular rupture, or stone movement through renal tissue [59]. Urinary abnormalities are the leading cause of ADPKD; people present low urinary volume, low pH, low ammonia excretion, low magnesium concentration, phosphate, potassium, hypocitraturia, hyperuricosuria, and hyperoxaluria; in this way, the lithos are composed of uric acid and oxalates [60]. Some individuals also reported nocturia and polyuria. It has been reported that magnesium and citrate are known crystallization stone inhibitors; moreover, low citrate is a risk factor for increased oxalate and uric acid deposition [61].

As we mentioned before, ADPKD patients present changes in urine composition; several studies have shown that vasopressin or antidiuretic hormone plays a fundamental role in the progression of renal diseases such as diabetic nephropathy or PKD. Clinical trials have shown that ADPKD patients exhibit impaired urine concentration and that urinary osmolality is lower in the ADPKD cohort than in the control population, with similar renal function in both groups. Additionally, the plasma levels of vasopressin were greater in ADPKD patients. Plasma sodium did not change; however, ADPKD patients had a 40% increase in plasma urea concentration, a risk factor for developing kidney stones or ESRD [62, 63].

Antidiuretic hormone or vasopressin is responsible for regulating fluid homeostasis. It is secreted after an osmotic stimulus, signaling through the V2 receptor that induces water and sodium reabsorption in the loop of Henle and the distal nephron by regulating aquaporin two and ENaC. As mentioned before, ADPKD patients have increased cAMP and vasopressin levels, which are factors associated with cytogenesis [64]. Recently, treatment with a selective inhibitor of the vasopressin V2 receptor tolvaptan has been associated with slow PKD progression [55, 60, 65, 66].

In addition to the direct signs of kidney growth and a reduced glomerular filtration rate, affected individuals might exhibit extrarenal manifestations, including hepatic and pancreatic cysts, colonic diverticulosis, intracranial aneurysms, abdominal hernias, cardiac valvular lesions, and endothelial dysfunction. Other possible complications related to chronic kidney disease development are anemia, secondary hyperparathyroidism, metabolic bone disorders, tubule interstitial fibrosis undernutrition, lipid abnormalities, and cardiovascular complications. Additionally, patients with ADPKD have an increased risk of developing cancer [10, 48, 52, 67]. The mechanisms of PKD are still not entirely known; however, below, we will describe some evidence found in animal and clinical trials.

Molecular Mechanisms

Polycystins have been described in the epithelial and endothelial renal cell cilia; they are expressed in embryogenesis and the adult kidney. The known normal function of both proteins is to form a tetrameric complex through the interaction of the coil-coil domain at the COOH end, with a stoichiometry of one molecule of PKD1 and three molecules of PKD2 to regulate Ca^{2+} influx [36]. The binding domain at the COOH end is the site of multiple interactors, such as tuberin, a regulator of mammalian target of rapamycin (mTOR) signaling that activates proliferation and cell cycle progression [25].

In cilia, polycystins are mechanosensors of shear stress and cytoskeleton signaling [38, 42]. Further studies demonstrated that the interaction between PKD1 and PKD2 is essential for the maturation and stability of PKD1 in epithelial cells [10]. However, it was also proven that PKD2 could work independently as a calcium channel [38]. Recently, in *PKD2* knockout mice, amino acid biosynthesis was reprogrammed by defective ER signaling through the protein kinase R-like eukaryotic initiator factor 2α-activating transcription 4 (PERK–eIF2α–ATF4) pathway, and the biosynthesis of serine, arginine, and cysteine was significantly reduced [68]. The complete functions and interactions of PKD1, PKD2, and PKHD1 remain unknown; however, it is well known that the lack of PKD genes is directly related to cytogenesis growth activating several signaling pathways, making their study complex [5].

Partial loss of *PKD1* and *PKD2*, or abnormal cilia function, can reduce intracellular Ca^{2+} levels, activating adenylyl cyclase and reducing phosphodiesterase I activity, leading to an increase in cAMP, which activates proliferation in renal collecting and distal tubules and promotes fluid accumulation. This affects tubular cells that proliferate continuously and results in increased cell numbers, tubular dilatation and growth of cysts into the interstice [10, 69, 70]. The direct consequence is renal parenchyma damage. Some authors believe that injured tubules and expanding cysts release inflammatory cytokines, causing fibrosis and eventual progression to ESRD [69]. Cyst growth could be due to the increase in cAMP, which induces the activation of extracellular signal-regulated kinase (ERK), leading to the activation of transcription factors such as EGF and the presence of TGFα that promote epithelial proliferation. Additionally, it has been observed that prostaglandin E_2 (PGE2) stimulates cAMP production and cyst growth [1, 71]. The hippo signaling cascade is also involved in ADPKD progression and is related to size, organ control, differentiation, and regeneration. Yes-associated protein 1/transcriptional coactivator with PDZ domain (YAP/TAZ) and proto-oncogene (cMYC) members of this cascade were upregulated in PKD1 knockout mice. With increased catenin activity, inhibition of TAZ delayed cyst growth, showing that Wnt signaling contributes to PKD pathogenesis [72]. Fluid accumulation plays a fundamental role in disease progression, and several transport proteins, such as cystic fibrosis transmembrane conductance regulator (CFTR) and calcium-activated potassium channel (KCa3.1), which are regulated by cAMP, are altered in ADPKD patients. Unmeasured proliferation leads to the accumulation of collagen, metalloproteases, integrins, catenin, and inflammatory molecules, among others [1].

Animal models and clinical trials are intended to identify common pathogenic mechanisms, elucidate specific targets, and identify new therapeutic agents that reduce disease progression and comorbidities. Recently, a meta-analysis of profile expression revealed that 92 transcription factors were differentially regulated in ADPKD patients, some of which involved TGFβ and estrogen modulation, apoptosis, oxidative stress, inflammation, adipogenesis, and cellular metabolism. Thirty-two were related to injury repair mechanisms, with more significant changes in STAT3 and RUNX1 molecular signaling, which are pathways involved in the cellular repair process [73].

Activation of the Janus kinase and signal transcription activator (JAK/STAT) pathway is upregulated in ADPKD disease; its activation induces epithelial cell proliferation and increases cytogenesis. In a murine model of ADPKD, an increase in STAT3 phosphorylation followed by a significant increase in JAK2 in the cyst lining was found; the authors showed that the inhibition of JAK2 with antioxidants such as curcumin or tofacitinib prevented these increases; these effects were associated with reduced cyst growth in mice as well as humans [74]. One of the mechanisms underlying the development of ADPKD in the early stages is the presence of oxidative stress. In a knockout mouse and human cell line of ADPKD patients, miR132-3p was upregulated; this increase was related to the inhibition of the transcription factor forkhead box protein O 3 (FOXO3) and decreased mitochondrial expression of glycine amidinotransferase (GATM), leading to an increase in reactive oxygen species (ROS). These effects are directly related to cyst formation [75]. Additionally, mitochondrial impairment is present in ADPKD; it was observed that PKD deficiency induces changes in energy production in mitochondria via AMPK inhibition. The inhibition of aerobic glycolysis reduces cyst growth, and fatty acid oxidation is impaired by PKD1 loss [76].

The presence of fibrosis is controversial in PKD, and fibrosis is due to an increase in extracellular matrix protein (ECM) deposition, leading to an increase in inflammatory markers and tissue damage. In ADPKD, cysts can be reversed by fibrosis; however, multiple studies have shown the presence of macrophages and myofibroblasts in ADPKD models, which leads to ECM accumulation and the inhibition of metalloproteases conducive to fibrosis. Hypoxia in ADPKD can increase the ECM mediated by TGFβ, bone morphogenetic proteins, and SMAD 2/3 proteins, activating the JAK/STAT pathway, which is important in mediating cyst growth [23, 77].

Epigenetic studies have shown that kidneys from patients with ADPKD have slight hypomethylation in the whole genome compared with those from patients without ADPKD [78]; also, when the *PKD1* promoter was analyzed, the authors observed decreased methylation in ADPKD patients compared with that in subjects without ADPKD [79]. In contrast, the *PKD1* gene from ADPKD patients presented highly methylated regions and was significantly different from that of non-ADPKD patients; this effect was directly correlated with higher mRNA levels of *PKD1* [78]. In cilia, histone deacetylases are involved in ciliary dissembling; specifically, histone deacetylase 6 (HDAC6) is upregulated in PKD cells, and the inhibition of HDAC6 in *PKD1* cell culture and knockout mice is related to reduced cyst growth and proliferation. The proposed mechanism involves reducing cAMP levels, CTF, and proliferation inhibition [80]. All these findings revealed the role of epigenetic regulation in ADPKD.

DIAGNOSIS

Ultrasonography is the preferred initial approach for diagnosing PKD because of its widespread availability, low cost, and noninvasiveness. Ultrasound has traditionally been limited to detecting cysts of 10 mm or greater in diameter; however, high-definition ultrasound in the hands of skilled operators can detect cysts as small as 2–3 mm across. T2-weighted magnetic resonance imaging (MRI) or computed tomography (CT) with contrast readily detects 2–3 mm diameter cysts. Thus, MRI can be beneficial in evaluating younger individuals at risk of disease because more than ten kidney cysts detected by MRI are sufficient to diagnose ADPKD with a specificity and sensitivity of 100%. Additionally, these procedures help determine the TKV adequately [48, 81]. In patients with an adverse family history, genetic testing should be considered to confirm the diagnosis of ADPKD.

The number of cortical and medullary cysts increased with age; the 97.5th percentile for cortical and medullary cysts greater than 5 mm was ten for men and four for women in the 60–69 years age group, whereas, in the 18–39 years age group, the 97.5th percentile was one to two for both men and women. Therefore, the presence of a few cysts should not lead to the exclusion of potential donors, and genetic testing or heavy T2-weighted MRI could be performed to clarify the status of the relatives considering donation [48, 54].

The current research demonstrates a new diagnostic test for PKD in humans; clinical whole-genome sequencing can overcome pseudogene homology and identify all types of variants in the *PKD1* gene and has proven to be sensitive and specific for meeting the specifications for a diagnostic test. Importantly, it enables the analysis of multiple genes associated with PKD [82, 83]. Several authors have shown that mutation screening of *PKD1* is arduous due to its size and complexity, making it both expensive and labor-intensive. Therefore, conventional Sanger sequencing-based genetic testing is limited in elucidating the causes of atypical polycystic kidney disease, such as within-family disease, atypical kidney imaging patterns, and discordant disease severity between the TKV and estimated glomerular filtration rate (eGFR) [83]. Nonetheless, approximately 85% of PKD mutations are detected by direct sequencing [84, 85]

Many research groups are interested in elucidating PKD's diagnosis, physiopathology, and symptomatology. Genetic history, environmental factors, family conditions, genetic modifiers, and somatic mosaicism contribute to disease variability. In this way, Jennifer Q.J. Zhang and collaborators showed that the DNA damage response (DDR) and signaling markers are increased in human and experimental ADPKD; these studies concluded that the constitutive expression of the DDR pathway in ADPKD may promote the survival of *PKD1*-mutated cells and contribute to kidney cyst growth [86]. In mice, Chao Zhang *et al.* showed the dysregulation of Cdk1, an early driver of cyst cell proliferation in ADPKD due to *PKD1* inactivation. Selective targeting of cyst cell proliferation could effectively slow ADPKD progression caused by the inactivation of *PKD1* [86].

CURRENT NOVEL STUDIES AND TREATMENT

As we mentioned before, PKD is a very complex disease with no cure. Health professionals focus on managing diverse symptoms to reduce disease progression and improve the quality of life of these patients. Investigators have made efforts to find therapies that may help reduce symptoms. Table **1** shows proposed treatments in experimental animals and human clinical trials to reduce ADPKD symptoms and progression.

Table 1. Treatments used in ADPKD. (TKV) total kidney volume, (GFR) Glomerular filtration rate, (PTH) Parathyroid hormone.

Study	Treatment	Model	Effects	Uses
Radadiya PS, *et al* [98]	Ciclopirox olamine (Cpx). Inhibits cell cycle progression	*PKD1*RC/RC *PKD2*$^{+/-}$ mice. Moderate cystic progression from birth until 6 weeks. Administration of CPX-O IP (10 mg/kg) from 21-49 postnatal day	Inhibited in vitro cytogenesis in human PKD culture cells. Decreased cell proliferation cyst area in *PKD2*$^{+/-}$ mice Improved GFR and ferritin levels in *PKD2*$^{+/-}$ mice Reduction of TKV	Research use
Radadiya PS, *et al* [99]	Quinomycin A Antibiotic with anti-neoplasia activity	*PKD1*$^{RC/RC}$; *PKD2*$^{+/-}$ mice with moderate cyst progression since birth. Mice of 21 days were treated with 10 µg/kg of Quinomycin for 27 days.	Decreased kidney weight Reduced renal cystic area and fibrosis. Reduced proliferation markers. Reduction of transdifferentiation markers Increased apoptosis index Normalization of cilia length	Research use

(Table 1) cont.....

Study	Treatment	Model	Effects	Uses
Sorohan BM, *et al.* [100]	Metformin. Gluconeogenesis inhibitor	ADPKD patients 18-60 years ESRD 1-5 Metformin 500mg/day 2 1 month, 1000mg/day Follow up 24 months	No changes in GFR, No presence of lactic acidosis No changes in body mass index Well tolerability, low side effects	Clinical use, No effects in advanced ADPKD
Heidi J, *et al* [101]	Tolvaptan Vasopressin receptor V2 inhibitor	A prospective and observational study included 31 ADPKD patients with a mean age of 42 ± 8.3 years and eGFR (33–51) ml/min/1.73 m². Tolvaptan administration 3:4 ratio 45mg morning/15 mg night 1 month Upgraded to 60/30 mg another month final dose 90/30 mg for one month	Polyuria Increase in plasma osmolality Metabolic alkalosis Increase of Na^+ and Cl^- in plasma Slight fall in GFR Increase HCO_3^- reabsorption	Clinical use
Priyanka S. Raina R, *et al.* [26]	Tolvaptan Vasopressin receptor V2 inhibitor	Post hoc double-blinded study including 51 Adolescents with ADPKD between 18–24 age Tolvaptan: 29, placebo: 22. Tolvaptan doses 45 mg morning/15 mg night 1 month Upgraded to 60/30 mg another month final dose 90/30 mg for one month 3 years follow up	tolvaptan targets the arginine vasopressin receptor AVP V2R leading to decreased cAMP production and inhibition of cell proliferation and cyst growth in ADPKD Lower TKV growth per year compared to the placebo group (3.9% vs. 6.5%, P = 0.0491) No changes in GFR No changes in liver damage marker No signs of hepatic toxicity	Clinical use
Nakatani S, *et al.* [92]	Cinacalcet. Calcium sensing receptor agonist	12 hemodialysis patients ADPKD patients with end-stage renal disease hemodialysis 7 Cinacalcet 5 placebo No dose reported 1 year follow up	TKV was reduced significantly compared to the placebo group at a rate of nearly 5% yearly. Decrease of intact PTH Decrease in Ca^{2+} and PO_4^-	Clinical use

(Table 1) cont.....

Study	Treatment	Model	Effects	Uses
Blazer BL, *et al.* [91]	Pioglitazone Agonist of peroxisome proliferator-activated receptor -γ	Patients with CKD stages 3b to 5, based on two or more estimated glomerular ☐filtration rate measurements less than 45 mL/min/1.73 m ^{2}, aged 40 years or older were identi☐ed. Double-blind –placebo crossover study 15 ADPKD patients were administered with 15 mg/day of pioglitazone for one year, two weeks of washout, and change the medication	Decrease of total body water determined by bioimpedance. No changes in TKV, No changes in Cyst growth	Clinical use. No effects in ADPKD
Serra A, *et al.* [102]	Sirolimus Mammalian target for rapamycin (mTOR) inhibitor	Open opopeen Open-label controlled trial 50 ADPKD patients 18-40 years old GFR > 70 ml/min Sirolimus 2 mg/day 18 months of follow up	No changes in TKV No changes in GFR Increase in albumin excretion	Clinical use. No effects in early ADPKD
Klawitter J, *et al.* [103]	Pravastatin HMG Co-A reductase inhibitor	Ch Children and young adults with ADPKD GFR>80ml/min 8-12 years: 20 mg pravastatin 13-23 years 40 mg pravastatin 3 years	Reduction of cyclooxygenase- and lipoxygenase in plasma	Clinical use. No effect on ADPKD

One of the main symptoms of PKD is pain; almost 60% of ADPKD patients experience costal or abdominal pain due to kidney enlargement, transient cyst rupture, and the presence of kidney infections, kidney stones, or the compression of adjacent organs. Pain can be treated with drugs; however, in severe cases, surgery, including nerve blockade and kidney denervation, is the last option. In nonsevere cases, cyst aspiration may be performed; in ARPKD patients, children, or young adults, nephrectomy could be an option; however, the risk of complications might be high, and surgical procedures involve renal transplantation [87, 88].

Blood pressure control has been demonstrated to be a critical factor in reducing albumin excretion and cardiovascular complications and slowing the progression of ESRD in PKD patients. The use of antihypertensives such as angiotensin-converting enzyme 2 (ACE2) inhibitors (enalapril ramipril or lisinopril) and angiotensin II receptor blockers (ARBs) has been successful in controlling blood pressure and delaying chronic disease in these populations [57]. Using lisinopril and telmisartan in stage 3 ADPKD patients with kidney disease results in the same blood pressure control and reduction in aldosterone; nonetheless, combining both therapies did not result in any additional improvement [89]. ACE or ARBs have also been associated with a reduction in albumin excretion and a decreased risk of developing cardiovascular complications without affecting the GFR or total kidney volume [90].

Moreover, different treatments are used to prevent the progression of human PKD; for example, small-dose thiazolidinediones, such as pioglitazone, effectively decrease cyst growth in experimental models [91]. In addition, an allosteric modulator of the calcium-sensing receptor decreases cAMP, an essential factor for kidney enlargement. In one study, 12 hemodialysis ADPKD patients were included. The activation of calcium-sensing receptors suppressed kidney enlargement, and the results showed that cinacalcet significantly reduced the annual rate of increase in TKV after treatment from $3.26 \pm 2.8\%$ before cinacalcet to $-4.71 \pm 6.42\%$ after 2.5 years of treatment initiation. Therefore, cinacalcet could be a novel therapeutic tool for suppressing kidney injury progression in ADPKD patients [92]. One of the known theories in ADPKD disease progression could be reduced cytosolic calcium levels with increased cAMP concentrations. In a study performed in *PKD1* knockdown epithelial cells from ADPKD patients, the intracellular calcium concentration was significantly lower than that in wild-type cells; furthermore, the authors added the calcimimetic NPS-R568 to monitor a significant decrease in cAMP levels and mTOR activity in these cells, suggesting that the activation of calcium sensors could be a key factor in ADPKD treatment and that the use of calcimimetic agents could be a therapeutic alternative [93].

At the same time, somatostatin analogs also decrease cyst growth in the kidney or liver during PKD. Somatostatin is an endogenous peptide that has endocrine and paracrine effects. Its signaling occurs through five known receptors, and its inhibition reduces cAMP levels by reducing adenylyl cyclase activity [94]; moreover, it has recently been shown to improve polycystic liver disease by reducing cell proliferation. Clinical trials investigating ALADIN and ALADIN2 in ADPKD patients in which octreotide, lanreotide, and pasireotide were administered significantly reduced cell proliferation [94, 95]. In ADPKD patients in the last stages of ESRD, octreotide reduced TKV after one and three years of follow-up; the GFR did not change [94]. Similar results were observed with pasireotide, another somatostatin analog, which slightly reduced the yearly total kidney or liver volume in ADPKD patients compared with that in non-ADPKD patients without affecting the yearly eGFR, albumin excretion or blood pressure. Unfortunately, the main secondary effect was that 79% of the pasireotide group had a significant increase in glucose and AC1 levels after one year of treatment [96]; finally, a meta-analysis showed that the main effect of somatostatin analogs is on liver disease, with no therapeutic improvement in polycystic kidneys, and the presence of adverse events such as diabetes limits their use [97].

As we mentioned, no treatment prevents PDK development or progression; however, due to high cAMP production in ADPKD patients and the presence of G protein-binding domain sites in polycystins, G proteins have recently received much attention [104, 105]. Knockout of adenylate cyclase in ADPKD rats reduces cytogenesis, revealing the importance of G proteins and their coupled receptors in PKD physiopathology [106]. GPRS belongs to the largest receptor protein family, with more than 100 members, one-third of which are used as therapeutic drugs for some GPRs [105], and PKD is not the exception; some medications used to treat it are GPRs, such as vasopressin V2 or somatostatin receptors. Recent studies have shown that the V2 receptor antagonists mozavaptan and tolvaptan reduce the progression of PKD in experimental models [84, 107]. The same results were observed with satavaptan, which induced the downregulation of frizzled-related protein 4, a protein involved in the cytogenesis of zebrafish pro-nephrons [108].

Recently, vasopressin V2 receptor antagonists have been approved for treating ADPKD in several countries [104]. The TEMPO 3:4, TEMPO 4:4, and REPRISE trials have proven that tolvaptan inhibits cell proliferation, electrolyte misbalance, and cyst growth [109 - 111]. In a study by Vicente Torres et al., ADPKD patients with high TKV were included. Patients were administered tolvaptan at different rates. The maximum tolerated dose was 3:2 daily in the morning and afternoon (90-30 mg) for 36 months. After three years, the annual increase in TKV was 2.8% in the tolvaptan group compared with 5.5% in the placebo group, with a decrease in the rate of kidney function loss of 2% vs. 5% per year, respectively, and a reduction in kidney pain of 5% vs. 7% each year. Tolvaptan reduced the rate of kidney disease after three years; however, side effects such as thirst, polyuria, nocturia, and high drug detachment were observed [109]. Studies using *in vitro* and *in vivo* models have shown that tolvaptan diminishes kidney proliferation and decreases the eGFR in all stages of kidney disease [109, 110]. Tolvaptan seems to be well tolerated; however, the authors suggest close monitoring to prevent toxicity and failure of the liver [112].

Some clinical trials are ongoing to test new analog drugs or drug combinations that might slow or reduce PKD progression, such as V2 receptor and somatostatin analogs, metformin, kinase inhibitors, and vitamin supplementation [10, 112]. Additionally, adequate diet management is essential for reducing or controlling the leading symptoms and complications of PKD and improving the welfare of PKD patients.

Finally, the last option for all patients with high total kidney volume, persistent urinary infections, intractable pain, cyst rupture, and repeated stone formation is nephrectomy, which could be possible by choice or urgency. Clinicians suggest unilateral or bilateral nephrectomy for patients with TKVs less than 1.5 kg, and laparoscopic surgery is the option because larger cysts are more favorable for open surgery. Laparotomy and laparoscopy have been shown to have similar risks associated with excessive bleeding and infection [113]. These procedures are more commonly used in children with ARPKD. It is frequently performed in the first years of life; therefore, many patients will need replacement therapy, such as hemodialysis or renal transplant [26]. Adults with stage 5 ADPKD renal disease have undergone nephrectomy simultaneously with kidney or liver transplant; however, the risks increase with surgery and recovery time, and physicians prefer to perform nephrectomy before transplant; additionally, uni-nephrectomy has a lower mortality rate. The graft survival rate was similar to that of non-ADPKD patients; the associated risks were bleeding, incisional hernia, pulmonary embolism, and death. The performance of this alternative should be discussed clearly with each patient and their family, indicating all the risks involved [7, 23, 87, 113].

CONCLUSION

As we reviewed here, PKD is a very complex disease with no cure and is generally accompanied by multiple but treatable symptoms due to the activation of numerous signaling pathways; the pathophysiological mechanisms involved are complicated and poorly studied. The diagnosis is limited by the high cost of sequencing or a lack of imaging technology; additionally, its progression and complication treatment represent a major challenge due to costs for patients and health systems. Many efforts have been made to improve patient's quality of life, beginning with early diagnosis and using available drugs to treat the main symptoms. Treating renal complications is fundamental for delaying the development of end-stage renal disease as much as possible. Further, it requires the use of nephrectomy, replacement therapy, or transplantation. Clinicians have enormous work to do, maintaining close monitoring of ADPKD patients because of the multiple symptoms and comorbidities present. Each patient must be carefully evaluated to introduce an adequate treatment scheme that fulfills all its necessities due to diverse clinical signs and various stratification statuses. Hopefully, some of these efforts will benefit PKD patients' well-being.

REFERENCES

[1]   Aukema HM. Prostaglandins as potential targets for the treatment of polycystic kidney disease. Prostaglandins Leukot Essent Fatty Acids 2021; 164: 102220.
[http://dx.doi.org/10.1016/j.plefa.2020.102220] [PMID: 33285393]

[2]   Kalatharan V, McArthur E, Nash DM, *et al.* Diagnostic accuracy of administrative codes for autosomal dominant polycystic kidney disease in clinic patients with cystic kidney disease. Clin Kidney J 2021; 14(2): 612-6.
[http://dx.doi.org/10.1093/ckj/sfz184] [PMID: 33623686]

[3]   Xue C, Mei CL. Polycystic Kidney Disease and Renal Fibrosis. Adv Exp Med Biol 2019; 1165: 81-100.
[http://dx.doi.org/10.1007/978-981-13-8871-2_5] [PMID: 31399962]

[4]   Bergmann C. Early and Severe Polycystic Kidney Disease and Related Ciliopathies: An Emerging Field of Interest. Nephron J 2019; 141(1): 50-60.
[http://dx.doi.org/10.1159/000493532] [PMID: 30359986]

[5]   Bergmann C, Guay-Woodford LM, Harris PC, Horie S, Peters DJM, Torres VE. Polycystic kidney disease. Nat Rev Dis Primers 2018; 4(1): 50.
[http://dx.doi.org/10.1038/s41572-018-0047-y] [PMID: 30523303]

[6]   Gallagher AR, Germino GG, Somlo S. Molecular advances in autosomal dominant polycystic kidney disease. Adv Chronic Kidney Dis 2010; 17(2): 118-30.
[http://dx.doi.org/10.1053/j.ackd.2010.01.002] [PMID: 20219615]

[7]   Liebau MC. Early clinical management of autosomal recessive polycystic kidney disease. Pediatr Nephrol 2021; 36(11): 3561-70.
[http://dx.doi.org/10.1007/s00467-021-04970-8] [PMID: 33594464]

[8]   Losekoot M, Meijer E, Hagen EC, *et al.* Polycystic Kidney Disease Caused by Bilineal Inheritance of Truncating *PKD1* as Well as *PKD2* Mutations. Kidney Int Rep 2020; 5(10): 1828-32.
[http://dx.doi.org/10.1016/j.ekir.2020.07.006] [PMID: 33102977]

[9]   Arroyo J, Escobar-Zarate D, Wells HH, *et al.* The genetic background significantly impacts the severity of kidney cystic disease in the Pkd1$^{RC/RC}$ mouse model of autosomal dominant polycystic kidney disease. Kidney Int 2021; 99(6): 1392-407.
[http://dx.doi.org/10.1016/j.kint.2021.01.028] [PMID: 33705824]

[10]   Cornec-Le Gall E, Alam A, Perrone RD. Autosomal dominant polycystic kidney disease. Lancet 2019; 393(10174): 919-35.
[http://dx.doi.org/10.1016/S0140-6736(18)32782-X] [PMID: 30819518]

[11]   Baliga MM, Klawitter J, Christians U, *et al.* Metabolic profiling in children and young adults with autosomal dominant polycystic kidney disease. Sci Rep 2021; 11(1): 6629.
[http://dx.doi.org/10.1038/s41598-021-84609-8] [PMID: 33758231]

[12]   Lanktree MB, Haghighi A, Guiard E, *et al.* Prevalence Estimates of Polycystic Kidney and Liver Disease by Population Sequencing. J Am Soc Nephrol 2018; 29(10): 2593-600.
[http://dx.doi.org/10.1681/ASN.2018050493] [PMID: 30135240]

[13]   Lanktree MB, Iliuta IA, Haghighi A, Song X, Pei Y. Evolving role of genetic testing for the clinical management of autosomal dominant polycystic kidney disease. Nephrol Dial Transplant 2019; 34(9): 1453-60.
[http://dx.doi.org/10.1093/ndt/gfy261] [PMID: 30165646]

[14]   Ekinci İ, Buyukkaba M, Cinar A, *et al.* Endothelial Dysfunction and Atherosclerosis in Patients With Autosomal Dominant Polycystic Kidney Disease. Cureus 2021; 13(2): e13561.
[http://dx.doi.org/10.7759/cureus.13561] [PMID: 33815976]

[15]   Willey C, Kamat S, Stellhorn R, Blais J. Analysis of nationwide data to determine the incidence and diagnosed prevalence of autosomal dominant polycystic kidney disease in the USA: 2013–2015.

Kidney Dis 2019; 5(2): 107-17.
[http://dx.doi.org/10.1159/000494923] [PMID: 31019924]

[16]   Willey CJ, Blais JD, Hall AK, Krasa HB, Makin AJ, Czerwiec FS. Prevalence of autosomal dominant polycystic kidney disease in the European Union. Nephrol Dial Transplant 2016; 32(8): gfw240.
[http://dx.doi.org/10.1093/ndt/gfw240] [PMID: 27325254]

[17]   Solazzo A, Testa F, Giovanella S, *et al.* The prevalence of autosomal dominant polycystic kidney disease (ADPKD): A meta-analysis of European literature and prevalence evaluation in the Italian province of Modena suggest that ADPKD is a rare and underdiagnosed condition. PLoS One 2018; 13(1): e0190430.
[http://dx.doi.org/10.1371/journal.pone.0190430] [PMID: 29338003]

[18]   Suwabe T, Shukoor S, Chamberlain AM, *et al.* Epidemiology of autosomal dominant polycystic kidney disease in olmsted county. Clin J Am Soc Nephrol 2020; 15(1): 69-79.
[http://dx.doi.org/10.2215/CJN.05900519] [PMID: 31791998]

[19]   Su Q, Hu F, Ge X, *et al.* Structure of the human PKD1-PKD2 complex. Science 2018; 361(6406): eaat9819.
[http://dx.doi.org/10.1126/science.aat9819] [PMID: 30093605]

[20]   Kasap Demïr B, Mutlubaş F, Soyaltin E, *et al.* Demographic and clinical characteristics of children with autosomal dominant polycystic kidney disease: a single center experience. Turk J Med Sci 2021; 51(2): 772-7.
[http://dx.doi.org/10.3906/sag-2009-79] [PMID: 33315352]

[21]   Ibraghimov-Beskrovnaya O, Bukanov N. Polycystic kidney diseases: From molecular discoveries to targeted therapeutic strategies. Cell Mol Life Sci 2008; 65(4): 605-19.
[http://dx.doi.org/10.1007/s00018-007-7362-x] [PMID: 17975706]

[22]   Bergmann C. Genetics of autosomal recessive polycystic kidney disease and its differential diagnoses. Front Pediatr 2018; 5: 221.
[http://dx.doi.org/10.3389/fped.2017.00221] [PMID: 29479522]

[23]   Spithoven EM, Kramer A, Meijer E, *et al.* Renal replacement therapy for autosomal dominant polycystic kidney disease (ADPKD) in Europe: prevalence and survival--an analysis of data from the ERA-EDTA Registry. Nephrol Dial Transplant 2014; 29(Suppl 4) (Suppl. 4): iv15-25.
[http://dx.doi.org/10.1093/ndt/gfu017] [PMID: 25165182]

[24]   Gorriz JL, Arroyo D, D'Marco L, *et al.* Cardiovascular risk factors and the impact on prognosis in patients with chronic kidney disease secondary to autosomal dominant polycystic kidney disease. BMC Nephrol 2021; 22(1): 110.
[http://dx.doi.org/10.1186/s12882-021-02313-1] [PMID: 33765945]

[25]   Paul BM, Vanden Heuvel GB. Kidney: polycystic kidney disease. Wiley Interdiscip Rev Dev Biol 2014; 3(6): 465-87.
[http://dx.doi.org/10.1002/wdev.152] [PMID: 25186187]

[26]   Raina R, DeCoy M, Chakraborty R, *et al.* Renal cystic diseases during the perinatal and neonatal period. J Neonatal Perinatal Med 2021; 14(2): 163-76.
[http://dx.doi.org/10.3233/NPM-200520] [PMID: 32986687]

[27]   Lu H, Galeano MCR, Ott E, *et al.* Mutations in DZIP1L, which encodes a ciliary-transition-zone protein, cause autosomal recessive polycystic kidney disease. Nat Genet 2017; 49(7): 1025-34.
[http://dx.doi.org/10.1038/ng.3871] [PMID: 28530676]

[28]   McConnachie DJ, Stow JL, Mallett AJ. Ciliopathies and the Kidney: A Review. Am J Kidney Dis 2021; 77(3): 410-9.
[http://dx.doi.org/10.1053/j.ajkd.2020.08.012] [PMID: 33039432]

[29]   Verghese P, Miyashita Y. Neonatal polycystic kidney disease. Clin Perinatol 2014; 41(3): 543-60.
[http://dx.doi.org/10.1016/j.clp.2014.05.005] [PMID: 25155726]

[30]   Adeva M, El-Youssef M, Rossetti S, *et al.* Clinical and molecular characterization defines a broadened spectrum of autosomal recessive polycystic kidney disease (ARPKD). Medicine (Baltimore) 2006; 85(1): 1-21.
[http://dx.doi.org/10.1097/01.md.0000200165.90373.9a] [PMID: 16523049]

[31]   foundation P. Autosomal dominant polycystic kidney disease: Mutation database. 2021. Available at: https://pkdb.mayo.edu/welcome

[32]   Ranjzad F, Aghdami N, Tara A, Mohseni M, Moghadasali R, Basiri A. Identification of Three Novel Frameshift Mutations in the PKD1 Gene in Iranian Families with Autosomal Dominant Polycystic Kidney Disease Using Efficient Targeted Next-Generation Sequencing. Kidney Blood Press Res 2018; 43(2): 471-8.
[http://dx.doi.org/10.1159/000488471] [PMID: 29590654]

[33]   PKHD1 Gene [Internet]. 2021 [cited June 2021]. Available from: https://www.genecards.org/cgi-bin/carddisp.pl?gene=PKHD1&keywords=PKHD1#snp

[34]   Autosomal Dominant Polycystic Kidney Disease: Mutation Database [Internet]. 2021. Available from: https://pkdb.mayo.edu/cgi-bin/v2_display_mutations.cgi?GENE=PKD1&apkd_mode=PROD&username=

[35]   Stelzer G, Rosen N, Plaschkes I, *et al.* The GeneCards Suite: From Gene Data Mining to Disease Genome Sequence Analyses. Curr Protoc Bioinformatics 2016; 54:1 30 1-1.
[http://dx.doi.org/10.1002/cpbi.5]

[36]   Hardy E, Tsiokas L. Polycystins as components of large multiprotein complexes of polycystin interactors. Cell Signal 2020; 72: 109640.
[http://dx.doi.org/10.1016/j.cellsig.2020.109640] [PMID: 32305669]

[37]   Streets A, Ong A. Post-translational modifications of the polycystin proteins. Cell Signal 2020; 72: 109644.
[http://dx.doi.org/10.1016/j.cellsig.2020.109644] [PMID: 32320857]

[38]   Douguet D, Patel A, Honoré E. Structure and function of polycystins: insights into polycystic kidney disease. Nat Rev Nephrol 2019; 15(7): 412-22.
[http://dx.doi.org/10.1038/s41581-019-0143-6] [PMID: 30948841]

[39]   Ramírez-Sagredo A, Quiroga C, Garrido-Moreno V, *et al.* Polycystin-1 regulates cardiomyocyte mitophagy. FASEB J 2021; 35(8): e21796.
[http://dx.doi.org/10.1096/fj.202002598R] [PMID: 34324238]

[40]   Jung SH, You JE, Choi SW, *et al.* Polycystin-1 Enhances Stemmness Potential of Umbilical Cord Blood-Derived Mesenchymal Stem Cells. Int J Mol Sci 2021; 22(9): 4868.
[http://dx.doi.org/10.3390/ijms22094868] [PMID: 34064452]

[41]   Song X, Haghighi A, Iliuta IA, Pei Y. Molecular diagnosis of autosomal dominant polycystic kidney disease. Expert Rev Mol Diagn 2017; 17(10): 885-95.
[http://dx.doi.org/10.1080/14737159.2017.1358088] [PMID: 28724316]

[42]   Adamiok-Ostrowska A, Piekiełko-Witkowska A. Ciliary Genes in Renal Cystic Diseases. Cells 2020; 9(4): 907.
[http://dx.doi.org/10.3390/cells9040907] [PMID: 32276433]

[43]   Kim DY, Park JH. Genetic Mechanisms of ADPKD. Adv Exp Med Biol 2016; 933: 13-22.
[http://dx.doi.org/10.1007/978-981-10-2041-4_2] [PMID: 27730431]

[44]   Mochizuki T, Wu G, Hayashi T, *et al.* PKD2, a gene for polycystic kidney disease that encodes an integral membrane protein. Science 1996; 272(5266): 1339-42.
[http://dx.doi.org/10.1126/science.272.5266.1339] [PMID: 8650545]

[45]   Bitarafan F, Garshasbi M. Molecular Genetic Analysis of PKHD1 Mutations in Pedigrees With Autosomal Recessive Polycystic Kidney Disease. Iran J Kidney Dis 2018; 12(6):

350-8.https://www.ijkd.org/index.php/ijkd/article/download/3931/1036/19460
[PMID: 30595564]

[46]   Ma M. Cilia and polycystic kidney disease. Semin Cell Dev Biol 2021; 110: 139-48.
[http://dx.doi.org/10.1016/j.semcdb.2020.05.003] [PMID: 32475690]

[47]   Guay-Woodford LM. Renal cystic diseases: diverse phenotypes converge on the cilium/centrosome complex. Pediatr Nephrol 2006; 21(10): 1369-76.
[http://dx.doi.org/10.1007/s00467-006-0164-9] [PMID: 16823577]

[48]   Cornec-Le Gall E, Olson RJ, Besse W, *et al.* Monoallelic Mutations to DNAJB11 Cause Atypical Autosomal-Dominant Polycystic Kidney Disease. Am J Hum Genet 2018; 102(5): 832-44.
[http://dx.doi.org/10.1016/j.ajhg.2018.03.013] [PMID: 29706351]

[49]   Colbert GB, Elrggal ME, Gaur L, Lerma EV. Update and review of adult polycystic kidney disease. Dis Mon 2020; 66(5): 100887.
[http://dx.doi.org/10.1016/j.disamonth.2019.100887] [PMID: 31582186]

[50]   Porath B, Gainullin VG, Cornec-Le Gall E, *et al.* Mutations in GANAB, Encoding the Glucosidase IIα Subunit, Cause Autosomal-Dominant Polycystic Kidney and Liver Disease. Am J Hum Genet 2016; 98(6): 1193-207.
[http://dx.doi.org/10.1016/j.ajhg.2016.05.004] [PMID: 27259053]

[51]   Higashihara E, Horie S, Muto S, Mochizuki T, Nishio S, Nutahara K. Renal disease progression in autosomal dominant polycystic kidney disease. Clin Exp Nephrol 2012; 16(4): 622-8.
[http://dx.doi.org/10.1007/s10157-012-0611-9] [PMID: 22526483]

[52]   Li M, Qin S, Wang L, Zhou J. Genomic instability in patients with autosomal-dominant polycystic kidney disease. J Int Med Res 2013; 41(1): 169-75.
[http://dx.doi.org/10.1177/0300060513475956] [PMID: 23569143]

[53]   Meijer E, Rook M, Tent H, *et al.* Early renal abnormalities in autosomal dominant polycystic kidney disease. Clin J Am Soc Nephrol 2010; 5(6): 1091-8.
[http://dx.doi.org/10.2215/CJN.00360110] [PMID: 20413443]

[54]   Chapman AB, Devuyst O, Eckardt KU, *et al.* Autosomal-dominant polycystic kidney disease (ADPKD): executive summary from a Kidney Disease: Improving Global Outcomes (KDIGO) Controversies Conference. Kidney Int 2015; 88(1): 17-27.
[http://dx.doi.org/10.1038/ki.2015.59] [PMID: 25786098]

[55]   Ryu H, Park HC, Oh YK, *et al.* RAPID-ADPKD (Retrospective epidemiological study of Asia-Pacific patients with rapId Disease progression of Autosomal Dominant Polycystic Kidney Disease): study protocol for a multinational, retrospective cohort study. BMJ Open 2020; 10(2): e034103.
[http://dx.doi.org/10.1136/bmjopen-2019-034103] [PMID: 32034027]

[56]   Srivastava A, Patel N. Autosomal dominant polycystic kidney disease. Am Fam Physician 2014; 90(5): 303-7.https://www.aafp.org/pubs/afp/issues/2014/0901/p303.pdf
[PMID: 25251090]

[57]   Hian CK, Lee CL, Thomas W. Renin-Angiotensin-Aldosterone System Antagonism and Polycystic Kidney Disease Progression. Nephron J 2016; 134(2): 59-63.
[http://dx.doi.org/10.1159/000448296] [PMID: 27476173]

[58]   McEneaney V, Harvey BJ, Thomas W. Aldosterone rapidly activates protein kinase D via a mineralocorticoid receptor/EGFR trans-activation pathway in the M1 kidney CCD cell line. J Steroid Biochem Mol Biol 2007; 107(3-5): 180-90.
[http://dx.doi.org/10.1016/j.jsbmb.2007.03.043] [PMID: 17681751]

[59]   Nishiura JCAAL, Neves RFCA, Eloi SRM, Cintra SMLF, Ajzen SA, Heilberg IP. Evaluation of nephrolithiasis in autosomal dominant polycystic kidney disease patients. Clin J Am Soc Nephrol 2009; 4(4): 838-44.
[http://dx.doi.org/10.2215/CJN.03100608] [PMID: 19339428]

[60]   Bargagli M, Dhayat NA, Anderegg M, *et al.* Urinary Lithogenic Risk Profile in ADPKD Patients Treated with Tolvaptan. Clin J Am Soc Nephrol 2020; 15(7): 1007-14.
[http://dx.doi.org/10.2215/CJN.13861119] [PMID: 32527945]

[61]   Grampsas SA, Chandhoke PS, Fan J, *et al.* Anatomic and metabolic risk factors for nephrolithiasis in patients with autosomal dominant polycystic kidney disease. Am J Kidney Dis 2000; 36(1): 53-7.
[http://dx.doi.org/10.1053/ajkd.2000.8266] [PMID: 10873872]

[62]   Bankir L, Bichet DG. An early urea-selective urine-concentrating defect in ADPKD. Nat Rev Nephrol 2012; 8(8): 437-9.
[http://dx.doi.org/10.1038/nrneph.2012.139] [PMID: 22735763]

[63]   Zittema D, Boertien WE, van Beek AP, *et al.* Vasopressin, copeptin, and renal concentrating capacity in patients with autosomal dominant polycystic kidney disease without renal impairment. Clin J Am Soc Nephrol 2012; 7(6): 906-13.
[http://dx.doi.org/10.2215/CJN.11311111] [PMID: 22516290]

[64]   van Gastel MDA, Torres VE. Polycystic Kidney Disease and the Vasopressin Pathway. Ann Nutr Metab 2017; 70 (Suppl. 1): 43-50.
[http://dx.doi.org/10.1159/000463063] [PMID: 28614813]

[65]   Borrego Utiel FJ, Merino García E. Glomerular filtration rate is the main predictor of urine volume in autosomal dominant polycystic kidney disease patients treated with tolvaptan when daily osmolar excretion is expressed as urinary osmolality/creatinine ratio. Clin Kidney J 2021; 14(3): 1031-3.
[http://dx.doi.org/10.1093/ckj/sfaa171] [PMID: 33777387]

[66]   Seliger SL, Watnick T, Althouse AD, *et al.* Baseline characteristics and patient-reported outcomes of ADPKD patients in the multicenter TAME-PKD clinical trial. Kidney360 2020; 1(12): 1363-72.
[http://dx.doi.org/10.34067/KID.0004002020] [PMID: 33768205]

[67]   Pirson Y. Extrarenal manifestations of autosomal dominant polycystic kidney disease. Adv Chronic Kidney Dis 2010; 17(2): 173-80.
[http://dx.doi.org/10.1053/j.ackd.2010.01.003] [PMID: 20219620]

[68]   Zhou X, Xiong H, Lu Y, *et al.* PKD2 deficiency suppresses amino acid biosynthesis in ADPKD by impairing the PERK–TBL2–eIF2α–ATF4 pathway. Biochem Biophys Res Commun 2021; 561: 73-9.
[http://dx.doi.org/10.1016/j.bbrc.2021.05.012] [PMID: 34015761]

[69]   Gaur P, Gedroyc W, Hill P. ADPKD—what the radiologist should know. Br J Radiol 2019; 92(1098): 20190078.
[http://dx.doi.org/10.1259/bjr.20190078] [PMID: 31039325]

[70]   Cowley BD Jr. Calcium, cyclic AMP, and MAP kinases: Dysregulation in polycystic kidney disease. Kidney Int 2008; 73(3): 251-3.
[http://dx.doi.org/10.1038/sj.ki.5002695] [PMID: 18195694]

[71]   Singh B, Carpenter G, Coffey RJ. EGF receptor ligands: recent advances. F1000Res 2016; 5.
[http://dx.doi.org/10.12688/f1000research.9025.1]

[72]   Lee EJ, Seo E, Kim JW, *et al.* TAZ/Wnt-β-catenin/c-MYC axis regulates cystogenesis in polycystic kidney disease. Proc Natl Acad Sci USA 2020; 117(46): 29001-12.
[http://dx.doi.org/10.1073/pnas.2009334117] [PMID: 33122431]

[73]   Formica C, Malas T, Balog J, Verburg L, 't Hoen PAC, Peters DJM. Characterisation of transcription factor profiles in polycystic kidney disease (PKD): identification and validation of STAT3 and RUNX1 in the injury/repair response and PKD progression. J Mol Med (Berl) 2019; 97(12): 1643-56.
[http://dx.doi.org/10.1007/s00109-019-01852-3] [PMID: 31773180]

[74]   Patera F, Cudzich-Madry A, Huang Z, Fragiadaki M. Renal expression of JAK2 is high in polycystic kidney disease and its inhibition reduces cystogenesis. Sci Rep 2019; 9(1): 4491.
[http://dx.doi.org/10.1038/s41598-019-41106-3] [PMID: 30872773]

[75] Choi S, Kim DY, Ahn Y, Lee EJ, Park JH. Suppression of *Foxo3-Gatm* by miR-132-3p Accelerates Cyst Formation by Up-Regulating ROS in Autosomal Dominant Polycystic Kidney Disease. Biomol Ther (Seoul) 2021; 29(3): 311-20.
[http://dx.doi.org/10.4062/biomolther.2020.197] [PMID: 33408288]

[76] Duong Phu M, Bross S, Burkhalter MD, Philipp M. Limitations and opportunities in the pharmacotherapy of ciliopathies. Pharmacol Ther 2021; 225: 107841.
[http://dx.doi.org/10.1016/j.pharmthera.2021.107841] [PMID: 33771583]

[77] Fragiadaki M, Macleod FM, Ong ACM. The controversial role of fibrosis in autosomal dominant polycystic kidney disease. Int J Mol Sci 2020; 21(23): 8936.
[http://dx.doi.org/10.3390/ijms21238936] [PMID: 33255651]

[78] Bowden SA, Rodger EJ, Bates M, Chatterjee A, Eccles MR, Stayner C. Genome-scale single nucleotide resolution analysis of DNA methylation in human autosomal dominant polycystic kidney disease. Am J Nephrol 2018; 48(6): 415-24.
[http://dx.doi.org/10.1159/000494739] [PMID: 30463078]

[79] Hajirezaei F, Ghaderian SMH, Hasanzad M, *et al.* Methylation of the *PKD1* promoter inversely correlates with its expression in autosomal dominant polycystic kidney disease. Rep Biochem Mol Biol 2020; 9(2): 193-8.
[http://dx.doi.org/10.29252/rbmb.9.2.193] [PMID: 33178869]

[80] Cebotaru L, Liu Q, Yanda MK, *et al.* Inhibition of histone deacetylase 6 activity reduces cyst growth in polycystic kidney disease. Kidney Int 2016; 90(1): 90-9.
[http://dx.doi.org/10.1016/j.kint.2016.01.026] [PMID: 27165822]

[81] Pei Y, Obaji J, Dupuis A, *et al.* Unified criteria for ultrasonographic diagnosis of ADPKD. J Am Soc Nephrol 2009; 20(1): 205-12.
[http://dx.doi.org/10.1681/ASN.2008050507] [PMID: 18945943]

[82] Mallawaarachchi AC, Lundie B, Hort Y, *et al.* Genomic diagnostics in polycystic kidney disease: an assessment of real-world use of whole-genome sequencing. Eur J Hum Genet 2021; 29(5): 760-70.
[http://dx.doi.org/10.1038/s41431-020-00796-4] [PMID: 33437033]

[83] Lanktree MB, Haghighi A, di Bari I, Song X, Pei Y. Insights into autosomal dominant polycystic kidney disease from genetic studies. Clin J Am Soc Nephrol 2021; 16(5): 790-9.
[http://dx.doi.org/10.2215/CJN.02320220] [PMID: 32690722]

[84] Torres VE, Harris PC, Pirson Y. Autosomal dominant polycystic kidney disease. Lancet 2007; 369(9569): 1287-301.
[http://dx.doi.org/10.1016/S0140-6736(07)60601-1] [PMID: 17434405]

[85] Irazabal MV, Torres VE. Experimental therapies and ongoing clinical trials to slow down progression of ADPKD. Curr Hypertens Rev 2013; 9(1): 44-59.
[http://dx.doi.org/10.2174/1573402111309010008] [PMID: 23971644]

[86] Zhang JQJ, Saravanabavan S, Chandra AN, *et al.* Up-regulation of dna damage response signaling in autosomal dominant polycystic kidney disease. Am J Pathol 2021; 191(5): 902-20.
[http://dx.doi.org/10.1016/j.ajpath.2021.01.011] [PMID: 33549515]

[87] El Chediak A, Degheili JA, Khauli RB. Genitourinary Interventions in Autosomal Dominant Polycystic Kidney Disease: Clinical Recommendations for Urologic and Transplant Surgeons. Exp Clin Transplant 2021; 19(2): 95-103.
[http://dx.doi.org/10.6002/ect.2020.0292] [PMID: 33494664]

[88] Collini A, Benigni R, Ruggieri G, Carmellini PM. Laparoscopic Nephrectomy for Massive Kidneys in Polycystic Kidney Disease. JSLS 2021; 25(1): e2020.00107.
[http://dx.doi.org/10.4293/JSLS.2020.00107] [PMID: 33879988]

[89] Torres VE, Abebe KZ, Chapman AB, *et al.* Angiotensin blockade in late autosomal dominant polycystic kidney disease. N Engl J Med 2014; 371(24): 2267-76.

[http://dx.doi.org/10.1056/NEJMoa1402686] [PMID: 25399731]

[90] Schrier RW, Abebe KZ, Perrone RD, *et al.* Blood pressure in early autosomal dominant polycystic kidney disease. N Engl J Med 2014; 371(24): 2255-66.
[http://dx.doi.org/10.1056/NEJMoa1402685] [PMID: 25399733]

[91] Blazer-Yost BL, Bacallao RL, Erickson BJ, *et al.* A randomized phase 1b cross-over study of the safety of low-dose pioglitazone for treatment of autosomal dominant polycystic kidney disease. Clin Kidney J 2021; 14(7): 1738-46.
[http://dx.doi.org/10.1093/ckj/sfaa232] [PMID: 34221381]

[92] Nakatani S, Nishide K, Okuno S, *et al.* Cinacalcet may suppress kidney enlargement in hemodialysis patients with autosomal dominant polycystic kidney disease. Sci Rep 2021; 11(1): 10014.
[http://dx.doi.org/10.1038/s41598-021-89480-1] [PMID: 33976330]

[93] Di Mise A, Tamma G, Ranieri M, *et al.* Activation of Calcium-Sensing Receptor increases intracellular calcium and decreases cAMP and mTOR in PKD1 deficient cells. Sci Rep 2018; 8(1): 5704.
[http://dx.doi.org/10.1038/s41598-018-23732-5] [PMID: 29632324]

[94] Perico N, Ruggenenti P, Perna A, *et al.* Octreotide-LAR in later-stage autosomal dominant polycystic kidney disease (ALADIN 2): A randomized, double-blind, placebo-controlled, multicenter trial. PLoS Med 2019; 16(4): e1002777.
[http://dx.doi.org/10.1371/journal.pmed.1002777] [PMID: 30951521]

[95] Caroli A, Perico N, Perna A, *et al.* Effect of longacting somatostatin analogue on kidney and cyst growth in autosomal dominant polycystic kidney disease (ALADIN): a randomised, placebo-controlled, multicentre trial. Lancet 2013; 382(9903): 1485-95.
[http://dx.doi.org/10.1016/S0140-6736(13)61407-5] [PMID: 23972263]

[96] Hogan MC, Chamberlin JA, Vaughan LE, *et al.* Pansomatostatin Agonist Pasireotide Long-Acting Release for Patients with Autosomal Dominant Polycystic Kidney or Liver Disease with Severe Liver Involvement. Clin J Am Soc Nephrol 2020; 15(9): 1267-78.
[http://dx.doi.org/10.2215/CJN.13661119] [PMID: 32843370]

[97] Griffiths J, Mills MT, Ong ACM. Long-acting somatostatin analogue treatments in autosomal dominant polycystic kidney disease and polycystic liver disease: a systematic review and meta-analysis. BMJ Open 2020; 10(1): e032620.
[http://dx.doi.org/10.1136/bmjopen-2019-032620] [PMID: 31924636]

[98] Radadiya PS, Thornton MM, Puri RV, *et al.* Ciclopirox olamine induces ferritinophagy and reduces cyst burden in polycystic kidney disease. JCI Insight 2021; 6(8): e141299.
[http://dx.doi.org/10.1172/jci.insight.141299] [PMID: 33784251]

[99] Radadiya PS, Thornton MM, Daniel EA, *et al.* Quinomycin A reduces cyst progression in polycystic kidney disease. FASEB J 2021; 35(5): e21533.
[http://dx.doi.org/10.1096/fj.202002490R] [PMID: 33826787]

[100] Sorohan BM, Ismail G, Andronesi A, *et al.* A single-arm pilot study of metformin in patients with autosomal dominant polycystic kidney disease. BMC Nephrol 2019; 20(1): 276.
[http://dx.doi.org/10.1186/s12882-019-1463-2] [PMID: 31337351]

[101] Heida JE, Gansevoort RT, Meijer E. Acid-Base Homeostasis During Vasopressin V2 Receptor Antagonist Treatment in Autosomal Dominant Polycystic Kidney Disease Patients. Kidney Int Rep 2021; 6(3): 839-41.
[http://dx.doi.org/10.1016/j.ekir.2020.12.021] [PMID: 33732999]

[102] Serra AL, Poster D, Kistler AD, *et al.* Sirolimus and kidney growth in autosomal dominant polycystic kidney disease. N Engl J Med 2010; 363(9): 820-9.
[http://dx.doi.org/10.1056/NEJMoa0907419] [PMID: 20581391]

[103] Klawitter J, McFann K, Pennington AT, *et al.* Pravastatin Therapy and Biomarker Changes in

Children and Young Adults with Autosomal Dominant Polycystic Kidney Disease. Clin J Am Soc Nephrol 2015; 10(9): 1534-41.
[http://dx.doi.org/10.2215/CJN.11331114] [PMID: 26224879]

[104]   Sussman CR, Wang X, Chebib FT, Torres VE. Modulation of polycystic kidney disease by G-protein coupled receptors and cyclic AMP signaling. Cell Signal 2020; 72: 109649.
[http://dx.doi.org/10.1016/j.cellsig.2020.109649] [PMID: 32335259]

[105]   Sriram K, Insel PA. G Protein-Coupled Receptors as Targets for Approved Drugs: How Many Targets and How Many Drugs? Mol Pharmacol 2018; 93(4): 251-8.
[http://dx.doi.org/10.1124/mol.117.111062] [PMID: 29298813]

[106]   Gurevich VV, Gurevich EV. Biased GPCR signaling: Possible mechanisms and inherent limitations. Pharmacol Ther 2020; 211: 107540.
[http://dx.doi.org/10.1016/j.pharmthera.2020.107540] [PMID: 32201315]

[107]   Wang X, Gattone V II, Harris PC, Torres VE. Effectiveness of vasopressin V2 receptor antagonists OPC-31260 and OPC-41061 on polycystic kidney disease development in the PCK rat. J Am Soc Nephrol 2005; 16(4): 846-51.
[http://dx.doi.org/10.1681/ASN.2004121090] [PMID: 15728778]

[108]   Romaker D, Puetz M, Teschner S, *et al.* Increased expression of secreted frizzled-related protein 4 in polycystic kidneys. J Am Soc Nephrol 2009; 20(1): 48-56.
[http://dx.doi.org/10.1681/ASN.2008040345] [PMID: 18945944]

[109]   Torres VE, Chapman AB, Devuyst O, *et al.* Tolvaptan in patients with autosomal dominant polycystic kidney disease. N Engl J Med 2012; 367(25): 2407-18.
[http://dx.doi.org/10.1056/NEJMoa1205511] [PMID: 23121377]

[110]   Torres VE, Chapman AB, Devuyst O, *et al.* Multicenter, open-label, extension trial to evaluate the long-term efficacy and safety of early versus delayed treatment with tolvaptan in autosomal dominant polycystic kidney disease: the TEMPO 4:4 Trial. Nephrol Dial Transplant 2018; 33(3): 477-89.
[http://dx.doi.org/10.1093/ndt/gfx043] [PMID: 28379536]

[111]   Reif GA, Yamaguchi T, Nivens E, Fujiki H, Pinto CS, Wallace DP. Tolvaptan inhibits ERK-dependent cell proliferation, Cl⁻ secretion, and in vitro cyst growth of human ADPKD cells stimulated by vasopressin. Am J Physiol Renal Physiol 2011; 301(5): F1005-13.
[http://dx.doi.org/10.1152/ajprenal.00243.2011] [PMID: 21816754]

[112]   Testa F, Magistroni R. ADPKD current management and ongoing trials. J Nephrol 2020; 33(2): 223-37.
[http://dx.doi.org/10.1007/s40620-019-00679-y] [PMID: 31853789]

[113]   Lubennikov AE, Petrovskii NV, Krupinov GE, *et al.* Bilateral Nephrectomy in Patients with Autosomal Dominant Polycystic Kidney Disease and End-Stage Chronic Renal Failure. Nephron J 2021; 145(2): 164-70.
[http://dx.doi.org/10.1159/000513168] [PMID: 33550285]

CHAPTER 8

Renal Lithiasis: Current Concepts about a Millenary Disease

Roberto Lugo[1,*] and **Martha Medina-Escobedo**[1]

¹ Research Division, Hospital Regional de Alta Especialidad de la Península de Yucatán IMSS-Bienestar, Mérida, Yucatán, Mexico

Abstract: Renal lithiasis has been a disease afflicting humankind since ancient times; epidemiological data worldwide show that its prevalence varies in different geographical areas, with a higher prevalence in a belt mainly encompassing tropical regions.

Initially, medicine focused on searching for and developing surgical strategies for treating renal lithiasis; currently, the application of minimally invasive surgical procedures predominates. The predominant clinical symptoms are hematuria and acute and intense pain.

Because of its high recurrence rate, research on renal lithiasis has focused on determining its causes and risk factors. Diagnostic methods for pathology have evolved significantly; currently, there are accessible and inexpensive methods (renal and urinary tract ultrasound), as well as more sophisticated methods; however, computed tomography is the gold standard method because it offers high sensitivity and specificity and allows us to pinpoint the location of the stone and suggest its composition. Even so, a percentage of patients are asymptomatic, and the diagnosis is made fortuitously.

New approaches to treating this disease are focused on metabolic studies to improve medical and nutritional therapy, minimally invasive surgical procedures, and the development of new wireless laparoscopic devices to obtain real-time images and biopsies to reduce the recurrence of the pathology.

Keywords: Hounsfield units, Kidney stones, Lithiasis belt, Risk factors, Stone composition.

INTRODUCTION

Renal lithiasis is a millenary disease. In Ancient Egypt, the first evidence dates from El–Amrah. In 1991, Elliot Smith found stones in the bladder in a mummy

---

* **Corresponding author Roberto Lugo:** Research Division Hospital Regional de Alta Especialidad de la Península de Yucatán IMSS-Bienestar, Altabrisa, 97130 Mérida, Yucatán, Mexico; E-mail: roberto.lugo.gomez@gmail.com.

Rafael Valdez-Ortiz, Katy Sánchez-Pozos, Ana Carolina Ariza & Enzo C. Vásquez-Jiménez (Eds.)

from 4800 B.C. The discovery of the oldest kidney stone has been attributed to Shattock. His reports describe a stone located next to the spinal column of a mummy from 3000 B.C. The first reports about the symptoms and prevention of lithiasis are found in the medical books of Asutu in Mesopotamia (320-1200 B.C.) [1]. In addition, the book Sushruta Samhita (600 B.C.) describes the first surgical procedures, including perineal lithotomy, used to treat bladder stones. However, this document does not mention kidney and ureteral stones [2].

Hippocrates (46-377 B.C.) described kidney diseases and symptoms of bladder lithiasis. He mentioned that specialists must perform stone extraction surgeries due to the high risk of death and due to neural stimulation of the bladder. Similarly, he was the first to issue some theories about the formation of kidney stones; he carried out a detailed macroscopic analysis of alterations in the urine and provided diagnostic interpretations and concepts currently in use [3]. After Hippocrates, advances were slow for a long time until Celsus' investigations. He described surgical techniques for stone removal; nonetheless, the origin of the stones was unknown [4].

In the 7th century, the Arab Rhazes proposed the theory of stone formation due to excess salts in urine [5]. Hildegard (1098–1179) was the first to identify modern "metabolic syndrome" and urinary tract infections as the causes of lithiasis [6].

Later, in the 18th century, hypercalciuria was recognized as the principal cause of lithiasis, and the importance of diet in treating lithiasis caused by uric acid was established. At the same time, several strategies have been developed to dissolve stones using alkaline salts, potassium carbonate, and others. Advances in treating lithiasis are related to the surgical treatment of the stones [5].

Over time, the frequency of bladder stones has decreased, and that of kidney stones has increased [7]. However, in the 19th century, studies on the surgical treatment of lithiasis focused on treating the disease. Multiple studies on metabolic disorders and the medical management of kidney stones have been performed in the last century, the most relevant of which will be addressed in the appropriate sections of this chapter.

EPIDEMIOLOGY

Urinary tract lithiasis is a global problem and is the third most common type of urological disorder after urinary tract infections and prostate disease. The incidence and prevalence can vary according to the geographic area and the socio-demographic aspects of the population. The first signs of the disease documented in the ancient population revealed a predominance of bladder lithiasis. Decades later, a progressive increase in renal lithiasis was observed, especially in industrialized countries, where significant changes in eating habits and lifestyle were established [8]. In the last 3-40 years, the prevalence of renal lithiasis has progressively increased globally. Between 1964 and 1972 [9], an increase of 200% was reported in the United States. Subsequent studies revealed an increase in the prevalence of 3.4% from 1976 to 1980 and an increase of 5.2% between 1988 and 1994 [10]. Between 2007 and 2010, an unadjusted prevalence of 8.8% was observed [11], and between 2013–2014, a 10.1% was reported [12].

An increase in the prevalence of renal lithiasis has also been reported in Europe. In Spain, the prevalence increased from 4.2% to 5.2% between 1986 and 2007. In Italy, renal lithiasis increased from 5.9% to 8.0% in 1986-1998. In Germany, the prevalence was 4.0% to 4.7% between 1979 and 2001 [13]. Reports from China showed a similar prevalence of renal lithiasis; they reported 6.0% in 1991–2000 to 10.6% in 2001–2011 [14].

A geographical belt of lithiasis has been identified, in which countries with the highest prevalence of renal lithiasis, such as Egypt, Sudan, Saudi Arabia, Iran, the United Arab Emirates, the Philippines, India, Pakistan, Thailand, Myanmar, and Indonesia, are found [7]. In 2015, Ahmad *et al.* reported the prevalence of urinary stones according to the origin of the patients. These countries included Egypt (29.5%), Pakistan (24.9%), India (23.3%), Yemen (20.5%), Sudan (17.6%), Bangladesh (16.2%), Eritrea (15.4%), and Saudi Arabia (7.4%). The mean prevalence in the population of this geographical area was 19.1%. Seventy-five percent of the urinary tract stones were found in the kidneys [15].

On the American continent, Canada has reported a greater prevalence of regional variations and a greater prevalence in New Brunswick than in other Canadian regions [16]. A similar situation has been reported in the United States, where a geographic belt in the southeast is also mentioned. It includes the states of Alabama, Arkansas, Florida, Georgia, Louisiana, Mississippi, North Carolina, South Carolina, Tennessee, Virginia, and Kentucky [17].

In Mexico, there are few epidemiological studies on this topic. Gomez *et al.* reported that the national prevalence of renal lithiasis was 2.4 per 10,000 patients at the Instituto Mexicano del Seguro Social (Public Hospitals of the Mexico Government) in 1984; this region refers to the lithogenic geographic areas of Yucatan, Puebla, and Quintana Roo [18]. In addition, Medina-Escobedo *et al.* reported that the prevalence of lithiasis in Yucatan, Mexico, was 550 per 10,000 inhabitants in 2002 [19]. The results confirmed the findings of Ortegon-Gallareta et al., who reported that Yucatan has an annual hospitalization rate for lithiasis of 12.5 per 1,000 inhabitants, which is higher than the national average estimated at 4.4 per 1,000 inhabitants [20].

Additionally, there are scarce epidemiological studies on Central and South American countries. The available studies generally include few cases and show some clinical and demographic data; however, they are not representative of the reality of the problem [8, 21].

Studies have shown that renal lithiasis is more prevalent in the population between 30 and 50 years old than in young people, and this prevalence increases with age [14, 16] (Fig. **1**). Furthermore, the disease has been predominantly observed in the male population [22].

Another interesting situation is the symptomatic recurrence of stones, which is observed in 11% of patients at two years after expulsion or surgical extraction, 20% at five years, and 31% at ten years [23]. In addition, observational studies have reported the spontaneous expulsion of localized stones in the proximal (12%), middle (22%), and distal (45%) portions of the ureter. According to their size, the frequency of the stones can vary: 55% are less than 4 mm, 35% are between 4-6 mm, and 8% are greater than 6 mm; those smaller than 5 mm tend to move in the urinary tract and cause many symptoms, particularly intense pain, and hematuria [24].

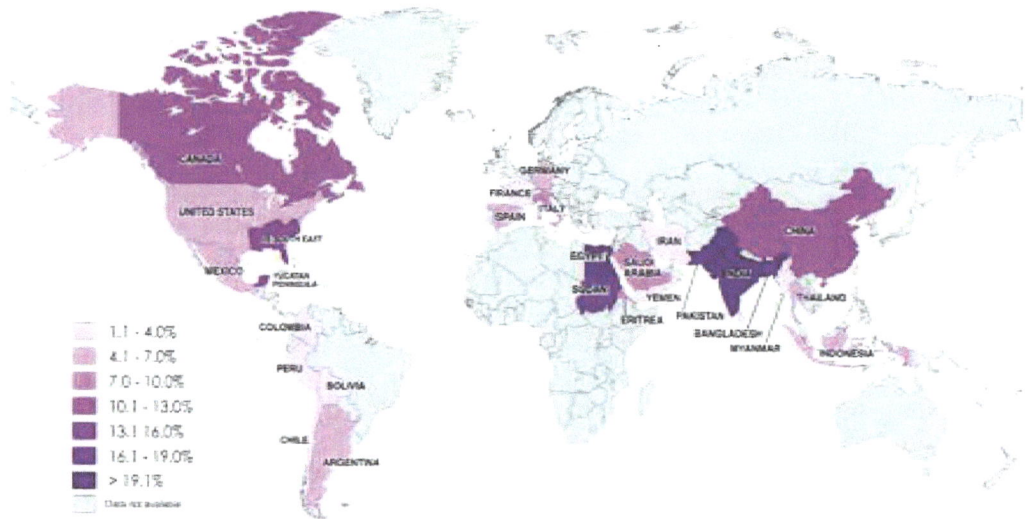

Fig. (1). The prevalence of renal lithiasis is expressed as a percentage.

PHYSIOPATHOLOGY

Renal lithiasis is related to several saline concretions in the kidneys. The size of formed stones can range from a few millimeters to several centimeters, and they can be located at any level of the urinary tract; however, renal stones are the most common (67.4%). The right kidney was usually the most affected (41.7%). In addition, bilateral stones can be observed in 26.2% of patients, and multiple stones or anatomical locations can be observed in 37% of affected patients [25].

Among the processes of kidney stone formation, various substances or elements that act as promoters and inhibitors of stone formation are involved. The physicochemical mechanisms that lead to their appearance in the urine are precipitation or nucleation, growth, aggregation, and retention. Tubular epithelial cells also play an essential role in stone formation, participating in adhesion and/or endocytosis [26]. Genetic, metabolic, environmental, and dietary factors participate in the formation of urinary stones, and all of these factors promote the crystallization of salts inside renal tubules through various processes [27 - 30].

- Supersaturation (excessive concentration). Calcium, oxalate, and uric acid are among the substances that stimulate crystallization (promoting factors), while cystine, xanthine, ammonium urate, and dihydroxyadenine are less frequent. In rare cases, the precipitation of drugs such as atazanavir, indinavir, acyclovir, sulfadiazine, methotrexate, triamterene, quinolones, or aminopenicillins is related to this phenomenon.
- An imbalance of factors promotes and inhibits crystallization in the urine. In contrast to supersaturation, reducing inhibitors such as citrate, magnesium, and potassium increases the formation of stones.
- Abnormalities in the epithelium increase crystal adhesion and growth. Crystal deposits in calcium phosphate nests at the level of renal papillae are called Randall's plaques. These plaques are formed by calcium phosphate precipitation on the basement membrane of the loops of Henle, which grow into the interstitium, accumulate in the subepithelial space of the renal papilla, and eventually erode through the papillary urothelium. This situation can be observed in patients with hypercalciuria.

Urinary volumes play an essential role in the processes involved in stone formation. If they are low, the urine is concentrated or saturated; when they remain normal or high, they favor the dilution of the urine. Crystals are common in the urine; however, if the concentration remains normal and there is no adherence to these crystals anywhere in the kidneys' collector system, the formation of stones is avoided [28].

The formation of stones begins with nucleation in the collector systems of kidneys, which is the formation of a solid crystalline phase in a solution and is the guideline for starting stone formation; in this phase, the composition is homogeneous. Once nucleation has started, other elements (epithelial cells, casts, red blood cells) can be added and undergo heterogeneous nucleation until they become large particles. After nucleation, the adhesion of the crystals continues on the heterogeneous nucleus formed, giving rise to a small hard rock mass called crystal growth. The growth of the stones is slow, and as time passes, they block the kidney tubules. In calcium oxalate stones, the leading growth promoters are the Tamm-Horsfall protein and osteopontin [31]. Aggregation, which occurs when the mass of a crystal in solution sticks together to form a stone, is the most critical step in stone formation and is likely involved in the retention of crystals in the kidneys [32]. Therefore, crystal retention may be due to the adhesion of crystals to epithelial cells. Thus, lithiasis requires the formation of crystals followed by their retention and accumulation in the kidney. Retention could also depend on the composition of the renal tubular epithelial cell surface [28].

Metabolic disorders are risk factors for developing lithiasis, as shown by various studies. Metabolic syndrome, particularly hypertriglyceridemia, is a risk factor for renal lithiasis in obese patients [33]. On the other hand, a direct relationship between the number of metabolic alterations and the increase in weight has been observed in patients with urolithiasis; hence, obesity is a risk factor for metabolic alterations in patients with urolithiasis [34]. Likewise, in patients with diabetes mellitus, a low pH has been observed in urine, which contributes to the production of uric acid stones; additionally, when the excretion of oxalates is significant, it predisposes patients to the formation of oxalate stones [27].

TYPES OF KIDNEY STONES

A central nucleus and concentric layers conform to kidney stones. They can be pure (45% of calcium oxalate). In this case, the nucleus and layers have only one component. Kidney stones are mixed when the nucleus and the layers have two or more compounds [35]. There are several components in the composition of the stones, among which are as follows:

Calcium oxalate. This compound is present in 7-80% of all calculi. Calcium oxalate stones have a low saturation concentration, and many stones may contain this compound as a nucleation center [36]. The formation of calcium oxalate stones results in hypercalciuria or deficient calcium reabsorption within renal tubes. In addition, it has an attenuation density between [496–1868] Hounsfield units. The variants of this compound are calcium oxalate monohydrate

$(CaC_2O_4 \cdot H_2O)$, which represents 40% of all stones, and calcium oxalate dihydrate $(CaC_2O_4 \cdot 2H_2O)$, which represents 60% of them [37 - 39].

Magnesium ammonium phosphate, also called struvite $(MgNH_4PO_4)$, is present in 15% to 20% of kidney stones. Stones are generally caused by bacterial urinary tract infections resulting from urea production. The compound has an attenuation density of [79-2143] Hounsfield units. Other less frequent compounds with similar characteristics include magnesium hydrogen phosphate trihydrate $(MgNPO_4 \cdot 3H_2O)$ and magnesium ammonium phosphate hexahydrate $(MgNH_4PO_4 \cdot 6H_2O)$ [36, 38].

Hydroxyapatite stones $(Ca_{10}(PO_4)_6(OH)_2)$ represent approximately 6-80% of stones; they have characteristics similar to those of calcium oxalates, but their formation differs from that of alkaline urine. The attenuation density is between [120-1600] Hounsfield units. Hydroxyapatite has a similar compound, carbonate apatite $(Ca_{10}(PO_4)_{6-x}(OH)_{2-y}(CO_3)_{x+y})$ [40, 41].

Uric acid $(C_5H_4N_4O_3)$ represents 5–10% of urinary stones and is usually caused by hyperuricosuria and urinary acidification. Uric acid has an attenuation density of [20-450] Hounsfield units. Similar structures are observed, such as uric acid dihydrate $(C_5H_4N_4O_3 \cdot 2H_2O)$, ammonium acid urate $(C_5H_3N_4O_3NH_4)$, and sodium acid urate $(C_5H_3N_4O_3Na)$ [38 - 40].

Cystine stones $([-SCH_2CHNH_2COOH]_2)$ represent 1–2% of kidney stones and are caused by a metabolic disorder resulting from a genetic defect in kidney transport. Cystine has an attenuation density of [60-1100] Hounsfield units [39, 42, 43]. Cystinuria is a complex hereditary problem secondary to the mutation of the *SLC3A1* and *SLC7A9* genes, which encode the subunits that transport dibasic amino acids such as cysteine, which leads to defects in the absorption of filtered cystine in the proximal tubule, with the consequent accumulation and precipitation of crystals [44] (Table **1**).

In addition, other kidney stones are less frequent (<1%), among which are the following:

Xanthine stones $(C_5H_4N_4O_2)$ are rare in people with inherited xanthinuria, myeloproliferative diseases, and Lesch-Nyhan syndrome. Although the stones are accompanied by xanthine oxidase deficiency, no reports indicate renal failure in patients with these conditions [45].

2,8–Dihydroxyadenine stones $(C_5H_5N_5O_2)$ result from the enzyme adenine-phosphoribosyl transferase deficiency. There are few reports of these types of stones, and they can be attributed to a misinterpretation of uric acid compounds. These types of stones can be confirmed by infrared spectrophotometry [46, 47].

Table 1. Attenuation density in Hounsfield Units of the main stone composition.

Stones Composition	Attenuation Density (HU)
Hydroxyapatite	[120-1600]
Magnesium ammonium phosphate	[79-2143]
Cystine	[60-1100]
Calcium oxalate	[496–1868]
Uric acid	[20-450]

RISK FACTORS FOR RENAL DISEASE IN LITHIASIS

Renal lithiasis is a multifactorial disease. Ferrari *et al.* described several factors that can lead to the development of this disease and its complications [48]:

Individual risk factors. Among them, genetic factors can be observed in 25–40% of people with first-degree relatives with kidney stones. Other risk factors are age and sex; for example, studies have shown that men over 50 years old are at high risk for developing kidney stones [19, 48]. Several genes are involved in urolithiasis genesis, such as a) Taq1, Apa1, and Fok1, which are also genetic variants of the vitamin D receptor gene; the latter are observed in patients with hypercalciuria. b) The variant I550V of the NaDC1 gene, related to hypocitraturia, and variants in the *SLC3A1* and *SLC7A9* genes related to cystinuria, to name a few [49].

Environmental factors. People who live in deserts, mountainous places, tropical climates, or areas with high temperatures may be prone to developing kidney stones. This phenomenon is probably due to the high concentration of minerals in the water in places with hot weather, high temperatures, and/or low fluid intake, which leads to the filtration of minerals, supersaturation of the urine, and precipitation of crystals [48].

Lifestyle can be another risk factor; excessive consumption of carbonated drinks and a diet rich in sodium, calcium, and animal protein can promote the formation of new stones in the urinary tract; in the same way, minor consumption of liquid, a sedentary lifestyle, or a lack of sports can predispose individuals to kidney stone formation [50].

There are also *systemic diseases* that are prevalent in the population and are associated with the formation of stones, such as diabetes mellitus, obesity, hypertension, and metabolic syndrome; however, they are not the only systemic diseases since malabsorption and inflammatory processes in the intestine can cause kidney stones, but they are sporadic cases [48, 51].

Drugs such as indinavir have also been associated with stone formation. Therefore, researching the history of drug intake is important. The stones may be indinavir crystals, calcium oxalate, or phosphate [52].

DIAGNOSTIC METHODS

Renal lithiasis can be diagnosed by clinical symptoms or by imaging techniques. In general, patients can experience severe low back pain that spreads through the iliac fossa. The specialists suggest biochemical analysis when the first symptoms of the disease are present: serum creatinine levels, ionic calcium, plasma electrolytes (Na, K), prothrombin time, and international normalized ratio (PT/INP). In addition, a general urine test that quantifies red blood cells and white blood cells, nitrites, urinary pH, and urine culture is needed to determine infections [53]. However, these results are insufficient to accurately diagnose renal lithiasis because biochemical analysis and medical exploration results can be confused with other pathologies, such as irritable bowel syndrome or appendicitis.

Diagnosis by imaging is the best method used by specialists. The method can identify stone length and diameter, determine the specific location of the stone in the kidney, and identify stone attenuation and the presence of staghorn stones for practical surgical procedures.

Clinical History of Renal Lithiasis

The characteristic clinical finding of renal lithiasis is intense and stabbing pain at the lumbar level, which does not subside with changes in position and can radiate toward the ipsilateral region of the abdomen, groin, scrotum, or labia majora, and the inner thigh; on many occasions, the pain is intense and may be accompanied by vomiting. Occasionally, the pain is continuous but not intense, often confused with muscular or spinal pain. Hematuria is observed in 14.3% of patients with lithiasis and pain, sometimes as an initial clinical finding, which further directs the diagnosis toward a problem of urinary origin. Hematuria can be micro- or macroscopic, so it can generally be an alarm signal, forcing the patient to seek immediate medical attention [54].

Other nonspecific clinical data of renal lithiasis, which causes persistent complications in patients, include fever and a general physical feeling of malaise, both of which suggest an infection. Urinary tract infections are observed in 40% of patients with lithiasis and are more frequent in patients with risk factors for developing kidney stones. The infection can be moderate or severe, causing septic shock (OR 1.80; 95% CI 1.08–3.02; p=0.025) and even leading to death [55, 56].

Some patients may have acute kidney injury (AKI) or chronic kidney disease (CKD) because of renal lithiasis. AKI is rare in adults (0.72–2.00%) and is usually secondary to tubular obstruction due to crystallization or bilateral ureteral, urethral, or unilateral obstruction in patients with a single kidney. The risk of AKI increases in patients with urolithiasis (OR 1.95; 95% CI 1.22–3.12; p=0.045); however, the clinical data are not specific and usually manifest as decreased urinary volumes [56, 57]. Therefore, lithiasis increases the risk of renal function deterioration (OR 1.82; 95% CI 1.63–2.02; p=0.031). CKD is usually observed after a mean period of 10 years of lithiasis evolution, with an incidence of 11.2% compared to that of subjects without lithiasis (6.1%) [58].

There are reports of renal lithiasis in asymptomatic patients (4.3% to 5.8%). These diagnoses are usually detected when the patient undergoes ultrasound studies for different pathologies [59].

Diagnoses by Imaging

Several imaging techniques are used to diagnose renal lithiasis. The following section describes the main radiology techniques used for this purpose.

Radiologists and urologists first selected ultrasound, radiography, and excretory urography to diagnose renal lithiasis.

Ultrasonography is the most common method used in the diagnosis of renal lithiasis. Ultrasonography provides easy access for urologists and patients, is inexpensive, has no deleterious effects, and allows the identification of radiolucent calculi [38]. In addition, the method shows 74% sensitivity and 90% specificity in diagnosing renal lithiasis; the sensitivity and specificity decrease when the calculi are less than 3 mm [60]. Ultrasonography has several advantages: high availability in many clinics and hospitals, good cost-effectiveness, no radiation, and no need for intravenous contrast agent injections. In addition, ultrasonography effectively detects stones at the ureteral and vesicoureteral junctions and the bladder. However, it does not help diagnose ureteral stones, especially those in the middle portion of the ureter [61]. Ultrasonography can identify hydronephrosis in patients.

Additionally, it is recommended for pediatric patients, pregnant patients, and patients who experience recurrence of lithiasis because the technique does not involve radiation. One of the main factors that make diagnosing renal lithiasis difficult is the size of the stones. Some studies have reported a sensitivity of 13%

for stones smaller than 3 mm, a sensitivity of 26% for stones between 3-7 mm, and a sensitivity of 71% for stones greater than 7 mm; in all cases, the specificity reached 98% [62]. Currently, some centers are using a combination of ultrasonography and radiography to reduce radiation in patients with renal lithiasis or patients with recurrence of this disease. In addition, the combination of these techniques can help monitor the calculus in the urinary tract [38].

Radiography is used when the patient shows acute onset flank pain and continues to experience signs of renal colic. This technique is accessible, low-cost, and does not require qualified personnel. Radiography provides the first approximation of the disease because 90% of urinary tract calculi are radiopaque [38]. In addition, the technique uses a relatively low radiation dose compared with other techniques. Unfortunately, the method is not specific; its sensitivity and specificity are only 60% and 70%, respectively [63], and the radiopaque structures observed can be confused with other soft, osseous, or gas forms that can interfere with the calculi observed. However, many health professionals use radiography to closely monitor the progression or obstruction of calculi in patients with renal lithiasis.

Excretory urography is a contrast study used to determine whether kidney stones obstruct the urinary tract, particularly at the upper level. In addition, the method allows for a better delimitation of the anatomy of the kidney compared with the X-ray. The sensitivity and specificity are 85% and 94%, respectively [64]. This technique helps identify radiolucent structures such as uric acid stones in the kidney. Unfortunately, exposure to the contrast agent does not delay the contrast agent's excretion or increase the study's duration [38]. Despite the new diagnostic methods, excretory urography is still a good technique that provides excellent details of the urinary tract, especially in the renal pelvis and ureters.

Other methods for detecting renal lithiasis exist; however, in many cases, they require high radiation doses, sophisticated equipment, and specialist personnel for surgery.

Magnetic resonance urography (MR) is used to identify secondary effects caused by renal lithiasis. MR urography does not use ionizing radiation, and high-quality urography images comparable to those of sophisticated techniques such as computed tomography can be obtained [65]. Unfortunately, MR has several limitations, such as the significant duration of exploration. However, it is possible to shorten this exposure time using complementary techniques. Rapid acquisition with relaxation enhancement (RARE) has reduced the exposure time and has allowed us to obtain urography imaging sequences in a single breath-hold without contrast.

Additionally, a single shot achieves a resolution between 20-80 mm thickness without further processing. Another complementary technique is half-Fourier acquisition single-shot turbo spin echo (HASTE), which uses multiple shots but only acquires half of the image lines to save time, calculating the other half by symmetry. The technique can acquire between 10-20 cuts of 3-5 mm in only one apnea [66]. MR urography can be used in combination with radiography in pediatric and pregnant patients with renal lithiasis recurrence [38, 65].

Computed tomography (CT) is the gold standard for detecting renal lithiasis. CT can detect kidney stones up to 1 mm in length due to its high sensitivity of approximately 98-100% and high specificity of 96-100% [36]. The technique consists of a quick procedure, which does not require a specific preparation of the patient or the injection of contrast solutions. In addition, image acquisition can measure calculi attenuation through Hounsfield units, assess the secondary effects of renal obstruction, show the anatomical aspects of surgical procedures, and detect other specific pain regions with abnormalities [38, 67]. For calculi detection, radiologists recommend making helicoidal cuts to reduce imaging artifacts due to respiratory movements that can mask small stones. The technique also allows multiplanar or curved reconstruction that better visualizes the exact position of the stone in the urinary tract [68]. CT is used to identify phleboliths or calcified structures that are usually confused with stones and could eventually provide more information on the urinary tract. The disadvantage of this technique lies mainly in ionizing radiation with significant doses on average of 10 mSv, equivalent to approximately the natural radiation accumulated in 4.5 years, or approximately 500 plain radiographs [69]. Similarly, it is contraindicated in pregnant women and pediatric patients. The high costs associated with this technique are also of concern compared to those associated with other imaging techniques, surgical personnel, and the insufficient availability of CT scanners with adequate resolution to carry out renal lithiasis studies in small hospitals or small populations.

Despite the drawbacks of the CT technique, its use has shown great utility for determining the attenuation of stones expressed in Hounsfield units. These units can predict kidney stone composition [39, 70].

In addition, the CT technique can reveal other interesting radiological aspects of renal lithiasis, such as a) the exact number of kidney stones, which depends on the metabolic state of each patient; b) the size of the stone; c) the anatomical location of the kidney, where the stone can be located in the upper, middle and/or lower collector of the kidney and/or the ureteral junction; and d) the relevant anatomy, the relationship of the kidney with other proximal organs (the gallbladder, pleural reflections, and the diaphragm), or with various anatomies (kidney transplantation, pelvic kidney, and diaphragm) [37, 38].

Recently, some studies have been published on detecting and diagnosing renal lithiasis using *dual-energy CT*. Dual-energy CT is a technique that uses two separate and independent X-ray photon energy spectra to read the projection data at different time points, which can provide spectral information in single-source systems but with different spectral sensitivities. The Compton effect causes X-ray attenuation, coherent scattering, and the photoelectric effect. The goal of the technique is to replace the protocol used in a single-dose test and to avoid an extra radiation dose to the patient. Therefore, the dual-energy CT technique may be a viable alternative for detecting stones, especially in patients who experience renal lithiasis recurrence [71, 72].

Methods to Determine the Stone Composition

Determining the composition of renal stones is one of the main objectives of urologists and nephrologists. Developing an adequate etiological diagnosis and specific treatment for each patient is possible. Some methods for detecting stone compounds range from chemical methods to those measured by imaging techniques. *Infrared spectroscopy* and *X-ray crystallography* are used to determine the chemical compounds of stones; however, CT or dual-energy CT techniques can determine the stone compounds through *Hounsfield units*.

X-ray crystallography is the most frequent method for determining proteins, viruses, immune complexes, protein-nuclei acids, and biological macromolecules. In addition, it is an excellent method used to determine stone composition because urinary calculi consist of an accumulation of crystals that precipitate and are compacted to form renal stones [73]. The composition of the stone can be in its nucleus or nucleation center. The principle of this method consists of passing the X-ray beam through a crystal of the sample. The diffraction beam splits in several directions, resulting in an intensity pattern that can be interpreted based on the location of the crystal atom. The intensities obtained can determine the structures of the crystals, generating a map of electron density that can construct the sample's molecular structure (stones in the case of renal lithiasis) [74].

The main compounds detected via X-ray crystallography are calcium oxalate monohydrate, calcium oxalate dihydrate, magnesium ammonium phosphate hexahydrate, magnesium hydrogen phosphate trihydrate, hydroxyapatite, carbonate-apatite, calcium hydrogen phosphate dihydrate, tricalcium phosphate, octacalcium phosphate, uric acid, uric acid dihydrate, ammonium acid urate, sodium acid urate monohydrate, cystine, xanthine, calcium sulfate dihydrate and 2,8-dihydroxyadenine [40].

The infrared spectroscopy method absorbs radiation in a wavelength range through a substance to identify structural differences. The infrared spectrum is described in terms of wavenumber and is expressed in cm^{-1}. The wavelength ranges of electromagnetic energy can be divided into near-infrared (NIR) [78-2500 nm, 1280-4000 cm^{-1}], mid-infrared (MIR) [2.5–25 mm, 400-400 cm^{-1}], and far infrared [25–400 mm, 40-25 cm^{-1}]. Among the three infrared regions, the NIR spectrum is the most commonly used for identifying compounds in urinary stones [75, 76]. The infrared spectroscopy principle states that infrared radiation is emitted in two parallel beams of equal intensity. One ray passes through the sample, and the other ray serves to compensate for the absorption of infrared radiation by water vapor and carbon dioxide from the source to the monochromator. The infrared spectrum was recorded with a sodium chloride prism in the monochromator. The pen system of the recorder directly indicates the transmittance as a percentage of the sample [76, 77].

The main compounds detected using infrared spectroscopy were calcium oxalate monohydrate, calcium oxalate dihydrate, tertiary calcium phosphate, uric acid, and cystine. The technique can also detect magnesium phosphate, hydroxyapatite, xanthine, calcium sulfate dihydrate, and 2,8-dihydroxyadenine, among others.

The Hounsfield units are the most common imaging method used to determine the possible composition of renal stones. As mentioned above, Hounsfield units are related to the density of the tissue or stone. Hounsfield units result from the linear X-ray attenuation scale, and its value is related to distilled water at standard pressure and temperature [78]. The Hounsfield units are obtained from the images generated by the CT. The images can generate grayscale intensities, called Hounsfield units; the scale is based on the attenuation of each sample. The range of the scale is from [1000] Hounsfield units to [−1000] Hounsfield units, with approximately [1000] units for solid structures such as bone and approximately [−1000] units for soft structures such as air. Zero Hounsfield units correspond to distilled water [70, 79].

Unfortunately, Hounsfield units do not show similar ranges at the same stone composition interlaboratory results. In other words, depending on the laboratory, when analyzing two fragments of the same stone, the range of the Hounsfield units could be different. This phenomenon is not observed with X-ray crystallography or infrared spectroscopy because the results are similar. Comparing the studies of Marchiñena et al., Zarse et al., and Gupta et al., when identifying the compounds involved in renal lithiasis, they observed that the intervals of the calcium oxalate monohydrate were [496–1865], [1707–1925], and [507–1639], respectively, and when they identified magnesium ammonium phosphate, their results were [79-2143], [862–944], and [549–869], respectively. Only the uric acid compound was well identified [30-450] [80 - 82]. The differences in the measurements could be because of the acquisition method and not because of the CT or energy-dual CT technique [83]. However, the results could be underestimated because they are operator-dependent.

Using Hounsfield units, it is possible to identify the following compounds: calcium oxalate monohydrate, calcium oxalate dihydrate, magnesium ammonium phosphate, hydroxyapatite, carbonate-apatite, calcium hydrogen phosphate dihydrate, uric acid, uric acid dihydrate, and ammonium acid urate. However, this technique has not been reported for cystine, xanthine, or 2,8-dihydroxyadenine; perhaps the limitation is associated with structures with similar attenuations or optical isomeric ions in the compounds that make up the renal stone.

CURRENT STUDIES OF RENAL LITHIASIS

As mentioned previously, renal lithiasis is a multifactorial disease. New studies in this field have focused on corrective treatment and less on preventive methods. In the past, exploratory and open surgeries were the primary treatments used by specialists; moreover, minimally invasive surgeries, endourological procedures, and specialized drugs are the new methods used for patients with this disease. In addition, the importance of the nutrition plan in patients with renal lithiasis can become increasingly important in the treatment of this disease.

TREATMENT OF KIDNEY STONES

The treatment of kidney stones should involve a multidisciplinary approach. The diagnosis of renal lithiasis must be established using the methods mentioned above. In this context, it is necessary to know the characteristics of the stones (location, size, number, Hounsfield units), define whether there are comorbidities or risk factors that could increase the probability of kidney stone diagnosis, and determine the presence of metabolic abnormalities.

Once clinical information is obtained, it must be determined whether surgical treatment is required and whether the procedure is urgent. The size of the stone, obstruction, or some complications (abscess, hydronephrosis) were considered for these decisions. The urologist defines the method used to remove the stones and the type of surgical approach (open surgery, endourology, minimally invasive surgery, among others), and it can vary depending on the patient [84]. If the stone is obtained, infrared spectroscopy studies are recommended, as there are components such as cystine, neuberite, xanthine, and 2-8-dihydroxyadenine, which conventional laboratory methods cannot determine [76, 77].

The treatment of this disease can be nutritional and/or pharmacological. These studies should focus on risk factors and the detection of metabolic abnormalities. In acute and intense pain cases, the patient should receive care for pain management in the emergency medical unit. If the patient shows an infection, adequate medication must be given to expel the stones [85]. The treatment goal is to control or correct risk factors and change the urine composition to prevent stone formation and/or growth. In most cases, treatment begins with drug induction before providing nutritional recommendations, which must be carried out jointly.

Nonmedical or nutritional treatment includes some general recommendations that apply to all patients with lithiasis, such as a) the intake of 2.5 to 3 liters of water per day to promote the excretion of diluted urine to prevent urine concentration; b) the intake of drinks with citrus fruits (oranges and lemons), which provide magnesium and natural citrates, substances that inhibit the crystallization of urine; and c) reducing the consumption of sodium or salt, since the excess of these substances increases the excretion of promoter substances and decreases the excretion of substances that inhibit crystallization. In general, eliminating high-sodium foods, snacks, and canned foods from the diet is recommended [86].

Therefore, a balanced diet rich in vegetables and fiber is recommended. Animal proteins should be restricted (to avoid acidifying the urine and decreasing the excretion of citrates), and calcium should be maintained at a regular daily intake. A decrease in calcium intake favors the intestinal absorption of oxalates and, eventually, the formation of new stones. In patients with oxalate stones, celery, spinach, radishes, and chocolates should be restricted [87].

It is important to remember that the etiology of kidney stones is multifactorial, and the comorbidities that patients may suffer (obesity, diabetes, hypertension) should not be overlooked, so the primary focus should be on nutritional aspects. This approach includes lifestyle, so it is recommended to perform physical activity regularly, manage stress, and stay well hydrated, especially in cases of excessive sweating, in climates with high temperatures, or due to intense sports or work activity. The nutritionist must be involved in managing patients with kidney stones to increase the chances of success in reducing recurrence or increasing the size of the stones.

Pharmacological treatment is usually adequate. For this, it is essential that the patient correctly follow the indications provided by the specialist. The following drugs have been used to treat metabolic disorders [85]:

Allopurinol. In some cases of hyperuricosuria and uric acid stones, uric acid crystals form a nucleation center to which calcium crystals are added to form calcium stones; this process works by lowering uric acid levels in urine.

Thiazides (hydrochlorothiazides) and *pseudothiazides (indapamines).* It is used when there is hypercalciuria to reduce the elimination of calcium in the urine.

Citrate solutions (sodium citrate and potassium citrate) are indicated for patients with hypocitraturia, urinary pH less than 5.5, and uric acid lithiasis. Citrate inhibits the growth and aggregation of crystals in the urine and forms complexes with calcium and phosphate, decreasing these substances in the urine. Other alkalizing substances used are sodium and potassium bicarbonate.

Drugs that are less commonly used include the following:

Magnesium. It inhibits the growth of calcium phosphate crystals and the formation of Brushite stones.

Pyridoxine (vitamin B6). It is indicated for patients with primary and idiopathic hyperoxaluria combined with orthophosphate.

D-penicillamine is indicated for cystinuria. It inhibits the crystallization of cystine, preventing the formation of stones. However, the associated costs and side effects limit its use.

Alpha-mercaptopropionyl glycine (thiopronine). Like D-penicillamine, it has fewer side effects but is less effective.

FUTURE PERSPECTIVES

Currently, studies are focused on new methods of diagnosis and treatment. However, several groups are working on early diagnosis through imaging techniques to identify the specific compound of urinary stones, on the design of systematized methods to obtain specific Hounsfield units, and on the design of new devices capable of separating resonant structures and objectively identifying the compound of the stone.

In the treatment, new minimally invasive surgical and laparoscopic procedures are used. The prototypes of medical robots for surgical procedures and the design of wireless laparoscopic microdevices for obtaining images and biopsies in real-time have attracted the attention of biomedical researchers, all of whom aim to obtain personalized and individualized treatment for patients. In addition, nanotechnologies such as lab-on-a-chip are being used to detect abnormalities (mutations, deletions, polymorphisms) at the cellular and molecular levels that could lead to possible kidney stones or possible complications.

It is crucial to form multidisciplinary teams (urologists, internists, nephrologists, researchers, and nutritionists) focused on managing patients with kidney stones. Workgroups must receive adequate training to contribute to the early diagnosis of the disease and prevent its progression, significantly improving patient's quality of life.

Finally, it is essential to create appropriate programs focused on preventing the disease, raising awareness of the secondary ailments that cause kidney stones, and generating campaigns for the most vulnerable population.

REFERENCES

[1]   Shah J, Whitfield HN. Urolithiasis through the ages. BJU Int 2002; 89(8): 801-10.
      [http://dx.doi.org/10.1046/j.1464-410X.2002.02769.x] [PMID: 11972501]

[2]   Chakravorty RC. Urinary stones their cause and treatment as described in the sushrutasamhita. Hist Sci Med 1982; 17(Spec 2): 328-32.
      [PMID: 11612318]

[3]   Dimopoulos C, Gialas A, Likourinas M, Androutsos G, Kostakopoulos A. Hippocrates: founder and pioneer of urology. Br J Urol 1980; 52(2): 73-4.
      [http://dx.doi.org/10.1111/j.1464-410X.1980.tb02931.x] [PMID: 7000221]

[4]   Tefekli A, Cezayirli F. The history of urinary stones: in parallel with civilization. ScientificWorldJournal 2013; 2013(1): 423964.
      [http://dx.doi.org/10.1155/2013/423964] [PMID: 24348156]

[5]   Gonzalo Rodríguez V, Pérez Albacete M, Pérez-Castro Ellendt E. El mal de la piedra . Archivos Españoles de Urología (Ed. impresa) 2009; 62: 623–629.

[6]   Riethe P. [Hildegards von Bingen 'Liber simplicis medicinae' in the Mainz 'Garden of Health']. Sudhoffs Arch Z Wissenschaftsgesch 2005; 89(1): 96-119. [Hildegards von Bingen 'Liber simplicis medicinae' in the Mainz 'Garden of Health'].
      [PMID: 16095070]

[7]   Sohgaura A, Bigoniya P. A Review on Epidemiology and Etiology of Renal Stone. American Journal of Drug Discovery and Development 2017; 7(2): 54-62.
      [http://dx.doi.org/10.3923/ajdd.2017.54.62]

[8]   Gamboa Gutiérrez E, Varela Villalobos M, Varela Briceño C. Litiasis renal en Costa Rica: bioquímica y epidemiología. Acta Med Costarric 2020; 62(2): 79-83.
      [http://dx.doi.org/10.51481/amc.v62i2.1065]

[9]   Romero V, Akpinar H, Assimos DG. Kidney stones: a global picture of prevalence, incidence, and associated risk factors. Rev Urol 2010; 12(2-3): e86-96.
      [PMID: 20811557]

[10] Stamatelou KK, Francis ME, Jones CA, Nyberg LM Jr, Curhan GC. Time trends in reported prevalence of kidney stones in the United States: 1976–199411.See Editorial by Goldfarb, p. 1951. Kidney Int 2003; 63(5): 1817-23.
      [http://dx.doi.org/10.1046/j.1523-1755.2003.00917.x] [PMID: 12675858]

[11] Scales CD Jr, Smith AC, Hanley JM, Saigal CS. Prevalence of kidney stones in the United States. Eur Urol 2012; 62(1): 160-5.

[http://dx.doi.org/10.1016/j.eururo.2012.03.052] [PMID: 22498635]

[12]   Chen Z, Prosperi M, Bird VY. Prevalence of kidney stones in the USA: The National Health and Nutrition Evaluation Survey. J Clin Urol 2019; 12(4): 296-302.
[http://dx.doi.org/10.1177/2051415818813820]

[13]   Osther PJS. Epidemiology of Kidney Stones in the European Union Urolithiasis – Basic Science and Clinical Practice. Springer 2012.

[14]   Wang W, Fan J, Huang G, *et al.* Prevalence of kidney stones in mainland China: A systematic review. Sci Rep 2017; 7(1): 41630.
[http://dx.doi.org/10.1038/srep41630] [PMID: 28139722]

[15]   Ahmad F, Nada M, Farid A, Haleem MA, Razack SMA. Epidemiology of urolithiasis with emphasis on ultrasound detection: A retrospective analysis of 5371 cases in Saudi Arabia. Saudi J Kidney Dis Transpl 2015; 26(2): 386-91.
[http://dx.doi.org/10.4103/1319-2442.152557] [PMID: 25758899]

[16]   Chen VY, Chen Y. The first epidemiology study of urolithiasis in New Brunswick. Can Urol Assoc J 2021; 15(7): E356-60.
[PMID: 33382373]

[17]   Sharma AP, Filler G. Epidemiology of pediatric urolithiasis. Indian journal of urology: IJU: journal of the Urological Society of India 2010; 26: 516–522.

[18]   Gomez-Orta F, Reyes-Sosa G, Espinosa-Said L, *et al.* Algunos aspectos epidemiologicos de la litiasis renal en Mexico. Cir Cir 1984; 52: 365-72.

[19]   Medina-Escobedo M, Zaidi M, Real-de León E, Orozco-Rivadeneyra S. Urolithiasis prevalence and risk factors in Yucatan, Mexico. Salud Publica Mex 2002; 44(6): 541-5.
[http://dx.doi.org/10.1590/S0036-36342002000600006] [PMID: 20383456]

[20]   Ortegón-Gallareta R, Aguilar-Moreno J, Álvarez-Baeza A, Méndez-Domínguez N, Pech-Cervantes PI. Perfil epidemiológico de las hospitalizaciones por urolitiasis en el Estado de Yucatán, México. Rev Mex Urol 2019; 79(5): 1-11.
[http://dx.doi.org/10.48193/revistamexicanadeurologa.v79i5.517]

[21]   Ruiz A, Pérez P, Ponte M, *et al.* Prevalencia de nefrolitiasis en pacientes que asisten al hospital nacional de clínicas de la provincia de Córdoba, Argentina. Consideraciones fisiopatológicas. Nephrol Argentina 2015; 13: 105-14.

[22]   Chewcharat A, Curhan G. Trends in the prevalence of kidney stones in the United States from 2007 to 2016. Urolithiasis 2021; 49(1): 27-39.
[http://dx.doi.org/10.1007/s00240-020-01210-w] [PMID: 32870387]

[23]   Eisner BH, Goldfarb DS. A nomogram for the prediction of kidney stone recurrence. J Am Soc Nephrol 2014; 25(12): 2685-7.
[http://dx.doi.org/10.1681/ASN.2014060631] [PMID: 25104802]

[24]   Peña-Rodríguez JC. Avances y retos en la fisiopatología y tratamiento de la nefrolitiasis. Acta Med Grupo Ángeles 2016; 14: 155-61.

[25]   Faridi M, Singh K. Preliminary study of prevalence of urolithiasis in North-Eastern city of India. J Family Med Prim Care 2020; 9(12): 5939-43.
[http://dx.doi.org/10.4103/jfmpc.jfmpc_1522_20] [PMID: 33681023]

[26]   Yasui T, Okada A, Hamamoto S, et al. Pathophysiology-based treatment of urolithiasis. International journal of urology: official journal of the Japanese Urological Association 2017; 24: 32–38.

[27]   Pfau A, Knauf F. Update on Nephrolithiasis: Core Curriculum 2016. Am J Kidney Dis 2016; 68(6): 973-85.
[http://dx.doi.org/10.1053/j.ajkd.2016.05.016] [PMID: 27497526]

[28]   Jayaram U, Gurusamy A. Review on Uro-Lithiasis Pathophysiology and Aesculapian Discussion.

IOSR J Pharm 2018; 8: 30-42.

[29]   García-Perdomo HA, Solarte PB, España PP. Pathophysiology associated with forming urinary stones. Urología Colombiana 2016; 25(2): 118-25.
[http://dx.doi.org/10.1016/j.uroco.2015.12.013]

[30]   Figueres L, Hourmant M, Lemoine S. Understanding and managing hypercalciuria in adults with nephrolithiasis: keys for nephrologists. Nephrol Dial Transplant 2020; 35(4): 573-5.
[http://dx.doi.org/10.1093/ndt/gfz099] [PMID: 31219589]

[31]   Alelign T, Petros B. Kidney Stone Disease: An Update on Current Concepts. Adv Urol 2018; 2018: 1-12.
[http://dx.doi.org/10.1155/2018/3068365] [PMID: 29515627]

[32]   Aggarwal KP, Narula S, Kakkar M, Tandon C. Nephrolithiasis: molecular mechanism of renal stone formation and the critical role played by modulators. BioMed Res Int 2013; 2013: 1-21.
[http://dx.doi.org/10.1155/2013/292953] [PMID: 24151593]

[33]   Sansores-España DJ, Medina-Escobedo MMLÁ, Rubio-Zapata HA, Romero-Campos SG, Leal-Ortega G. Metabolic syndrome and urolithiasis: a case-control study. Rev Med Inst Mex Seguro Soc 2020; 58(6): 657-65.
[PMID: 34705397]

[34]   Medina-Escobedo M, Alcocer-Dzul R, López-López J, Salha-Villanueva J. Obesity as a risk factor for metabolic disorders in adults with urolithiasis. Rev Med Inst Mex Seguro Soc 2015; 53(6): 692-7.
[PMID: 26506485]

[35]   Kravdal G, Helgø D, Moe MK. Kidney stone compositions and frequencies in a Norwegian population. Scand J Urol 2019; 53(2-3): 139-44.
[http://dx.doi.org/10.1080/21681805.2019.1606031] [PMID: 31070078]

[36]   Smith CL. Renal stone analysis. Curr Opin Nephrol Hypertens 1998; 7(6): 703-10.
[http://dx.doi.org/10.1097/00041552-199811000-00014] [PMID: 9864669]

[37]   Enríquez G, Viramontes T. Lo que no debe faltar en una interpretación de… "litiasis renal". Anales de Radiología México 2006; 5: 184-7.

[38]   Cheng PM, Moin P, Dunn MD, Boswell WD, Duddalwar VA. What the radiologist needs to know about urolithiasis: part 1--pathogenesis, types, assessment, and variant anatomy. AJR Am J Roentgenol 2012; 198(6): W540-7.
[http://dx.doi.org/10.2214/AJR.10.7285] [PMID: 22623568]

[39]   Chávez NC, Castillo JO, Serrato AM, *et al.* Utilidad de las unidades Hounsfield en la predicción de la composición química de los cálculos urinarios. 2014.

[40]   Sutor DJ, Scheidt S. Identification standards for human urinary calculus components, using crystallographic methods. Br J Urol 1968; 40(1): 22-8.
[http://dx.doi.org/10.1111/j.1464-410X.1968.tb11808.x] [PMID: 5642759]

[41]   Liu Y, Qu M, Carter RE, *et al.* Differentiating calcium oxalate and hydroxyapatite stones in vivo using dual-energy CT and urine supersaturation and pH values. Acad Radiol 2013; 20(12): 1521-5.
[http://dx.doi.org/10.1016/j.acra.2013.08.018] [PMID: 24200478]

[42]   Rutchik SD, Resnick MI. Cystine calculi. Diagnosis and management. Urol Clin North Am 1997; 24(1): 163-71.
[http://dx.doi.org/10.1016/S0094-0143(05)70361-X] [PMID: 9048859]

[43]   Bhatta KM, Prien EL Jr, Dretler SP. Cystine calculi--rough and smooth: a new clinical distinction. J Urol 1989; 142(4): 937-40.
[http://dx.doi.org/10.1016/S0022-5347(17)38946-2] [PMID: 2795746]

[44]   Øbro LF, Pedersen KV, Lildal SK, *et al.* The challenges of cystinuria in the twenty-first century: a mini review. 2016.

[45]   Pais VM Jr, Lowe G, Lallas CD, Preminger GM, Assimos DG. Xanthine urolithiasis. Urology 2006; 67(5): 1084.e9-1084.e11.
[http://dx.doi.org/10.1016/j.urology.2005.10.057] [PMID: 16698380]

[46]   Simmonds HA. 2,8-Dihydroxyadenine lithiasis--epidemiology, pathogenesis and therapy. Verh Dtsch Ges Inn Med 1986; 92: 503-8.
[http://dx.doi.org/10.1007/978-3-642-85459-0_96] [PMID: 3492830]

[47]   Manyak MJ, Frensilli FJ, Miller HC. 2,8-Dihydroxyadenine urolithiasis: report of an adult case in the United States. J Urol 1987; 137(2): 312-4.
[http://dx.doi.org/10.1016/S0022-5347(17)43993-0] [PMID: 3806829]

[48]   Ferrari P, Piazza R, Ghidini N, Bisi M, Galizia G, Ferrari G. Lithiasis and risk factors. Urol Int 2007; 79 (Suppl. 1): 8-15.
[http://dx.doi.org/10.1159/000104435] [PMID: 17726346]

[49]   Vasudevan V, Samson P, Smith AD, Okeke Z. The genetic framework for development of nephrolithiasis. Asian J Urol 2017; 4(1): 18-26.
[http://dx.doi.org/10.1016/j.ajur.2016.11.003] [PMID: 29264202]

[50]   Shah S, Calle JC. Dietary and medical management of recurrent nephrolithiasis. Cleve Clin J Med 2016; 83(6): 463-71.
[http://dx.doi.org/10.3949/ccjm.83a.15089] [PMID: 27281259]

[51]   Taylor EN, Stampfer MJ, Curhan GC. Obesity, weight gain, and the risk of kidney stones. JAMA 2005; 293(4): 455-62.
[http://dx.doi.org/10.1001/jama.293.4.455] [PMID: 15671430]

[52]   Izzedine H, Lescure FX, Bonnet F. HIV medication-based urolithiasis. Clin Kidney J 2014; 7(2): 121-6.
[http://dx.doi.org/10.1093/ckj/sfu008] [PMID: 25852859]

[53]   Susaeta R, Benavente D, Marchant F, Gana R. Diagnóstico y manejo de litiasis renales en adultos y niños. Rev Med Clin Las Condes 2018; 29(2): 197-212.
[http://dx.doi.org/10.1016/j.rmclc.2018.03.002]

[54]   Spivacow, del Valle EE L, Negri A. Hematuria as First Sign of Presentation in Urolithiasis. 2016.

[55]   Sarla G. An Association between Urolithiasis and Urinary Tract Infection. Int J Innov Med Health Sci 2018; 10: 6-11.

[56]   Hsiao CY, Chen TH, Lee YC, *et al.* Urolithiasis Is a Risk Factor for Uroseptic Shock and Acute Kidney Injury in Patients With Urinary Tract Infection. Front Med (Lausanne) 2019; 6: 288.
[http://dx.doi.org/10.3389/fmed.2019.00288] [PMID: 31867338]

[57]   Tang X, Lieske JC. Acute and chronic kidney injury in nephrolithiasis. Curr Opin Nephrol Hypertens 2014; 23(4): 385-90.
[http://dx.doi.org/10.1097/01.mnh.0000447017.28852.52] [PMID: 24848936]

[58]   Chuang TF, Hung HC, Li SF, Lee MW, Pai JY, Hung CT. Risk of chronic kidney disease in patients with kidney stones—a nationwide cohort study. BMC Nephrol 2020; 21(1): 292.
[http://dx.doi.org/10.1186/s12882-020-01950-2] [PMID: 32698782]

[59]   Bansal AD, Hui J, Goldfarb DS. Asymptomatic nephrolithiasis detected by ultrasound. Clin J Am Soc Nephrol 2009; 4(3): 680-4.
[http://dx.doi.org/10.2215/CJN.05181008] [PMID: 19261817]

[60]   Fowler KAB, Locken JA, Duchesne JH, Williamson MR. US for detecting renal calculi with nonenhanced CT as a reference standard. Radiology 2002; 222(1): 109-13.
[http://dx.doi.org/10.1148/radiol.2221010453] [PMID: 11756713]

[61]   Pais VM Jr, Payton AL, LaGrange CA. Urolithiasis in Pregnancy. Urol Clin North Am 2007; 34(1): 43-52.

[http://dx.doi.org/10.1016/j.ucl.2006.10.011] [PMID: 17145360]

[62]   Masch WR, Cronin KC, Sahani DV, Kambadakone A. Imaging in Urolithiasis. Radiol Clin North Am 2017; 55(2): 209-24.
[http://dx.doi.org/10.1016/j.rcl.2016.10.002] [PMID: 28126212]

[63]   Dyer RB, Munitz HA, Bechtold R, Choplin RH. The abnormal nephrogram. Radiographics 1986; 6(6): 1039-63.
[http://dx.doi.org/10.1148/radiographics.6.6.3685518] [PMID: 3685518]

[64]   Warshauer DM, McCarthy SM, Street L, *et al.* Detection of renal masses: sensitivities and specificities of excretory urography/linear tomography, US, and CT. Radiology 1988; 169(2): 363-5.
[http://dx.doi.org/10.1148/radiology.169.2.3051112] [PMID: 3051112]

[65]   Geva T. Magnetic resonance imaging: historical perspective. J Cardiovasc Magn Reson 2006; 8: 573–580.

[66]   Balci NC, Mueller-Lisse UG, Holzknecht N, Gauger J, Waidelich R, Reiser M. Breathhold MR urography: comparison between HASTE and RARE in healthy volunteers. Eur Radiol 1998; 8(6): 925-32.
[http://dx.doi.org/10.1007/s003300050489] [PMID: 9683694]

[67]   Türk C, Petřík A, Sarica K, *et al.* EAU Guidelines on Diagnosis and Conservative Management of Urolithiasis. Eur Urol 2016; 69(3): 468-74.
[http://dx.doi.org/10.1016/j.eururo.2015.07.040] [PMID: 26318710]

[68]   Heneghan JP, McGuire KA, Leder RA, DeLong DM, Yoshizumi T, Nelson RC. Helical CT for nephrolithiasis and ureterolithiasis: comparison of conventional and reduced radiation-dose techniques. Radiology 2003; 229(2): 575-80.
[http://dx.doi.org/10.1148/radiol.2292021261] [PMID: 14526095]

[69]   Moore CL, Daniels B, Singh D, *et al.* Ureteral stones: Implementation of a reduced-dose CT protocol in patients in the emergency department with moderate to high likelihood of calculi on the basis of stone score. Radiology 2016; 280(3): 743-51.
[http://dx.doi.org/10.1148/radiol.2016151691] [PMID: 26943230]

[70]   Kijvikai K, de la Rosette JJM. Assessment of stone composition in the management of urinary stones. Nat Rev Urol 2011; 8(2): 81-5.
[http://dx.doi.org/10.1038/nrurol.2010.209] [PMID: 21135879]

[71]   Johnson TRC. Dual-Energy CT: General Principles. AJR Am J Roentgenol 2012; 199(5_supplement) (Suppl.): S3-8.
[http://dx.doi.org/10.2214/AJR.12.9116] [PMID: 23097165]

[72]   Fung GSK, Kawamoto S, Matlaga BR, *et al.* Differentiation of kidney stones using dual-energy CT with and without a tin filter. AJR Am J Roentgenol 2012; 198(6): 1380-6.
[http://dx.doi.org/10.2214/AJR.11.7217] [PMID: 22623552]

[73]   Smyth MS, Martin JH. X ray crystallography. Molecular pathology: MP 2000; 53: 8–14.

[74]   Rodgers AL. Analysis of renal calculi by X-ray diffraction and electron microprobe: a comparison of two methods. Invest Urol 1981; 19(1): 25-8.
[PMID: 7251321]

[75]   Ng LM, Simmons R. Infrared Spectroscopy. Anal Chem 1999; 71(12): 343-50.
[http://dx.doi.org/10.1021/a1999908r] [PMID: 10384791]

[76]   Ferrari M, Mottola L, Quaresima V. Principles, techniques, and limitations of near infrared spectroscopy. Canadian journal of applied physiology = Revue canadienne de physiologie appliquee 2004; 29: 463–487.

[77]   Lehmann CA, McClure GL, Smolens I. Identification of renal calculi by computerized infrared spectroscopy. Clin Chim Acta 1988; 173(2): 107-16.

[http://dx.doi.org/10.1016/0009-8981(88)90248-3] [PMID: 3378352]

[78]   Ito H, Kawahara T, Terao H, *et al.* Predictive value of attenuation coefficients measured as Hounsfield units on noncontrast computed tomography during flexible ureteroscopy with holmium laser lithotripsy: a single-center experience. J Endourol 2012; 26(9): 1125-30.
[http://dx.doi.org/10.1089/end.2012.0154] [PMID: 22519718]

[79]   Kuwahara M, Kageyama S, Kurosu S, Orikasa S. Computed tomography and composition of renal calculi. Urol Res 1984; 12(2): 111-3.
[http://dx.doi.org/10.1007/BF00257175] [PMID: 6740833]

[80]   García Marchiñena P, Billordo Peres N, Liyo J, *et al.* CT SCAN as a predictor of composition and fragility of urinary lithiasis treated with extracorporeal shock wave lithotripsy *in vitro.* Arch Esp Urol 2009; 62(3): 215-22.
[PMID: 19542594]

[81]   Zarse CA, Hameed TA, Jackson ME, *et al.* CT visible internal stone structure, but not Hounsfield unit value, of calcium oxalate monohydrate (COM) calculi predicts lithotripsy fragility in vitro. Urol Res 2007; 35(4): 201-6.
[http://dx.doi.org/10.1007/s00240-007-0104-6] [PMID: 17565491]

[82]   Gupta NP, Ansari MS, Kesarvani P, Kapoor A, Mukhopadhyay S. Role of computed tomography with no contrast medium enhancement in predicting the outcome of extracorporeal shock wave lithotripsy for urinary calculi. BJU Int 2005; 95(9): 1285-8.
[http://dx.doi.org/10.1111/j.1464-410X.2005.05520.x] [PMID: 15892818]

[83]   Gallioli A, De Lorenzis E, Boeri L, *et al.* Clinical utility of computed tomography Hounsfield characterization for percutaneous nephrolithotomy: a cross-sectional study. BMC Urol 2017; 17(1): 104.
[http://dx.doi.org/10.1186/s12894-017-0296-1] [PMID: 29145836]

[84]   Streeper NM. Asymptomatic Renal Stones—to Treat or Not to Treat. Curr Urol Rep 2018; 19(5): 29.
[http://dx.doi.org/10.1007/s11934-018-0782-3] [PMID: 29550897]

[85]   Fontenelle LF, Sarti TD. Kidney Stones: Treatment and Prevention. Am Fam Physician 2019; 99(8): 490-6.
[PMID: 30990297]

[86]   Ng DM, Haleem M, Mamuchashvili A, *et al.* Medical evaluation and pharmacotherapeutical strategies in management of urolithiasis. Ther Adv Urol 2021; 13: 1756287221993300.
[http://dx.doi.org/10.1177/1756287221993300] [PMID: 33708261]

[87]   Guha M, Banerjee H, Mitra P, Das M. The Demographic Diversity of Food Intake and Prevalence of Kidney Stone Diseases in the Indian Continent. Foods 2019; 8(1): 37. Epub ahead of print
[http://dx.doi.org/10.3390/foods8010037] [PMID: 30669549]

CHAPTER 9

Sodium Imbalance and Hypertension: An Old and Current Disease

Mercedes Aguilar-Soto[1] and **Fabio Solis-Jiménez**[2,*]

[1] *Instituto Nacional de Ciencias Médicas y Nutrición" Salvador Zubirán", Mexico City, Mexico*

[2] *Instituto Nacional de Cardiología Ignacio Chávez, Tlalpan 14080, Mexico City, Mexico*

Abstract: The global prevalence of hypertension in adults ranges between 30-40% of the population, with an age-standardized global prevalence between 24 and 20 in women and men, respectively. Individuals with hypertension face approximately 2,000 dollars higher annual healthcare expenditure compared to an individual who does not suffer from it. Although it is considered a disease of multifactorial origin, there is broad agreement that excess salt in the diet is the most important controllable factor in the increase in blood pressure. In the study of arterial hypertension and sensitivity to sodium, the sodium intake in humans in developed countries is subject to important variations from day to day. The balance in sodium is controlled almost entirely by the ability of the kidney to vary urinary sodium excretion. The immediate effect of ingested sodium in the diet is to modify plasma sodium and extracellular volume. The increase in plasma sodium is rapidly dampened by the increase in osmolarity that tends to move fluid from the intracellular space to the extracellular space. Small increases in plasma sodium also strongly stimulate the thirst center, causing increased water intake and vasopressin secretion. These mechanisms return sodium levels to baseline but increase extracellular volume, which stimulates other compensatory mechanisms involved in the regulation of vascular tone. More research with a better diagnostic definition and a higher number of participants should be conducted to improve outcomes in this group of patients.

Keywords: Cardiovascular disease, Diastolic blood pressure, Diet, Osmolality, Salt, Sodium, Systolic blood pressure.

INTRODUCTION

Hypertension is currently recognized as the leading cause of cardiovascular disease worldwide. Based on blood pressure measurements in 2015, it was estimated that approximately 1.13 billion people in the world suffer from hypertension [1]. The global prevalence of hypertension in adults ranges between

* **Corresponding author Fabio Solís Jiménez:** Instituto Nacional de Cardiología Ignacio Chávez, Tlalpan 14080, Mexico City, Mexico; E-mail: fabiosolisjimenez@gmail.com.

Rafael Valdez-Ortiz, Katy Sánchez-Pozos, Ana Carolina Ariza & Enzo C. Vásquez-Jiménez (Eds.)

30% and 40% of the population, with an age-standardized global prevalence between 24% and 20% in women and men, respectively [2]. The mortality of hypertension reaches approximately 10.4 million people a year [3]. The prevalence increases with age and is more frequent in older adults (over 60% of people over 60 years) [4].

The burden of disease varies widely according to the level of awareness, accessibility to treatment, and level of hypertension control when comparing developing and developed countries [5].

Individuals with hypertension face approximately 2,000 dollars higher annual healthcare expenditure than people with no hypertension; hence, it is also a burden for the health system [6]. In addition, it affects the global economy, as it implies a lower number of productive life years per individual, which translates into a decrease in gross domestic product [7, 8].

Although it is considered a disease of multifactorial origin, there is broad agreement that excess salt in the diet is the most important factor controlling the increase in blood pressure with age in our culture [9].

Until 5000 years ago, when the Chinese discovered that salt could serve as a food preservative, we used to ingest low amounts of salt since less than 500 milligrams of sodium is required in adults to maintain homeostasis [10]. The salt began to become popular and commercialized even at high costs, reaching a peak in consumption in approximately 1870 when it was estimated that each person was ingesting approximately 9 to 12 g per day [11]. This approximately 50-fold increase in basal sodium intake in such a short evolutionary period did not allow adaptive changes to emerge to excrete these amounts, which are produced through different routes, such as the sustained increase in blood pressure that we currently know [12]. Since the middle of the last century, epidemiological studies have shown that there is a strong correlation between the consumption of salt and the development of hypertension in individuals, as well as the incidence of hypertension in populations [13, 14]. It has also been shown that a restriction in sodium consumption substantially lowers blood pressure [15].

On the other hand, high salt intake is associated with an increased risk of cerebrovascular disease [16], left ventricular hypertrophy [17], chronic kidney disease progression, and proteinuria, independent of the effect of blood pressure on these complications [18].

The increase in blood pressure and the adverse cardiovascular effects resulting from the increase in salt intake in the diet are related, at least initially, to the kidney's inability to excrete excess sodium [19]. The study of this and other pathophysiological mechanisms that explain the relationship between sodium consumption and hypertension led to the description of a condition called salt sensitivity, which is defined as the behavior of blood pressure parallel to changes in sodium intake; therefore, if salt intake increases, blood pressure increases, and the opposite occur when salt intake decreases [20].

Although the diagnostic criteria have not been well standardized, it is estimated that approximately 30% to 50% of hypertensive patients are sensitive to salt and that approximately 25% of normotensive patients are also sensitive to salt [21]. The clinical importance of salt-sensitive hypertension has been questioned for several years because there is a strong belief among some authors about whether it truly represents an abnormal condition. This finding contradicts the physiological basis that salt balance *via* natriuretic and antinatriuretic mechanisms is independent of blood pressure. However, more recent studies have shown that it is a risk factor for cardiovascular morbidity and mortality independent of blood pressure [22].

PATHOPHYSIOLOGY

In the study of arterial hypertension and sensitivity to sodium, sodium intake in humans in developed countries is subject to important daily variations. The balance in sodium is controlled almost entirely by the ability of the kidney to vary urinary sodium excretion. The immediate effect of ingested sodium in the diet is to modify plasma sodium and extracellular volume. These first changes are responsible for the immediate changes in blood pressure [23]. The increase in plasma sodium is rapidly dampened by the increase in osmolarity, which tends to move fluid from the intracellular space to the extracellular space. Small increases in plasma sodium also strongly stimulate the thirst center, causing increased water intake and vasopressin secretion, resulting in fluid retention. These mechanisms return sodium levels to baseline but increase extracellular volume, stimulating other compensatory mechanisms that regulate vascular tone [24].

Blood pressure must increase to increase the filtration pressure in the glomeruli and thus increase the filtered load and urinary sodium excretion. Under normal conditions, there is a balance between renal perfusion pressure (approximately 100 mmHg) and urinary sodium excretion (approximately 100-120 mEq). This balance is disrupted by the excessive consumption of sodium associated with different factors that affect the anatomical and functional integrity of the kidneys, resulting in hypertension [25].

When mineralocorticoids are given continuously, they cause sodium retention, which consequently causes natriuresis (sodium excretion through the urine) when sodium levels reach the cut-off point. This phenomenon is known as 'mineralocorticoid escape'. The two main phenomena that cause natriuresis are an increase in the glomerular filtration rate and a decrease in aldosterone levels, but neither is involved in mineralocorticoid escape. The determining factor of this phenomenon is known as the third factor, which is the endogenous factor similar to digitalis (EDLF), which causes inhibition of the activity of the renal tubular Na^+K^+-ATPase; this factor increases circulation and decreases the desire to eat salt [26, 27].

In the event of any increase in serum sodium, the kidney reacts by activating the natriuretic system (atrial natriuretic peptide, nitric oxide) and suppressing the antinatriuretic system (renin-angiotensin-aldosterone, sympathetic nervous system). In salt-sensitive patients, the first mechanism is not sufficiently activated, and the latter is not effectively suppressed [28].

Compared with patients with salt sensitivity, the renin-angiotensin-aldosterone axis is disproportionately suppressed in patients on a high-sodium diet. Studies have demonstrated that in patients who are subjected to a low sodium diet, blood pressure levels decrease, as does natriuresis, which is accompanied by an increase in renin and aldosterone levels [29]. In patients with severe hypertension, these dietary changes are accompanied by lower plasma renin activity and lower plasma aldosterone concentration compared to normotensive subjects, thus modifying the renin-angiotensin-aldosterone axis [30].

Sympathetic nervous activity is increased in salt-sensitive patients. Studies have shown that salt-sensitive patients who ingest a load of salt have higher plasma and urinary norepinephrine levels than normotensive or salt-resistant patients [31]. In addition, there is evidence that even small increases in plasma osmolality result in an increase in the sensitivity of the muscle baroreflex controlled by sympathetic activity [32].

The antinatriuretic activity of the sympathetic nervous system has been demonstrated through three different mechanisms: an increase in plasma renin, a decrease in renal blood flow, and an increase in tubular sodium reabsorption. Sodium suppresses aldosterone production and the expression of Ras-related C3 botulinum toxin substrate 1 (Rac1), which is required for corticosteroid receptor expression in epithelial sodium channels in the distal convoluted and collecting ducts of tubules to produce natriuresis and normal blood pressure. Paradoxically, Rac1 is activated in salt-sensitive patients and activates the action of aldosterone, which reabsorbs sodium [33].

Furthermore, salt normally suppresses the activity of the sympathetic nervous system, which activates With-no-lysine kinase 4 (WNK4 kinase), which is a negative regulator of the thiazide-sensitive sodium channel in the distal convoluted tubule, resulting in increased natriuresis. In patients with salt sensitivity, WNK4 is paradoxically suppressed [34]. At the cerebrospinal fluid level, patients with salt sensitivity who are subjected to a high sodium diet have more significant sodium reabsorption and type 1 angiotensin receptor levels than those fed a regular diet. This effect appears to release the local production of aldosterone and angiotensin II, which activate neural pathways in the periventricular nucleus, increasing the activity of the sympathetic nervous system [35].

Another important contributing factor in patients with salt sensitivity is insulin resistance. This factor is frequently found in obese patients, who have been shown to have significantly lower blood pressure when subjected to low-salt diets than in patients with a normal body mass index [36]. Similarly, other studies have shown that patients with central obesity have much greater sodium uptake in the proximal convoluted tubule than those with a normal weight [37].

From a pathophysiological point of view, there are theories that explain the close relationship between insulin resistance and salt sensitivity. One of the most accepted theories describes the influence of sodium on nitric oxide production and vascular reactivity, as well as on the sympathetic nervous system and the activation of the renin-angiotensin-aldosterone axis. On the other hand, oxidative stress modulates the NLRP3 inflammasome, a key factor for IL-1B secretion, which plays a central role in initiating and spreading insulin resistance [38].

According to Guyton's theory, an increase in sodium intake increases stroke volume, which in turn causes an increase in peripheral vascular resistance to protect tissues from overirrigation. However, this increase maintains or intensifies hypertension. The increase in stroke volume justifies the immediate but not sustained increase in blood pressure, for which a theory involving endothelial dysfunction has been postulated [39].

Studies on monozygotic and dizygotic twins have shown that approximately 50% of the genetic components influence hypertension, and the rest can be attributed to the environment [40].

Some characteristic mechanisms of rare diseases are related to an increase in sodium reabsorption, both directly and indirectly. Mutations that cause gain or loss of the function of genes that regulate sodium absorption (Liddle or Gordon syndrome), deficiencies of enzymes that regulate adrenal steroid hormone synthesis or their deactivation (apparent mineralocorticoid excess), and excess aldosterone synthesis lead to volume-dependent hypertension in the presence of suppression of renin secretion [41] (Fig. **1**).

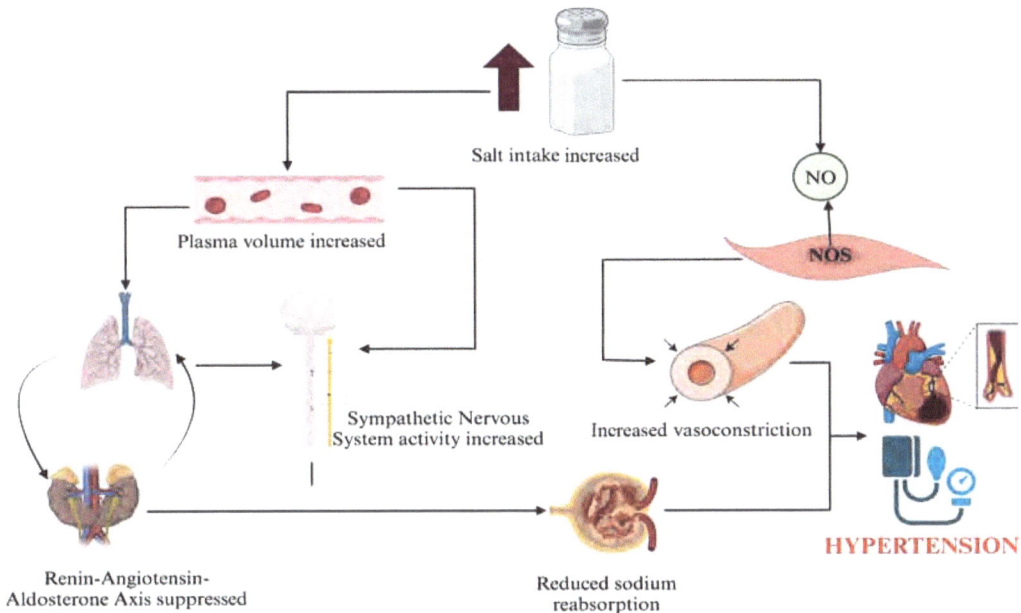

Fig. (1). Relationship between salt intake and hypertension. An increase in salt intake produces an increase in plasma volume, which in turn causes the suppression of the renin-angiotensin-aldosterone axis and an increase in the activity of the sympathetic nervous system. Both mechanisms produce a decrease in sodium reabsorption, contributing to increased blood pressure. On the other hand, an increase in salt decreases the peripheral production of nitric oxide (NO), which increases vasoconstriction and is a contributing factor to hypertension.

DIAGNOSIS

Because the relationship between blood pressure levels and adverse renal and cardiovascular outcomes is linear and becomes apparent at relatively low thresholds, the cut-off points for defining hypertension can be considered arbitrary [42]. Hypertension is defined as the blood pressure at which the benefits of implementing a treatment (pharmacological or nonpharmacological) outweigh its risks [43]. This cut-off point has been ≥ 140/90 mmHg for many years [44]; however, recently, the American College of Cardiology/American Heart Association postulated in their most recent clinical practice guidelines a cut-off value of ≥ 130/80 mmHg, which was highly criticized because various authors have postulated that the evidence regarding the reduction in cardiovascular and renal adverse events with this new value is contradictory [45, 46].

The American Heart Association provides some recommendations on how to diagnose salt sensitivity with two different types of protocols [20]:

• Outpatient diet-based protocols, which require a total of 2 weeks to directly measure blood pressure's response to changes in sodium intake.

- Protocols for hospitalized patients should be interpreted as indirect tests of salt sensitivity in which salt is strictly restricted in the diet for a relatively short period of 3 days, and the pressure response is observed to the administration of furosemide and the intravenous and oral administration of sodium.

According to this statement, no evidence exists to determine the best method for measuring salt sensitivity in humans [20].

However, evidence suggests that a well-conducted protocol based on controlled dietary variations in sodium intake, which is generally ambulatory, might be the best option for diagnosing this disease [47 - 49].

The protocols based on sodium dietary variations used in different clinical trials vary concerning duration, indicated salt intake, and dietary control [50 - 56]. However, there are some characteristics that they have in common and that are necessary for an appropriate protocol. Consequently, the diagnosis of sodium sensitivity has been described [57]:

- One week of low sodium intake (no more than 50 mmol NaCl per day)
- One week of high sodium intake (approximately 250 mmol NaCl per day).
- Adequate prescription and monitoring of diet during the study
- Serial 24-hour urinary sodium measurements to confirm NaCl consumption
- Appropriate blood pressure measurement technique according to the protocol used
- Cut-off points were established according to the type of patient to classify the patient as salt-sensitive:
  1. Normotensive patients: delta in mean arterial pressure equal to or greater than 3-5 mmHg
  2. Hypertensive patients: delta in mean arterial pressure equal to or greater than 8-10 mmHg

Despite these recommendations, performing this type of test continues to be difficult at present because, as mentioned above, the patient must be hospitalized for 3 days or strictly regulate sodium intake on an outpatient basis, which often results in complications.

For this reason, a biomarker that identifies patients in whom sodium reduction in the diet can significantly decrease blood pressure has been sought without success. On the other hand, there are several biometric parameters that can serve as surrogates of sensitivity to salt, among which are the maintenance of a heart rate above 70 beats per minute for 24 h and a decrease in the mean arterial pressure during the nights. A group of researchers classified hypertensive patients based on the presence of these traits. High-risk patients suffer from both characteristics, namely, moderate risk if they suffer from one of the two characteristics and low risk if they do not suffer either. Although good sensitivity was observed, it was also observed that up to 25% of patients classified as low risk suffered from salt sensitivity [58]. The combination of nighttime means arterial pressure drop and pulse pressure was used to improve this prediction. With this new method, misclassification within the low-risk group ranged from 25% to 5%, and a sensitivity of 74% and a specificity of 78% for the high-risk group were demonstrated [59].

Although these surrogates may show acceptable diagnostic performance, it is advisable to use demographic data and clinical phenotypes to make recommendations for even more strict restriction of salt intake in populations where salt resistance has been most common, such as African Americans, women, individuals older than 45 years, and those with metabolic syndrome [60].

CURRENT AND NOVEL STUDIES (THE STATE OF THE ART)

In recent years, interest in tailoring therapy to patients has increased. The different phenotypes have increased the need for studies conducted in specific populations with precise therapeutic targets. Salt-sensitive hypertension is not the exception. Since the pathophysiological mechanisms of hypertension might differ from those of other types of hypertension, different treatment targets are currently being evaluated.

Novel physiopathological mechanisms have been evaluated to identify new therapeutic targets. For instance, Cuevas *et al.* demonstrated that salt sensitivity might be related to a failure to increase hydrogen peroxide production in renal cells in response to an increase in salt intake. Although this study was conducted on rats, if proven in humans, it could suggest a harmful role of antioxidants and vitamins because they prevent H_2O_2 production in renal proximal tubules, which would result in sodium retention and increased blood pressure when consumed in high quantities [61].

Another breakthrough in the physiopathological pathway of salt-sensitive hypertension is the involvement of the amiloride-sensitive epithelial sodium channel (ENaC). Under normal conditions, when salt intake is increased, the expansion of body fluid volume is prevented by lower ENaC expression due to lower levels of aldosterone; however, it has been shown that salt-sensitive rats tend to gain weight when given high-sodium diets [62]. Although plasma aldosterone levels decreased in salt-sensitive and salt-resistant rats fed high-sodium diets, the expression of ENaC mRNA increased only in salt-sensitive rats. This elevation in ENaC mRNA might be one of the mechanisms causing high blood pressure in salt-sensitive patients [62, 63].

Other physiopathological targets that might create alternatives for therapeutic targets have been evaluated. For instance, Zheng *et al.* assigned 38 patients to low-sodium and high-sodium diets. They defined salt sensitivity as an increase of at least 10% in mean arterial blood pressure from a low-salt to a high-salt diet. Among the enrolled patients, 13 were salt-sensitive [64].

Recent studies have also emphasized the role of the brain protein Gαi2 (guanine nucleotide-binding protein alpha-inhibiting activity polypeptide 2) in salt-sensitive hypertension. These proteins facilitate the natriuretic response to acute volume expansion *via* a renal nerve-dependent mechanism. With chronically elevated dietary sodium intake, these proteins are essential for counteracting renal nerve-dependent salt-sensitive hypertension. Thus, selective targeting and activation of the paraventricular nucleus Gαi2 protein should be a novel therapeutic approach for the treatment of salt-sensitive hypertension [65].

As expected, a significant decrease in blood pressure was observed in salt-sensitive patients when they switched to low-sodium diets. Interestingly, salt-sensitive patients presented higher levels of GLP-1 when receiving low-salt diets, with an inverse correlation between serum GLP-1 levels and mean arterial pressure (r=-0.621, p < 0.01), suggesting that GLP-1 plays a role in the pathophysiological pathway in salt-sensitive patients. This change was not observed in salt-resistant individuals [64, 66]. In agreement with these findings, in salt-sensitive Dahl rats, compared with vehicle, recombinant glucagon-like peptide-1(7-36) amide had an ameliorating effect on the development of hypertension in rats fed an 8% sodium chloride diet. The causative mechanism is likely an increase in natriuresis and renal flow [67]. In healthy male humans, an increase in sodium fraction excretion was observed when given oral or intravenous salt loads and an infusion of GLP-1 compared with a placebo [66]. These findings suggest that GLP-1 agonists could be a treatment option for salt-sensitive patients.

An interesting finding regarding the treatment of salt-sensitive hypertension has been the role of fenofibrate as a blood pressure regulator, probably through mechanisms associated with the activation of PPAR-α, which leads to decreased volume or reduced vascular resistance. A study conducted in Tennessee assigned 31 patients to low- and subsequent high-salt diets. Afterwards, patients were randomized to receive fenofibrate or placebo for 5 days. When patients ended the first period of a high-salt diet, they received one week of washout. After they received another high-salt diet, they crossed the other drug (placebo or fenofibrate, according to the drug received first). There was no difference in systolic, diastolic, or mean arterial blood pressure in the salt-resistant group; nonetheless, a decrease in diastolic and mean arterial blood pressure was observed during high salt intake in the fenofibrate group in salt-sensitive volunteers (p=0.02 and p=0.04 for diastolic blood pressure and mean arterial pressure, respectively). This latter remained true after adjusting for the type of prestudy antihypertensive medication (p for effect >0.035 for ACEis, ARBs, beta-blockers, or thiazide diuretics). They also observed that renal plasma flow increased in both groups during high salt intake; however, this increase was significant only in the salt-sensitive group. A decrease in plasma renin activity was also observed in the salt-sensitive group, with a decrease in the mean arterial pressure. Previous findings suggest that salt-sensitive patients might also benefit from fenofibrate treatment for hyperlipidemia in hypertensive individuals [68].

One of the substances recently studied as a factor that could contribute to the treatment of salt sensitivity is caffeine. In the short term, its effects are contradictory because, despite diuresis and natriuresis, it increases the sympathetic system's activity and can produce a transitory increase in blood pressure. However, chronic administration of caffeine can increase the urinary expression of sodium in a sustained way. The mechanisms involved are increased AMPK phosphorylation and decreased alpha-ENaC expression in collecting duct cortical cells [69].

Another drug of interest for the treatment of salt-sensitive hypertension is the combination of sacubitril/valsartan, which has been shown to improve outcomes in other cardiovascular conditions, such as heart failure, with reduced ejection fraction. Wang *et al.* conducted a randomized, double-blind crossover study to prove that sacubitrate/valsartan induced increased rates of natriuresis and diuresis and therefore decreased blood pressure in salt-sensitive patients. A total of 72 patients with salt-sensitive hypertension were randomized to receive sacubitril/valsartan or valsartan only and then switched to the opposite treatment group with an intertreatment washout period of 1 to 2 weeks. After treatment with sacubitril/valsartan, an increase in natriuresis at 6 and 24 h was observed but not with valsartan only ($p < 0.001$). A significant reduction in blood pressure from baseline was observed with sacubitril/valsartan compared with valsartan alone, with an adjusted mean difference between treatments of -7.6 mmHg. Therefore, sacubitril/valsartan seems more beneficial than valsartan alone for blood pressure control in salt-sensitive patients through increased natriuresis. It is important to mention that these reductions have not been observed in salt-resistant patients [70].

The use of salbutamol has recently been associated with the development of hypertension in salt-sensitive patients. This drug appears to increase the activity of the NaCl cotransporter in the distal convoluted tubule. Of course, there is insufficient evidence to recommend disuse in patients with respiratory diseases, but this recently described mechanism should be studied to corroborate its clinical relevance [71].

An attempt has been made to elucidate whether there is a more effective treatment for salt-sensitive hypertensive patients, with interesting results. A meta-analysis that included 25 studies, including hypertensive patients with salt sensitivity under different treatments with antihypertensive drugs, revealed that for patients with salt sensitivity, the best treatment option was calcium channel blockers plus hydrochlorothiazide and a moderate reduction in the consumption of salt, while for those patients who, in addition to hypertension, suffered from obesity, adding metformin to the treatment resulted in a more effective treatment [72].

CONCLUSION

Even if advances have been made regarding the pathophysiological mechanisms and different therapeutic options for understanding and treating salt-sensitive hypertension, studies on humans are scarce and usually include a small number of patients. It is also important to consider that since the diagnosis of salt-sensitive hypertension is not uniform across studies, the results lack external validation. More research with a better diagnostic definition and a greater number of participants should be conducted to improve outcomes in this group of patients.

REFERENCES

[1]   Zhou B, Bentham J, Di Cesare M, *et al.* Worldwide trends in blood pressure from 1975 to 2015: a pooled analysis of 1479 population-based measurement studies with 19·1 million participants. Lancet 2017; 389(10064): 37-55.
[http://dx.doi.org/10.1016/S0140-6736(16)31919-5] [PMID: 27863813]

[2]   Chow CK, Teo KK, Rangarajan S, *et al.* Prevalence, awareness, treatment, and control of hypertension in rural and urban communities in high-, middle-, and low-income countries. JAMA 2013; 310(9): 959-68.
[http://dx.doi.org/10.1001/jama.2013.184182] [PMID: 24002282]

[3]   Unger T, Borghi C, Charchar F, *et al.* 2020 International Society of Hypertension global hypertension practice guidelines. J Hypertens 2020; 38(6): 982-1004.
[http://dx.doi.org/10.1097/HJH.0000000000002453] [PMID: 32371787]

[4]   Pinto E. Blood pressure and ageing. Postgrad Med J 2007; 83(976): 109-14.
[http://dx.doi.org/10.1136/pgmj.2006.048371] [PMID: 17308214]

[5]   Mills KT, Bundy JD, Kelly TN, *et al.* Global Disparities of Hypertension Prevalence and Control. Circulation 2016; 134(6): 441-50.
[http://dx.doi.org/10.1161/CIRCULATIONAHA.115.018912] [PMID: 27502908]

[6]   Kirkland EB, Heincelman M, Bishu KG, *et al.* Trends in Healthcare Expenditures Among US Adults With Hypertension: National Estimates, 2003–2014. J Am Heart Assoc 2018; 7(11): e008731.
[http://dx.doi.org/10.1161/JAHA.118.008731] [PMID: 29848493]

[7]   Hird TR, Zomer E, Owen AJ, *et al.* Productivity Burden of Hypertension in Australia. Hypertension (Dallas, Tex: 1979) 2019; 73: 777–784.
[http://dx.doi.org/10.1161/HYPERTENSIONAHA.118.12606]

[8]   Wierzejska E, Giernaś B, Lipiak A, Karasiewicz M, Cofta M, Staszewski R. A global perspective on the costs of hypertension: a systematic review. Arch Med Sci 2020; 16(5): 1078-91.
[http://dx.doi.org/10.5114/aoms.2020.92689] [PMID: 32863997]

[9]   Blaustein MP, Leenen FHH, Chen L, *et al.* How NaCl raises blood pressure: a new paradigm for the pathogenesis of salt-dependent hypertension. Am J Physiol Heart Circ Physiol 2012; 302(5): H1031-49.
[http://dx.doi.org/10.1152/ajpheart.00899.2011] [PMID: 22058154]

[10]   Bernstein AM, Willett WC. Trends in 24-h urinary sodium excretion in the United States, 1957–2003: a systematic review. Am J Clin Nutr 2010; 92(5): 1172-80.
[http://dx.doi.org/10.3945/ajcn.2010.29367] [PMID: 20826631]

[11]   He FJ, MacGregor GA. A comprehensive review on salt and health and current experience of worldwide salt reduction programmes. J Hum Hypertens 2009; 23(6): 363-84.
[http://dx.doi.org/10.1038/jhh.2008.144] [PMID: 19110538]

[12]   Afshin A, Sur PJ, Fay KA, *et al.* Health effects of dietary risks in 195 countries, 1990–2017: a systematic analysis for the Global Burden of Disease Study 2017. Lancet 2019; 393(10184): 1958-72.
[http://dx.doi.org/10.1016/S0140-6736(19)30041-8] [PMID: 30954305]

[13]   Dahl LK, Love RA. Evidence for relationship between sodium (chloride) intake and human essential hypertension. Arch Intern Med 1954; 94(4): 525-31.
[http://dx.doi.org/10.1001/archinte.1954.00250040017003] [PMID: 13196737]

[14]   Swales JD. Studies of salt intake in hypertension. What can epidemiology teach us? Am J Hypertens 1990; 3(8_Pt_1): 645-9.
[http://dx.doi.org/10.1093/ajh/3.8.645] [PMID: 2222958]

[15]   Onaka U, Miyata E. Long-Term Compliance of Salt Restriction and Blood Pressure Control Status in Hypertensive Outpatients. Clin Exp Hypertens 2010; 32(4): 234-8.
[http://dx.doi.org/10.3109/10641963.2010.491888]

[16]   Li Y, Huang Z, Jin C, *et al.* Longitudinal Change of Perceived Salt Intake and Stroke Risk in a Chinese Population. Stroke 2018; 49(6): 1332-9.
[http://dx.doi.org/10.1161/STROKEAHA.117.020277] [PMID: 29739913]

[17]   Kupari M, Koskinen P, Virolainen J. Correlates of left ventricular mass in a population sample aged 36 to 37 years. Focus on lifestyle and salt intake. Circulation 1994; 89(3): 1041-50.
[http://dx.doi.org/10.1161/01.CIR.89.3.1041] [PMID: 8124789]

[18]   Cirillo M, Bilancio G, Cavallo P, Palladino R, Terradura-Vagnarelli O, Laurenzi M. Sodium intake and kidney function in the general population: an observational, population-based study. Clin Kidney J 2021; 14(2): 647-55.
[http://dx.doi.org/10.1093/ckj/sfaa158] [PMID: 33623691]

[19]   De Wardener HE. The primary role of the kidney and salt intake in the aetiology of essential hypertension: Part I. Clin Sci (Lond) 1990; 79(3): 193-200.
[http://dx.doi.org/10.1042/cs0790193] [PMID: 2169366]

[20]   Elijovich F, Weinberger MH, Anderson CAM, *et al.* Salt Sensitivity of Blood Pressure: A Scientific Statement From the American Heart Association. Hypertension (Dallas, Tex: 1979) 2016; 68: e7–e46.
[http://dx.doi.org/10.1161/HYP.0000000000000047]

[21]   Kotchen TA, Cowley AW Jr, Frohlich ED. Salt in health and disease--a delicate balance. N Engl J Med 2013; 368(13): 1229-37.
[http://dx.doi.org/10.1056/NEJMra1212606] [PMID: 23534562]

[22]   Weinberger MH, Fineberg NS, Fineberg SE, *et al.* Salt sensitivity, pulse pressure, and death in normal and hypertensive humans. Hypertension (Dallas, Tex: 1979) 2001; 37: 429–432.
[http://dx.doi.org/10.1161/01.HYP.37.2.429]

[23]   He FJ, MacGregor GA, MacGregor GA. Plasma sodium and hypertension. Kidney Int 2004; 66(6): 2454-66.
[http://dx.doi.org/10.1111/j.1523-1755.2004.66018.x] [PMID: 15569339]

[24]   He FJ, Markandu ND, Sagnella GA, *et al.* Effect of salt intake on renal excretion of water in humans. Hypertension (Dallas, Tex: 1979) 2001; 38: 317–320.
[http://dx.doi.org/10.1161/01.HYP.38.3.317]

[25]   Guyton AC, Coleman TG, Cowley AW Jr, Scheel KW, Manning RD Jr, Norman RA Jr. Arterial pressure regulation. Am J Med 1972; 52(5): 584-94.
[http://dx.doi.org/10.1016/0002-9343(72)90050-2] [PMID: 4337474]

[26]   Francis J, Weiss RM, Wei SG, *et al.* Central mineralocorticoid receptor blockade improves volume regulation and reduces sympathetic drive in heart failure. Am J Physiol Heart Circ Physiol 2001; 281(5): H2241-51.
[http://dx.doi.org/10.1152/ajpheart.2001.281.5.H2241] [PMID: 11668089]

[27]   Takahashi H, Yoshika M, Komiyama Y, Nishimura M. The central mechanism underlying hypertension: a review of the roles of sodium ions, epithelial sodium channels, the renin–angiotensin–aldosterone system, oxidative stress and endogenous digitalis in the brain. Hypertens Res 2011; 34(11): 1147-60.
[http://dx.doi.org/10.1038/hr.2011.105] [PMID: 21814209]

[28]   Balafa O, Kalaitzidis RG. Salt sensitivity and hypertension. J Hum Hypertens 2021; 35(3): 184-92.
[http://dx.doi.org/10.1038/s41371-020-00407-1] [PMID: 32862203]

[29]   Parfrey PS, Markandu ND, Roulston JE, Jones BE, Jones JC, MacGregor GA. Relation between arterial pressure, dietary sodium intake, and renin system in essential hypertension. BMJ 1981; 283(6284): 94-7.
[http://dx.doi.org/10.1136/bmj.283.6284.94] [PMID: 6789950]

[30]   Yatabe MS, Yatabe J, Yoneda M, *et al.* Salt sensitivity is associated with insulin resistance, sympathetic overactivity, and decreased suppression of circulating renin activity in lean patients with essential hypertension. Am J Clin Nutr 2010; 92(1): 77-82.
[http://dx.doi.org/10.3945/ajcn.2009.29028] [PMID: 20444953]

[31]   Guild S-J, McBryde FD, Malpas SC, *et al.* High dietary salt and angiotensin II chronically increase renal sympathetic nerve activity: a direct telemetric study. Hypertension (Dallas, Tex: 1979) 2012; 59: 614–620.
[http://dx.doi.org/10.1161/HYPERTENSIONAHA.111.180885]

[32]   Charkoudian N, Eisenach JH, Joyner MJ, Roberts SK, Wick DE. Interactions of plasma osmolality with arterial and central venous pressures in control of sympathetic activity and heart rate in humans. Am J Physiol Heart Circ Physiol 2005; 289(6): H2456-60.
[http://dx.doi.org/10.1152/ajpheart.00601.2005] [PMID: 16199481]

[33]   Nishimoto M, Fujita T. Renal mechanisms of salt-sensitive hypertension: contribution of two steroid receptor-associated pathways. Am J Physiol Renal Physiol 2015; 308(5): F377-87.
[http://dx.doi.org/10.1152/ajprenal.00477.2013] [PMID: 25520008]

[34]   Ando K, Fujita T. Pathophysiology of salt sensitivity hypertension. Ann Med 2012; 44(sup1) (Suppl. 1): S119-26.
[http://dx.doi.org/10.3109/07853890.2012.671538] [PMID: 22713140]

[35]   Iovino M, Messana T, Lisco G, *et al.* Signal Transduction of Mineralocorticoid and Angiotensin II Receptors in the Central Control of Sodium Appetite: A Narrative Review. Int J Mol Sci 2021; 22(21): 11735.
[http://dx.doi.org/10.3390/ijms222111735] [PMID: 34769164]

[36]   Rocchini AP, Key J, Bondie D, *et al.* The effect of weight loss on the sensitivity of blood pressure to sodium in obese adolescents. N Engl J Med 1989; 321(9): 580-5.

[http://dx.doi.org/10.1056/NEJM198908313210905] [PMID: 2668763]

[37]   Strazzullo P, Barba G, Cappuccio FP, *et al.* Altered renal sodium handling in men with abdominal adiposity: a link to hypertension. J Hypertens 2001; 19(12): 2157-64.
[http://dx.doi.org/10.1097/00004872-200112000-00007] [PMID: 11725158]

[38]   Wan Z, Wen W, Ren K, *et al.* Involvement of NLRP3 inflammasome in the impacts of sodium and potassium on insulin resistance in normotensive Asians. Br J Nutr 2018; 119(2): 228-37.
[http://dx.doi.org/10.1017/S0007114517002926] [PMID: 29359681]

[39]   Sullivan JM, Rafts TE, Reed SW, Banna A, Riddle JC, Jordan C. Evidence for altered vascular reactivity in sodium-sensitive young subjects with borderline hypertension. Am J Med Sci 1984; 288(2): 65-73.
[http://dx.doi.org/10.1097/00000441-198409000-00004] [PMID: 6385702]

[40]   Levy D, Ehret GB, Rice K, *et al.* Genome-wide association study of blood pressure and hypertension. Nat Genet 2009; 41(6): 677-87.
[http://dx.doi.org/10.1038/ng.384] [PMID: 19430479]

[41]   Luft FC. Molecular genetics of salt-sensitivity and hypertension. Drug Metab Dispos 2001; 29(4 Pt 2): 500-4. https://www.sciencedirect.com/science/article/pii/S0090955624041746
[PMID: 11259340]

[42]   Ettehad D, Emdin CA, Kiran A, *et al.* Blood pressure lowering for prevention of cardiovascular disease and death: a systematic review and meta-analysis. Lancet 2016; 387(10022): 957-67.
[http://dx.doi.org/10.1016/S0140-6736(15)01225-8] [PMID: 26724178]

[43]   Williams B, Mancia G, Spiering W, *et al.* 2018 ESC/ESH Guidelines for the management of arterial hypertension. Eur Heart J 2018; 39(33): 3021-104.
[http://dx.doi.org/10.1093/eurheartj/ehy339] [PMID: 30165516]

[44]   Chobanian AV, Bakris GL, Black HR, *et al.* The Seventh Report of the Joint National Committee on Prevention, Detection, Evaluation, and Treatment of High Blood Pressure: the JNC 7 report. JAMA 2003; 289(19): 2560-72.
[http://dx.doi.org/10.1001/jama.289.19.2560] [PMID: 12748199]

[45]   Whelton PK, Carey RM, Aronow WS, *et al.* 2017 ACC/AHA/AAPA/ABC/ACPM/AGS/APhA/ ASH/ASPC/NMA/PCNA Guideline for the Prevention, Detection, Evaluation, and Management of High Blood Pressure in Adults: A Report of the American College of Cardiology/American Heart Association Task Force on Clinical Practice Guidelines. Hypertension (Dallas, Tex: 1979) 2018; 71: e13–e115.
[http://dx.doi.org/10.1161/HYP.0000000000000065]

[46]   Schiffrin EL. New blood pressure cut-offs, prevalence of hypertension and control, and mood disorders: are patients benefitting from lower cut-offs for defining hypertension? Eur Heart J 2019; 40(9): 739-42.
[http://dx.doi.org/10.1093/eurheartj/ehy891] [PMID: 30624628]

[47]   Sharma AM, Schorr U, Cetto C, Distler A. Dietary v intravenous salt loading for the assessment of salt sensitivity in normotensive men. Am J Hypertens 1994; 7(12): 1070-5.
[http://dx.doi.org/10.1093/ajh/7.12.1070] [PMID: 7702801]

[48]   Galletti F, Ferrara I, Stinga F, Iacone R, Noviello F, Strazzullo P. Evaluation of a rapid protocol for the assessment of salt sensitivity against the blood pressure response to dietary sodium chloride restriction. Am J Hypertens 1997; 10(4): 462-6.
[http://dx.doi.org/10.1016/S0895-7061(96)00491-8] [PMID: 9128214]

[49]   Galletti F, Strazzullo P. The blood pressure–salt sensitivity paradigm: pathophysiologically sound yet of no practical value. Nephrol Dial Transplant 2016; 31(9): 1386-91.
[http://dx.doi.org/10.1093/ndt/gfw295] [PMID: 27521374]

[50]   Sharma AM, Schattenfroh S, Kribben A, Distler A. Reliability of salt-sensitivity testing in

normotensive subjects. Klin Wochenschr 1989; 67(12): 632-4.
[http://dx.doi.org/10.1007/BF01718145] [PMID: 2671475]

[51]   Overlack A, Ruppert M, Kolloch R, *et al.* Divergent hemodynamic and hormonal responses to varying salt intake in normotensive subjects. Hypertension (Dallas, Tex: 1979) 1993; 22: 331–338.
[http://dx.doi.org/10.1161/01.HYP.22.3.331]

[52]   Draaijer P, de Leeuw P, Maessen J, van Hooff J, Leunissen K. Salt-sensitivity testing in patients with borderline hypertension: reproducibility and potential mechanisms. J Hum Hypertens 1995; 9(4): 263-9.
[http://dx.doi.org/10.3389/fphys.2022.1001434] [PMID: 7595909]

[53]   Gerdts E, Lund-Johansen P, Omvik P. Reproducibility of salt sensitivity testing using a dietary approach in essential hypertension. J Hum Hypertens 1999; 13(6): 375-84.
[http://dx.doi.org/10.1038/sj.jhh.1000814] [PMID: 10408587]

[54]   Mattes RD, Falkner B. Salt-sensitivity classification in normotensive adults. Clinical science (London, England: 1979) 1999; 96: 449–459.
[http://dx.doi.org/10.1042/CS19980301]

[55]   Obarzanek E, Proschan MA, Vollmer WM, *et al.* Individual blood pressure responses to changes in salt intake: results from the DASH-Sodium trial. Hypertension (Dallas, Tex: 1979) 2003; 42: 459–467.
[http://dx.doi.org/10.1161/01.HYP.0000091267.39066.72]

[56]   Gu D, Zhao Q, Chen J, *et al.* Reproducibility of blood pressure responses to dietary sodium and potassium interventions: the GenSalt study. Hypertension (Dallas, Tex: 1979) 2013; 62: 499–505.
[http://dx.doi.org/10.1161/HYPERTENSIONAHA.113.01034]

[57]   Kurtz TW, DiCarlo SE, Pravenec M, Morris RC Jr. An Appraisal of Methods Recently Recommended for Testing Salt Sensitivity of Blood Pressure. J Am Heart Assoc 2017; 6(4): e005653.
[http://dx.doi.org/10.1161/JAHA.117.005653] [PMID: 28365569]

[58]   Castiglioni P, Parati G, Brambilla L, *et al.* Detecting sodium-sensitivity in hypertensive patients: information from 24-hour ambulatory blood pressure monitoring. Hypertension (Dallas, Tex: 1979) 2011; 57: 180–185.
[http://dx.doi.org/10.1161/HYPERTENSIONAHA.110.158972]

[59]   Castiglioni P, Parati G, Brambilla L, *et al.* A new index of sodium sensitivity risk from arterial blood pressure monitoring during habitual salt intake. Int J Cardiol 2013; 168(4): 4523-5.
[http://dx.doi.org/10.1016/j.ijcard.2013.06.104] [PMID: 23886536]

[60]   Sacks FM, Svetkey LP, Vollmer WM, *et al.* Effects on blood pressure of reduced dietary sodium and the Dietary Approaches to Stop Hypertension (DASH) diet. N Engl J Med 2001; 344(1): 3-10.
[http://dx.doi.org/10.1056/NEJM200101043440101] [PMID: 11136953]

[61]   Cuevas S, Asico LD, Jose PA, Konkalmatt P. Renal Hydrogen Peroxide Production Prevents Salt☐Sensitive Hypertension. J Am Heart Assoc 2020; 9(1): e013818.
[http://dx.doi.org/10.1161/JAHA.119.013818] [PMID: 31902320]

[62]   Aoi W, Niisato N, Sawabe Y, *et al.* Abnormal expression of ENaC and SGK1 mRNA induced by dietary sodium in Dahl salt☐sensitively hypertensive rats. Cell Biol Int 2007; 31(10): 1288-91.
[http://dx.doi.org/10.1016/j.cellbi.2007.03.036] [PMID: 17485228]

[63]   Pavlov TS, Staruschenko A. Involvement of ENaC in the development of salt-sensitive hypertension. Am J Physiol Renal Physiol 2017; 313(2): F135-40.
[http://dx.doi.org/10.1152/ajprenal.00427.2016] [PMID: 28003189]

[64]   Zheng WL, Chu C, Lv YB, *et al.* Effect of Salt Intake on Serum Glucagon-Like Peptide-1 Levels in Normotensive Salt-Sensitive Subjects. Kidney Blood Press Res 2017; 42(4): 728-37.
[http://dx.doi.org/10.1159/000484152] [PMID: 29050005]

[65]   Carmichael CY, Kuwabara JT, Pascale CL, *et al.* Hypothalamic Paraventricular Nucleus Gαi(2) (Guanine Nucleotide-Binding Protein Alpha Inhibiting Activity Polypeptide 2) Protein-Mediated

Neural Control of the Kidney and the Salt Sensitivity of Blood Pressure. Hypertension (Dallas, Tex: 1979) 2020; 75: 1002–1011.
[http://dx.doi.org/10.1161/HYPERTENSIONAHA.119.13777]

[66]   Gutzwiller JP, Hruz P, Huber AR, *et al.* Glucagon-like peptide-1 is involved in sodium and water homeostasis in humans. Digestion 2006; 73(2-3): 142-50.
[http://dx.doi.org/10.1159/000094334] [PMID: 16809911]

[67]   Yu M, Moreno C, Hoagland KM, *et al.* Antihypertensive effect of glucagon-like peptide 1 in Dahl salt-sensitive rats. J Hypertens 2003; 21(6): 1125-35.
[http://dx.doi.org/10.1097/00004872-200306000-00012] [PMID: 12777949]

[68]   Gilbert K, Nian H, Yu C, Luther JM, Brown NJ. Fenofibrate lowers blood pressure in salt-sensitive but not salt-resistant hypertension. J Hypertens 2013; 31(4): 820-9.
[http://dx.doi.org/10.1097/HJH.0b013e32835e8227] [PMID: 23385647]

[69]   Yu H, Yang T, Gao P, *et al.* Caffeine intake antagonizes salt sensitive hypertension through improvement of renal sodium handling. Sci Rep 2016; 6(1): 25746.
[http://dx.doi.org/10.1038/srep25746] [PMID: 27173481]

[70]   Wang T-D, Tan R-S, Lee H-Y, *et al.* Effects of Sacubitril/Valsartan (LCZ696) on Natriuresis, Diuresis, Blood Pressures, and NT-proBNP in Salt-Sensitive Hypertension. Hypertension (Dallas, Tex: 1979) 2017; 69: 32–41.
[http://dx.doi.org/10.1161/HYPERTENSIONAHA.116.08484]

[71]   Poulsen SB, Cheng L, Penton D, *et al.* Activation of the kidney sodium chloride cotransporter by the β2-adrenergic receptor agonist salbutamol increases blood pressure. Kidney Int 2021; 100(2): 321-35.
[http://dx.doi.org/10.1016/j.kint.2021.04.021] [PMID: 33940111]

[72]   Qi H, Liu Z, Cao H, *et al.* Comparative efficacy of antihypertensive agents in salt-sensitive hypertensive patients: A network meta-analysis. Am J Hypertens 2018; 31(7): 835-46.
[http://dx.doi.org/10.1093/ajh/hpy027] [PMID: 29438454]

CHAPTER 10

Diabetic Kidney Disease: A Versatile Disease

María De Los Ángeles Granados-Silvestre[1], **Guadalupe Ortiz-López**[1] and **Katy Sánchez-Pozos**[1,*]

[1] *Research Division, Hospital Juárez de México, Gustavo A. Madero 07760, Mexico City, Mexico*

Abstract: Diabetic kidney disease (DKD) is a microvascular complication of diabetes characterized by elevated urine albumin excretion, a decrease in the glomerular filtration rate (GFR), or both. Type 2 diabetes (T2D) accounts for approximately 20%–40% of DKD cases. There are two main risk factors for progression to DKD: modifiable and nonmodifiable. Modifiable factors include hyperglycemia, a long duration of diabetes, a sedentary lifestyle, high blood pressure, obesity, metabolic syndrome, smoking, and dyslipidemia. Nonmodifiable factors include ethnicity, age, genetics, and sex. For many decades, albuminuria was considered the main clinical sign of DKD; however, many patients with diabetes do not follow the classic course of DKD. Approximately 9.0%-39.0% of patients with diabetes and a GFR < 60 mL/min/1.73 m2 do not present albuminuria. In this context, the effectiveness of diagnosis and early treatment for DKD is limited by the lack of accessible and safe biomarkers with high sensitivity. Hence, there is an urgent need to identify biomarkers to diagnose and monitor DKD. The use of different omics technologies can be helpful.

Keywords: DKD (Diabetic Kidney Disease), Diabetic nephropathy, Microvascular complication, Type 2 diabetes, Type 1 diabetes.

INTRODUCTION

Type 2 diabetes (T2D) is a metabolic disease characterized by chronic hyperglycemia as a consequence of defects in insulin secretion, insulin action, or both [1]. According to the International Diabetes Federation (IDF), global diabetes incidence continues to increase, and projections predict that 745 million adults will have diabetes by 2045 [2]. Among affected people, 30% to 40% will develop diabetic kidney disease (DKD), and approximately 30% will progress to end-stage renal disease (ESRD) [3]. Compared with Caucasians, Native Americans, Hispanics, and African Americans have a greater risk of developing DKD [4].

* **Corresponding author Katy Sánchez Pozos:** Research Division, Hospital Juárez de México, Gustavo A. Madero 07760, Mexico City, Mexico; E-mail: katypozos@gmail.com.

Rafael Valdez-Ortiz, Katy Sánchez-Pozos, Ana Carolina Ariza & Enzo C. Vásquez-Jiménez (Eds.)

According to the International Organization for Kidney Disease Improving Global Outcomes (KDIGO), DKD is defined as chronic kidney disease (CKD) in patients with diabetes. In contrast, diabetic nephropathy is the histological diagnosis of glomerular structural alterations detected through biopsy [5]. Therefore, DKD is a microvascular complication of diabetes characterized by elevated urine albumin excretion, a decrease in the glomerular filtration rate (GFR), or both [6]. DKD is infrequent if the duration of diabetes is less than one decade. An incidence of 3% per year occurs 10 to 20 years after diabetes begins, after which the incidence of DKD decreases (Table **1**). It is important to note that patients with 20 to 25 years of diabetes without clinical signs of DKD have a low risk of developing such complications. The progression of diabetes to DKD has become a health burden, not only because of costs but also because of the deterioration of patient quality of life and its consequences. As shown in Table **1**, the epidemiology of DKD in T1D and T2D patients is similar. T2D accounts for approximately 20%–40% of DKD cases [7 - 9].

Table 1. Epidemiology of DKD in patients with T1D and T2D.

-	T1D	T2D	References
Prevalence of DKD (%)	9.6 20.2 (After 30 years of postpubertal diabetes)	14.0-30.6 45.0 (40 years of duration of T2D)	[10 - 17]
Incidence of eGFR < 60 ml/min/1.73 m² (%)	2.1	2.2-4.3	
Prevalence of eGFR < 60 ml/min/1.73 m² (%)	11.4-15.0	28.0-29.6	
Microalbuminuria (%)	25.4-27.2	25.0-35.0	
Annual microalbuminuria and albuminuria incidence (%)	1.3-3.8	3.8-12.7	
Macroalbuminuria incidence (%)	1.1-1.8	1.0-4.8	
Macroalbuminuria (proteinuria) (%)	25.0-40.0	3.4-20.5	
Dialysis (%)	0.3 – 1.5	0.2 – 1.0	
Annual incidence of ESRD (%)	0.04-4.5		
ESRD (%)	3.3-7.8	19.5	
Microvascular complications (%)	35.5 – 60.1	38.8 – 65.1	
Macrovascular complications (%)	5.9 – 12.4	16.0 – 28.1	

There are two main risk factors for progression to DKD: modifiable and nonmodifiable. Modifiable factors included hyperglycemia, a long duration of diabetes, a sedentary lifestyle, high blood pressure, obesity, metabolic syndrome, smoking, and dyslipidemia (Tables **2** and **3**). Hyperglycemia and hypertension, either in combination or separately, are the principal risk factors for DKD development. Nonmodifiable factors include ethnicity, age, genetics, and sex. Most of these factors are variable and depend on drugs or modifications in lifestyle. Consequently, controlling modifiable risk factors is crucial for preventing and delaying the decrease in renal function. Clinical guidelines recommend managing numerous risk factors concurrently to ameliorate kidney outcomes in patients with T2D. These measures include smoking cessation, weight loss, increased physical activity, glycemia, blood pressure, and dyslipidemia control [18 - 20].

Table 2. Causal factors of DKD.

-	Type 1 Diabetes	Type 2 Diabetes
Causal factors (frequency, %)	Hyperglycemia Glomerular hyperfiltration (70%)	Hyperglycemia Glomerular hyperfiltration (50%) Obesity Hypertension Dyslipidemia

Table 3. Risk factors for DKD.

-	Odd ratios	References
HbA1c variability	1.43 (1.24-1.64)	[21]
Hypertension	1.67 (13.1–2.14)	[22]
Obesity	2.87 (1.24–6.66), $P = 0.014$ 3.76 (1.88-7.53), $P < 0.001$	[23, 24]
Triglycerides ≥150 mg/dL	1.71 (1.35-2.16), $P < 0.001$ 1.20 (1.06–1.36), $P = 0.004$	[25, 26]
HDL-C <40 mg/dL (men) or <50 mg/dL (women)	1.20 (1.06–1.36), $P = 0.005$	[26]
Smoking	1.33 (1.22, 1.46), $P < 0.001$	[27]

PATHOPHYSIOLOGY

For many decades, albuminuria was considered the main clinical sign of DKD; however, many patients with diabetes do not follow the classic course of DKD, which includes hyperfiltration, which begins with microalbuminuria, followed by proteinuria and ongoing renal function decline, leading to ESRD [28]. Nonetheless, approximately 9.0%-39.0% of patients with diabetes and a GFR < 60 mL/min/1.73 m^2 did not present albuminuria [29 - 32]. Hence, DKD can occur independently of the prior proteinuria development and microalbuminuria's onset. In this sense, several studies have proposed two pathways for the progression to renal impairment: with and without the progression from microalbuminuria to albuminuria. Nonproteinuric DKD was defined as an eGFR <60 mL/min/1.73 m^2 with a UACR <300 mg/g [7, 9].

The clinical characteristics of patients with albuminuric and nonalbuminuric DKD were very similar, except those patients with nonalbuminuric DKD who presented lower HbA1c levels, blood pressure, and incidence of retinopathy, as well as a shorter diabetes duration, than patients with DKD and albuminuria (Table **4**). However, smoking frequency and history of CVD were not different between these groups. The lower incidence of microvascular injury and slower decrease in the GFR have led scientists to hypothesize that macroangiopathy significantly contributes to the pathophysiology of nonalbuminuric DKD [33]. Three studies investigating pathological changes in nonalbuminuric DKD patients revealed that these changes are associated with advanced tubulointerstitial and vascular lesions and mild typical glomerular lesions compared with those in patients with albuminuria DKD [34 - 36]. A study by Chang *et al.* showed no significant difference between nonproteinuric and proteinuric DKD patients. Additionally, the patients were followed up for 24 months, and the authors observed progression to ESRD. None of the nonproteinuric DKD patients progressed to ESRD, while 61.3% of the patients in the proteinuric DKD group progressed to ESRD [37].

Table 4. Pathways involved in DKD development.

-	With proteinuria	Without proteinuria	References
BMI	↑	↓	
HbA1c	↑	↓	
Dyslipidemia	↑ sdLDL-C ↑ LDL-C	↓LDL-C	[38]
Glomerular lesions	↑	↓	

The classical histological changes observed in DKD patients are shown in Table **5** [39]. The most characteristic pathological modifications recognized in renal biopsies of DKD patients are glomerular lesions such as diffuse and nodular mesangial expansion and glomerular basement membrane (GMB) thickening [40]. Diffuse mesangial expansion is the first observable change by light microscopy that develops as early as the 5th year after the onset of diabetes. In addition, the mesangial fractional volume is correlated with the albumin excretion rate (AER) and glomerular filtration rate (GFR) in both T1D and T2D patients [41]. Along with the progression of the disease, diffuse mesangial expansion gradually progresses into nodular accumulations of mesangial matrix in the late phase of

DKD. Such nodular injuries, identified as Kimmelstiel–Wilson nodules, can be seen in nearly 25% of patients with advanced DKD. The two phases of DKD are the nodular and diffuse lesion phases. Patients with nodular diabetic glomerulosclerosis present severe renal damage, a longer duration of diabetes, and a poorer renal prognosis compared to patients with diffuse mesangial expansion [42].

Table 5. Classification of histological changes in DKD.

-	Histological changes [39]
Class I	GBM: isolated GMB thickening and mild, generic alterations by light microscopy
Class II	Mesangial expansion, mild (IIa) or severe (IIb): glomeruli categorized as mild or severe mesangial expansion but without Kimmelstiel-Wilson lesions or global glomerulosclerosis in more than 50% of glomeruli.
Class III	Kimmelstiel-Wilson lesions: at least one glomerulus with a nodular increase in the mesangial matrix (Kimmelstiel-Wilson)
Class IV	Advanced diabetic glomerulosclerosis: More than 50% of global glomerulosclerosis with other clinical or pathological evidence attributable to diabetic nephropathy

DIAGNOSIS

Early diagnosis of DKD is essential for the management of diabetes and its complications. The American Diabetes Association (ADA) endorses regular examinations for DKD patients [43]. The broadly accepted guidelines of the National Kidney Foundation involve determining GFR and CKD stages by means of serum creatinine in patients [18]. Nevertheless, because creatinine undergoes tubular secretion in addition to glomerular filtration and suffers extrarenal elimination *via* the gastrointestinal tract, especially in advanced renal failure, the GFR can be overstimulated [44, 45]. The techniques used to estimate the GFR are very invasive, and the use of certain markers is challenging. One indicator used in the diagnosis is microalbuminuria; in most patients, the first sign of DKD is a modest increase in urinary albumin excretion, i.e., 30-300 mg/g creatinine in a urine sample (microalbuminuria). Patients who progress to macroalbuminuria (>30-300 mg/g creatinine) are at high risk for developing DKD [46]. Nonetheless, up to 40% of patients with moderate albuminuria return to normoalbuminuria [47 - 49]. Furthermore, up to 50% of patients with T1D or T2D experience a decrease in the eGFR, notwithstanding moderate albuminuria or even normoalbuminuria [7, 32, 50]. In this sense, the current markers available for diagnosis are inaccurate; hence, the discovery of new markers that will allow the identification of patients at high risk for developing DKD is urgently needed to delay the progression of complications.

Biomarkers

The lack of accessible and safe biomarkers with high sensitivity limits the effectiveness of diagnosis and early treatment for DKD. Some classic biomarkers, such as serum creatinine or blood urea nitrogen (BUN), vary with muscle mass and overestimate glomerular filtration in advanced stages of the disease or may be linked to diseases not related to the kidney. Currently, cystatin C is used as a biomarker because it is not affected by muscle mass or diet; however, inflammation could modify it. Urine total protein and urine ALB are the classic diagnostic and prognostic markers of DKD. However, they are nonspecific and do not indicate the best time to start the corresponding treatment. Studies looking for biomarkers targeting specific DKD disorders hold great promise because the results will improve the diagnosis and treatment of patients [51]. The ideal biomarker must meet the following attributes: (a) can be assessed by rapid testing of available samples (urine or blood); (b) can be measured by a cost-effective and physiologically conceivable test with high sensitivity and specificity; (c) has dynamic and rapidly varying counts that correlate with disease evolution; and (d) has prognostic value [52]. To date, some promising biomarkers have been identified, taking into account molecules recognized from in vitro studies, cell-based studies, or animal models. This is the case for neutrophil gelatinase-associated lipocalin (NGAL) and molecule-1 (KIM-1), which were identified in animal models of kidney injury. Searching for biomarkers, pathways of inflammation and fibrosis were considered; therefore, soluble TNF-1 receptor and fibroblast growth factors 21 and 23 (FGF21, FGF23) were associated with an elevated risk of incident end-stage renal disease. Biomarkers of endothelial dysfunction, including the midregional fragment of pro-adrenomedullin (MR-proADM), and cardiac injury, including the pro-N-terminal B-type natriuretic peptide (NT-proBNP), improve the risk of renal function loss in patients with T2D [53]. Some of these biomarkers are shown in Table **6**.

Table 6. Recent biomarkers for DKD detection.

Biomarker	Function	Odd ratios	Advantages	-
Galectin-3 (Gal-3)	Regulates gene expression and inhibits apoptosis. In the extracellular milieu, Gal-3 has a role in organogenesis, tumorigenesis, and cell-cell and cell-matrix adhesion. In macrophages, Gal-3 is linked to their ability to phagocyte in response to noninfectious inflammatory agents.	2.2 (95% CI 1.89–2.60)	Its absence is associated with the reduced extent of renal injury through diminished macrophage function.	[54, 55]

(Table 6) cont.....

Biomarker	Function	Odd ratios	Advantages	-
Growth differentiation factor-15 (GDF-15)	Cytokine-induced as a stress response in inflammatory states, after tissue injury, and as a response to oxidative stress	1.40 (95% CI 1.16–1.69)	It is associated with the occurrence of cardiovascular events	[56, 57]
Neutrophil gelatinase-associated lipocalin (NGAL)	Released by neutrophils at sites of infection and inflammation to sequester bacterial ferric siderophores, contributing to the antibacterial iron-depletion strategy of the innate immune system.	$\beta = -0.287$, $P = 0.008$	Indicator of tubule-interstitial damage	[58, 59]
Fibroblast growth factor-23 (FGF-23)	Promotion of urinary phosphate excretion and the inhibition of the hydroxylation of 25-hydroxyvitamin D to reduce the production of the active 1,25-dihydroxy vitamin D	2.10 (95% CI, 1.31 to 3.36, $P<0.001$)	It is associated with an elevated risk of incident End Stage Renal Disease, independent of demographic characteristics, kidney disease risk factors, baseline eGFR, and mineral metabolism	[60, 61]
Platelet-derived growth factor (PDGF)	PDGF belongs to the family of mitogens, the growth factor superfamily has differentiating, proliferating, and migrating roles in developing and developed cell conditions.	$\beta = -0.03$, $P < 0.001$	Urinary PDGF-BB correlated positively with urinary albumin and negatively with creatinine clearance in diabetic patients	[62, 63]
Kidney injury Molecule-1 (KIM-1)	Phosphatidylserine receptor that confers a phagocytic phenotype on kidney epithelial cells	1.7-2.4 (95% CI 1.5 (1.7) - 2.1 (3.5))	Indicator of glomerular hyperfiltration	[64, 65]

CURRENT AND NOVEL STUDIES (THE STATE OF THE ART)

Genetic Variants Associated with DKD

DKD is a complex disease, and genetic and environmental factors determine its development and progression. In relatives of patients with DKD or ESRD, the risk of developing DKD is 43% and 58%, respectively [66]. According to genome-wide genotyping data, the estimated heritability of DKD is 29% to 35% [67, 68]. The contribution to genetics has also been shown through the different prevalence in various ethnic groups around the world.

Since genome-wide association studies (GWASs), advances in knowledge about genetic contributions to DKD have increased. GWASs are studies that search for genetic variants in the whole genome that could be associated with a specific disease [69]. A recent meta-analysis of available genetic association studies in the literature that included data on approximately 606 polymorphisms (228 genes) revealed 51 loci significantly associated with DKD. These loci are involved in inflammation and hemodynamic and metabolic pathways [70].

The largest meta-analysis of GWAS in 26,785 individuals identified a significant association of a variant in the TENM2 gene, which encodes a protein involved in cell-cell adhesion in podocytes. Other genes were identified from pathways involved in renal fibrosis, glomerular width, mesangial volume, and the podocyte foot process [71].

Transcriptomics

The emergence of novel technologies in the omics era has accelerated advances in biology systems, as well as in information systems, and, consequently, in the generation of knowledge on renal function, kidney homeostasis, and renal disease. In this sense, transcriptome signatures associated with a specific disease can provide extensive information about pathogenic mechanisms and identify high-priority gene expression biomarker candidates [72]. In addition, a comparison of transcriptome signatures can permit the identification of DEGs in distinct populations. Transcriptomics can be performed by RNA sequencing (RNAseq) [73]. In a study that used RNAseq on microdissected glomerular and tubulointerstitial tissue from patients with diabetic nephropathy (with chronic kidney disease stages 1-4) and living kidney donors, inflammation and extracellular matrix (ECM) organization pathways in the glomeruli and immune and apoptosis pathways in the tubulointerstitium were found to be upregulated. The gene modules were associated with renal function. Additionally, increased mRNA expression of renal injury markers, such as lipocalin 2 (LCN) and hepatitis A virus cellular receptor 1 (HAVCR1), in the tubulointerstitial segment was detected together with increased urinary concentrations of NGAL and KIM-1 [74].

Another study involving in vitro model RNA-Seq data described a subset of 179 coregulated genes. The differentially expressed genes represented pathways involved in renal fibrosis due to exposure to TGF-β1. These findings suggest that the primary genes involved in DN are related to fibrosis. According to the results obtained from DN biopsy analysis, TGF-β1 was implicated in renal tubule injury in DN patients. Finally, RNA-seq identified a TGF-β1-driven signal in renal tubule epithelial cells [75].

Epigenetics

Multiple factors, such as hyperglycemia, reactive oxygen species, and inflammation, can trigger epigenetic modifications in patients with diabetes. Epigenetic mechanisms can inhibit protective genes and activate pathological pathways associated with kidney damage. Studies on human and animal models have shown the contribution of epigenetics to the development of DKD. Hasegawa *et al.* demonstrated that differentially methylated genes correlated with fibrogenesis in microdissected tubules obtained from patients with DKD [76].

The development of DNA methylation arrays, high-throughput sequencing technologies, and robust methods for data analysis have allowed us to perform epigenome-wide association studies (EWASs) in DKD patients. One of the first EWAS studies on kidney biopsy samples revealed differentially methylated regions located habitually at enhancers and enriched in binding sites for specific transcription factors. Additionally, central genes related to renal fibrosis, such as genes that encode collagens, displayed differential methylation patterns associated with gene expression between patients and controls [77]. Nonetheless, because epigenetic signatures impact gene expression in a cell-specific way, early EWASs are often confounded by the cellular heterogeneity of the samples. Therefore, the integration of the results of EWAs with whole blood genomic DNA with candidate DNA methylation and gene expression changes in the same patient has been considered to determine whether different histological changes in biopsies are reflected in peripheral blood. These strategies aim to identify early diagnostic biomarkers that could help in the timely treatment of DKD patients [78].

CONCLUSION

There is an urgent need to identify biomarkers to diagnose and monitor DKD. The use of different omics technologies can be helpful. Currently, the most important challenge has been the integration of the data obtained by these strategies. Although many efforts have been made, we are still far from able to predict the incidence of DKD, and we still do not know why some patients develop the disease faster than others or why some do not. We can see common pathways among the three strategies: renal fibrosis, inflammation, and hemodynamic and metabolic pathways. This latter has gained importance due to the high prevalence of metabolic disorders in the population; however, despite preventive measures, the incidence of metabolic disorders is increasing. Thus, more studies that consider different strategies to integrate the information obtained, such as gene-gene interactions and network-assisted algorithms, will be helpful.

REFERENCES

[1]   Diagnosis and classification of diabetes mellitus. Diabetes Care 2013; 36(Suppl 1) (Suppl. 1): S67-74.
        [http://dx.doi.org/10.2337/dc13-S067] [PMID: 23264425]

[2]   International Diabetes Federation. IDF Diabetes Atlas. 10ᵗʰ ed. Brussels, Belgium, 2021. ISBN: 978--930229-98-0.

[3]   Koye DN, Magliano DJ, Nelson RG, Pavkov ME. The global epidemiology of diabetes and kidney
        disease. Adv Chronic Kidney Dis 2018; 25(2): 121-32.
        [http://dx.doi.org/10.1053/j.ackd.2017.10.011] [PMID: 29580576]

[4]   de Boer IH. Kidney disease and related findings in the diabetes control and complications
        trial/epidemiology of diabetes interventions and complications study. Diabetes Care 2014; 37(1): 24-30.
        [http://dx.doi.org/10.2337/dc13-2113] [PMID: 24356594]

[5]   de Boer IH, Caramori ML, Chan JCN, *et al.* Executive summary of the 2020 KDIGO Diabetes
        Management in CKD Guideline: evidence-based advances in monitoring and treatment. Kidney Int
        2020; 98(4): 839-48.
        [http://dx.doi.org/10.1016/j.kint.2020.06.024] [PMID: 32653403]

[6]   KDOQI clinical practice guidelines and clinical practice recommendations for diabetes and chronic
        kidney disease. Am J Kidney Dis 2007; 49(2): S12-S154.
        [http://dx.doi.org/10.1053/j.ajkd.2006.12.005]

[7]   MacIsaac RJ, Tsalamandris C, Panagiotopoulos S, Smith TJ, McNeil KJ, Jerums G. Nonalbuminuric
        renal insufficiency in type 2 diabetes. Diabetes Care 2004; 27(1): 195-200.
        [http://dx.doi.org/10.2337/diacare.27.1.195] [PMID: 14693989]

[8]   Kramer CK, Leitão CB, Pinto LC, Silveiro SP, Gross JL, Canani LH. Clinical and laboratory profile of
        patients with type 2 diabetes with low glomerular filtration rate and normoalbuminuria. Diabetes Care
        2007; 30(8): 1998-2000.
        [http://dx.doi.org/10.2337/dc07-0387] [PMID: 17468344]

[9]   Yamanouchi M, Furuichi K, Hoshino J, *et al.* Nonproteinuric Versus Proteinuric Phenotypes in
        Diabetic Kidney Disease: A Propensity Score–Matched Analysis of a Nationwide, Biopsy-Based
        Cohort Study. Diabetes Care 2019; 42(5): 891-902.
        [http://dx.doi.org/10.2337/dc18-1320] [PMID: 30833372]

[10]   Mbanya JC, Aschner P, Gagliardino JJ, *et al.* Screening, prevalence, treatment and control of kidney
        disease in patients with type 1 and type 2 diabetes in low-to-middle-income countries (2005–2017):
        the International Diabetes Management Practices Study (IDMPS). Diabetologia 2021; 64(6): 1246-55.
        [http://dx.doi.org/10.1007/s00125-021-05406-6] [PMID: 33594476]

[11]   Reutens AT. Epidemiology of diabetic kidney disease. Med Clin North Am 2013; 97(1): 1-18.
        [http://dx.doi.org/10.1016/j.mcna.2012.10.001] [PMID: 23290726]

[12]   Gheith O, Farouk N, Nampoory N, Halim MA, Al-Otaibi T. Diabetic kidney disease: world wide
        difference of prevalence and risk factors. J Nephropharmacol 2015; 5(1): 49-56.
        [http://dx.doi.org/10.4103/1110-9165.197379] [PMID: 28197499]

[13]   Abdel-Motal UM, G A, Abdelalim EM, *et al.* Prevalence of nephropathy in type 1 diabetes in the Arab
        world: A systematic review and meta-analysis. Diabetes Metab Res Rev 2018; 34(7): e3026.
        [http://dx.doi.org/10.1002/dmrr.3026] [PMID: 29774648]

[14]   Rabieenia E, Jalali R, Mohammadi M. Prevalence of nephropathy in patients with type 2 diabetes in
        Iran: A systematic review and meta-analysis based on geographic information system (GIS). Diabetes
        Metab Syndr 2020; 14(5): 1543-50.
        [http://dx.doi.org/10.1016/j.dsx.2020.08.007] [PMID: 32947753]

[15]   Parving HH, Lewis JB, Ravid M, Remuzzi G, Hunsicker LG. Prevalence and risk factors for
        microalbuminuria in a referred cohort of type II diabetic patients: A global perspective. Kidney Int

2006; 69(11): 2057-63.
[http://dx.doi.org/10.1038/sj.ki.5000377] [PMID: 16612330]

[16] Piscitelli P, Viazzi F, Fioretto P, *et al.* Predictors of chronic kidney disease in type 1 diabetes: a longitudinal study from the AMD Annals initiative. Sci Rep 2017; 7(1): 3313.
[http://dx.doi.org/10.1038/s41598-017-03551-w] [PMID: 28607417]

[17] Yokoyama H, Okudaira M, Otani T, *et al.* Higher incidence of diabetic nephropathy in type 2 than in type 1 diabetes in early-onset diabetes in Japan. Kidney Int 2000; 58(1): 302-11.
[http://dx.doi.org/10.1046/j.1523-1755.2000.00166.x] [PMID: 10886575]

[18] Stevens PE, Levin A. Evaluation and management of chronic kidney disease: synopsis of the kidney disease: improving global outcomes 2012 clinical practice guideline. Ann Intern Med 2013; 158(11): 825-30.
[http://dx.doi.org/10.7326/0003-4819-158-11-201306040-00007] [PMID: 23732715]

[19] Clinical Practice Guideline on management of patients with diabetes and chronic kidney disease stage 3b or higher (eGFR 45 mL/min). Nephrol Dial Transplant Off Publ Eur Dial Transpl Assoc - Eur Ren Assoc 2015; 30 Suppl 2: ii1-142.
[http://dx.doi.org/10.1093/ndt/gfv100]

[20] Eckardt KU, Bansal N, Coresh J, *et al.* Improving the prognosis of patients with severely decreased glomerular filtration rate (CKD G4+): conclusions from a Kidney Disease: Improving Global Outcomes (KDIGO) Controversies Conference. Kidney Int 2018; 93(6): 1281-92.
[http://dx.doi.org/10.1016/j.kint.2018.02.006] [PMID: 29656903]

[21] Cheng D, Fei Y, Liu Y, *et al.* HbA1C variability and the risk of renal status progression in Diabetes Mellitus: a meta-analysis. PLoS One 2014; 9(12): e115509.
[http://dx.doi.org/10.1371/journal.pone.0115509] [PMID: 25521346]

[22] Wagnew F, Eshetie S, Kibret GD, *et al.* Diabetic nephropathy and hypertension in diabetes patients of sub-Saharan countries: a systematic review and meta-analysis. BMC Res Notes 2018; 11(1): 565.
[http://dx.doi.org/10.1186/s13104-018-3670-5] [PMID: 30081966]

[23] Chen HM, Shen WW, Ge YC, Zhang YD, Xie HL, Liu ZH. The relationship between obesity and diabetic nephropathy in China. BMC Nephrol 2013; 14(1): 69.
[http://dx.doi.org/10.1186/1471-2369-14-69] [PMID: 23521842]

[24] Lu J, Liu X, Jiang S, *et al.* Body Mass Index and Risk of Diabetic Nephropathy: A Mendelian Randomization Study. J Clin Endocrinol Metab 2022; 107(6): 1599-608.
[http://dx.doi.org/10.1210/clinem/dgac057] [PMID: 35191949]

[25] Gong L, Wang C, Ning G, *et al.* High concentrations of triglycerides are associated with diabetic kidney disease in new-onset type 2 diabetes in C hina: Findings from the C hina C ardiometabolic D isease and C ancer C ohort (4C) S tudy. Diabetes Obes Metab 2021; 23(11): 2551-60.
[http://dx.doi.org/10.1111/dom.14502] [PMID: 34322974]

[26] Russo GT, De Cosmo S, Viazzi F, *et al.* Plasma Triglycerides and HDL-C Levels Predict the Development of Diabetic Kidney Disease in Subjects With Type 2 Diabetes: The AMD Annals Initiative. Diabetes Care 2016; 39(12): 2278-87.
[http://dx.doi.org/10.2337/dc16-1246] [PMID: 27703024]

[27] Yang L, Chu TK, Lian J, *et al.* Risk factors of chronic kidney diseases in Chinese adults with type 2 diabetes. Sci Rep 2018; 8(1): 14686.
[http://dx.doi.org/10.1038/s41598-018-32983-1] [PMID: 30279452]

[28] Tonneijck L, Muskiet MHA, Smits MM, *et al.* Glomerular Hyperfiltration in Diabetes: Mechanisms, Clinical Significance, and Treatment. J Am Soc Nephrol 2017; 28(4): 1023-39.
[http://dx.doi.org/10.1681/ASN.2016060666] [PMID: 28143897]

[29] Molitch ME, Steffes M, Sun W, *et al.* Development and progression of renal insufficiency with and without albuminuria in adults with type 1 diabetes in the diabetes control and complications trial and

the epidemiology of diabetes interventions and complications study. Diabetes Care 2010; 33(7): 1536-43.
[http://dx.doi.org/10.2337/dc09-1098] [PMID: 20413518]

[30]   Shikata K, Kodera R, Utsunomiya K, *et al.* Prevalence of albuminuria and renal dysfunction, and related clinical factors in Japanese patients with diabetes: The Japan Diabetes Complication and its Prevention prospective study 5. J Diabetes Investig 2020; 11(2): 325-32.
[http://dx.doi.org/10.1111/jdi.13116] [PMID: 31317670]

[31]   Garg AX, Kiberd BA, Clark WF, Haynes RB, Clase CM. Albuminuria and renal insufficiency prevalence guides population screening: Results from the NHANES III. Kidney Int 2002; 61(6): 2165-75.
[http://dx.doi.org/10.1046/j.1523-1755.2002.00356.x] [PMID: 12028457]

[32]   Kramer HJ, Nguyen QD, Curhan G, Hsu CY. Renal insufficiency in the absence of albuminuria and retinopathy among adults with type 2 diabetes mellitus. JAMA 2003; 289(24): 3273-7.
[http://dx.doi.org/10.1001/jama.289.24.3273] [PMID: 12824208]

[33]   Shi S, Ni L, Gao L, Wu X. Comparison of nonalbuminuric and albuminuric diabetic kidney disease among patients with type 2 diabetes: a systematic review and meta-analysis. Front Endocrinol (Lausanne) 2022; 13: 871272.
[http://dx.doi.org/10.3389/fendo.2022.871272] [PMID: 35721745]

[34]   Gao B, Wu S, Wang J, *et al.* Clinical features and long-term outcomes of diabetic kidney disease – A prospective cohort study from China. J Diabetes Complications 2019; 33(1): 39-45.
[http://dx.doi.org/10.1016/j.jdiacomp.2018.09.019] [PMID: 30482493]

[35]   Ekinci EI, Jerums G, Skene A, *et al.* Renal structure in normoalbuminuric and albuminuric patients with type 2 diabetes and impaired renal function. Diabetes Care 2013; 36(11): 3620-6.
[http://dx.doi.org/10.2337/dc12-2572] [PMID: 23835690]

[36]   Shimizu M, Furuichi K, Yokoyama H, *et al.* Kidney lesions in diabetic patients with normoalbuminuric renal insufficiency. Clin Exp Nephrol 2014; 18(2): 305-12.
[http://dx.doi.org/10.1007/s10157-013-0870-0] [PMID: 24081589]

[37]   Chang DY, Li MR, Yu XJ, Wang SX, Chen M, Zhao MH. Clinical and pathological characteristics of patients with nonproteinuric diabetic nephropathy. Front Endocrinol (Lausanne) 2021; 12: 761386. Epub ahead of print
[http://dx.doi.org/10.3389/fendo.2021.761386] [PMID: 34764941]

[38]   Hirano T, Satoh N, Kodera R, *et al.* Dyslipidemia in diabetic kidney disease classified by proteinuria and renal dysfunction: A cross-sectional study from a regional diabetes cohort. J Diabetes Investig 2022; 13(4): 657-67.
[http://dx.doi.org/10.1111/jdi.13697] [PMID: 34665936]

[39]   Tervaert TWC, Mooyaart AL, Amann K, *et al.* Pathologic classification of diabetic nephropathy. J Am Soc Nephrol 2010; 21(4): 556-63.
[http://dx.doi.org/10.1681/ASN.2010010010] [PMID: 20167701]

[40]   Maezawa Y, Takemoto M, Yokote K. Cell biology of diabetic nephropathy: Roles of endothelial cells, tubulointerstitial cells and podocytes. J Diabetes Investig 2015; 6(1): 3-15.
[http://dx.doi.org/10.1111/jdi.12255] [PMID: 25621126]

[41]   Nosadini R, Velussi M, Brocco E, *et al.* Course of renal function in type 2 diabetic patients with abnormalities of albumin excretion rate. Diabetes 2000; 49(3): 476-84.
[http://dx.doi.org/10.2337/diabetes.49.3.476] [PMID: 10868971]

[42]   Hong D, Zheng T, Jia-qing S, Jian W, Zhi-hong L, Lei-shi L. Nodular glomerular lesion: A later stage of diabetic nephropathy? Diabetes Res Clin Pract 2007; 78(2): 189-95.
[http://dx.doi.org/10.1016/j.diabres.2007.03.024] [PMID: 17683824]

[43]   *Standards of Medical Care in Diabetes—2020* Abridged for Primary Care Providers. Clin Diabetes

2020; 38(1): 10-38.
[http://dx.doi.org/10.2337/cd20-as01] [PMID: 31975748]

[44] Stevens LA, Coresh J, Greene T, Levey AS. Assessing kidney function--measured and estimated glomerular filtration rate. N Engl J Med 2006; 354(23): 2473-83.
[http://dx.doi.org/10.1056/NEJMra054415] [PMID: 16760447]

[45] Stevens LA, Levey AS. Measurement of kidney function. Med Clin North Am 2005; 89(3): 457-73.
[http://dx.doi.org/10.1016/j.mcna.2004.11.009] [PMID: 15755462]

[46] Levin A, Stevens PE. Summary of KDIGO 2012 CKD Guideline: behind the scenes, need for guidance, and a framework for moving forward. Kidney Int 2014; 85(1): 49-61.
[http://dx.doi.org/10.1038/ki.2013.444] [PMID: 24284513]

[47] de Boer IH, Rue TC, Cleary PA, et al. Long-term renal outcomes of patients with type 1 diabetes mellitus and microalbuminuria: an analysis of the Diabetes Control and Complications Trial/Epidemiology of Diabetes Interventions and Complications cohort. Arch Intern Med 2011; 171(5): 412-20.
[http://dx.doi.org/10.1001/archinternmed.2011.16] [PMID: 21403038]

[48] Hovind P, Tarnow L, Rossing P, et al. Predictors for the development of microalbuminuria and macroalbuminuria in patients with type 1 diabetes: inception cohort study. BMJ 2004; 328(7448): 1105.
[http://dx.doi.org/10.1136/bmj.38070.450891.FE] [PMID: 15096438]

[49] Vaidya VS, Niewczas MA, Ficociello LH, et al. Regression of microalbuminuria in type 1 diabetes is associated with lower levels of urinary tubular injury biomarkers, kidney injury molecule-1, and N-acetyl-β-D-glucosaminidase. Kidney Int 2011; 79(4): 464-70.
[http://dx.doi.org/10.1038/ki.2010.404] [PMID: 20980978]

[50] Perkins BA, Ficociello LH, Silva KH, Finkelstein DM, Warram JH, Krolewski AS. Regression of microalbuminuria in type 1 diabetes. N Engl J Med 2003; 348(23): 2285-93.
[http://dx.doi.org/10.1056/NEJMoa021835] [PMID: 12788992]

[51] Konvalinka A, Scholey JW, Diamandis EP. Searching for new biomarkers of renal diseases through proteomics. Clin Chem 2012; 58(2): 353-65.
[http://dx.doi.org/10.1373/clinchem.2011.165969] [PMID: 21980170]

[52] Bennett MR, Devarajan P. Chapter one - characteristics of an ideal biomarker of kidney diseases. In: Second E, Ed. Edelstein CLBT-B of KD. 1-20.
[http://dx.doi.org/10.1016/B978-0-12-375672-5.10001-5]

[53] Colhoun HM, Marcovecchio ML. Biomarkers of diabetic kidney disease. Diabetologia 2018; 61(5): 996-1011.
[http://dx.doi.org/10.1007/s00125-018-4567-5] [PMID: 29520581]

[54] Fernandes Bertocchi AP, Campanhole G, Wang PHM, et al. A Role for galectin-3 in renal tissue damage triggered by ischemia and reperfusion injury. Transpl Int 2008; 21(10): 999-1007.
[http://dx.doi.org/10.1111/j.1432-2277.2008.00705.x] [PMID: 18657091]

[55] Rebholz CM, Selvin E, Liang M, et al. Plasma galectin-3 levels are associated with the risk of incident chronic kidney disease. Kidney Int 2018; 93(1): 252-9.
[http://dx.doi.org/10.1016/j.kint.2017.06.028] [PMID: 28865675]

[56] Adela R, Banerjee SK. GDF-15 as a target and biomarker for diabetes and cardiovascular diseases: A translational prospective. J Diabetes Res 2015; 2015: 1-14.
[http://dx.doi.org/10.1155/2015/490842] [PMID: 26273671]

[57] Carlsson AC, Nowak C, Lind L, et al. Growth differentiation factor 15 (GDF-15) is a potential biomarker of both diabetic kidney disease and future cardiovascular events in cohorts of individuals with type 2 diabetes: a proteomics approach. Ups J Med Sci 2020; 125(1): 37-43.
[http://dx.doi.org/10.1080/03009734.2019.1696430] [PMID: 31805809]

[58]   Goetz DH, Holmes MA, Borregaard N, Bluhm ME, Raymond KN, Strong RK. The neutrophil lipocalin NGAL is a bacteriostatic agent that interferes with siderophore-mediated iron acquisition. Mol Cell 2002; 10(5): 1033-43.
[http://dx.doi.org/10.1016/S1097-2765(02)00708-6] [PMID: 12453412]

[59]   Li A, Yi B, Liu Y, *et al.* Urinary NGAL and RBP are biomarkers of normoalbuminuric renal insufficiency in type 2 diabetes mellitus. J Immunol Res 2019; 2019: 1-11.
[http://dx.doi.org/10.1155/2019/5063089] [PMID: 31637265]

[60]   Rebholz CM, Grams ME, Coresh J, *et al.* Serum fibroblast growth factor-23 is associated with incident kidney disease. J Am Soc Nephrol 2015; 26(1): 192-200.
[http://dx.doi.org/10.1681/ASN.2014020218] [PMID: 25060052]

[61]   Shimada T, Hasegawa H, Yamazaki Y, et al. FGF-23 is a potent regulator of vitamin D metabolism and phosphate homeostasis. J bone Miner Res Off J Am Soc Bone Miner Res 2004; 19: 429–435.
[http://dx.doi.org/10.1359/JBMR.0301264]

[62]   Farooqi A, Shoaib S, Nawaz A, *et al.*   https://www.researchgate.net/profile/Shahzad-Bhatti/ publication/268261806_Platelet-derived_growth_factor_PDGF_signaling_Detailed_mechanistic_ insights/links/55ae28b608aed614b09893ca/Platelet-derived-growth-factor-PDGF-signaling-Detailed-mechanistic-insights.pdf

[63]   Bessa SSED, Hussein TA, Morad MA, Amer AM. Urinary platelet-derived growth factor-BB as an early marker of nephropathy in patients with type 2 diabetes: an Egyptian study. Ren Fail 2012; 34(6): 670-5.
[http://dx.doi.org/10.3109/0886022X.2012.674438] [PMID: 22486214]

[64]   Ichimura T, Asseldonk EJP, Humphreys BD, Gunaratnam L, Duffield JS, Bonventre JV. Kidney injury molecule–1 is a phosphatidylserine receptor that confers a phagocytic phenotype on epithelial cells. J Clin Invest 2008; 118(5): 1657-68.
[http://dx.doi.org/10.1172/JCI34487] [PMID: 18414680]

[65]   Coca SG, Nadkarni GN, Huang Y, *et al.* Plasma Biomarkers and Kidney Function Decline in Early and Established Diabetic Kidney Disease. J Am Soc Nephrol 2017; 28(9): 2786-93.
[http://dx.doi.org/10.1681/ASN.2016101101] [PMID: 28476763]

[66]   Harjutsalo V, Katoh S, Sarti C, Tajima N, Tuomilehto J. Population-based assessment of familial clustering of diabetic nephropathy in type 1 diabetes. Diabetes 2004; 53(9): 2449-54.
[http://dx.doi.org/10.2337/diabetes.53.9.2449] [PMID: 15331558]

[67]   Sandholm N, Van Zuydam N, Ahlqvist E, *et al.* The Genetic Landscape of Renal Complications in Type 1 Diabetes. J Am Soc Nephrol 2017; 28: 557 LP – 574.
[http://dx.doi.org/10.1681/ASN.2016020231]

[68]   Kim J, Jensen A, Ko S, *et al.* Systematic Heritability and Heritability Enrichment Analysis for Diabetes Complications in UK Biobank and ACCORD Studies. Diabetes 2022; 71(5): 1137-48.
[http://dx.doi.org/10.2337/db21-0839] [PMID: 35133398]

[69]   Bush WS, Moore JH. Chapter 11: Genome-wide association studies. PLOS Comput Biol 2012; 8(12): e1002822.
[http://dx.doi.org/10.1371/journal.pcbi.1002822] [PMID: 23300413]

[70]   Tziastoudi M, Stefanidis I, Zintzaras E. The genetic map of diabetic nephropathy: evidence from a systematic review and meta-analysis of genetic association studies. Clin Kidney J 2020; 13(5): 768-81.
[http://dx.doi.org/10.1093/ckj/sfaa077] [PMID: 33123356]

[71]   Sandholm N, Cole JB, Nair V, *et al.* Genome-wide meta-analysis and omics integration identifies novel genes associated with diabetic kidney disease. Diabetologia 2022; 65(9): 1495-509.
[http://dx.doi.org/10.1007/s00125-022-05735-0] [PMID: 35763030]

[72]   Napierala JS, Li Y, Lu Y, *et al.* Comprehensive analysis of gene expression patterns in Friedreich's ataxia fibroblasts by RNA sequencing reveals altered levels of protein synthesis factors and solute

carriers. Dis Model Mech 2017; 10(11): 1353-69.
[http://dx.doi.org/10.1242/dmm.030536] [PMID: 29125828]

[73] Wang Z, Gerstein M, Snyder M. RNA-Seq: a revolutionary tool for transcriptomics. Nat Rev Genet 2009; 10(1): 57-63.
[http://dx.doi.org/10.1038/nrg2484] [PMID: 19015660]

[74] Levin A, Reznichenko A, Witasp A, *et al.* Novel insights into the disease transcriptome of human diabetic glomeruli and tubulointerstitium. Nephrol Dial Transplant 2020; 35(12): 2059-72.
[http://dx.doi.org/10.1093/ndt/gfaa121] [PMID: 32853351]

[75] Brennan EP, Morine MJ, Walsh DW, *et al.* Next-generation sequencing identifies TGF-β1-associated gene expression profiles in renal epithelial cells reiterated in human diabetic nephropathy. Biochim Biophys Acta Mol Basis Dis 2012; 1822(4): 589-99.
[http://dx.doi.org/10.1016/j.bbadis.2012.01.008] [PMID: 22266139]

[76] Hasegawa K, Wakino S, Simic P, *et al.* Renal tubular Sirt1 attenuates diabetic albuminuria by epigenetically suppressing Claudin-1 overexpression in podocytes. Nat Med 2013; 19(11): 1496-504.
[http://dx.doi.org/10.1038/nm.3363] [PMID: 24141423]

[77] Ko YA, Mohtat D, Suzuki M, *et al.* Cytosine methylation changes in enhancer regions of core pro-fibrotic genes characterize kidney fibrosis development. Genome Biol 2013; 14(10): R108.
[http://dx.doi.org/10.1186/gb-2013-14-10-r108] [PMID: 24098934]

[78] Kato M, Natarajan R. Epigenetics and epigenomics in diabetic kidney disease and metabolic memory. Nat Rev Nephrol 2019; 15(6): 327-45.
[http://dx.doi.org/10.1038/s41581-019-0135-6] [PMID: 30894700]

CHAPTER 11

The Nephrotoxicity by Chemicals

Estefani Yaquelin Hernández-Cruz[1,2]**, Estefany Ingrid Medina-Reyes**[1] **and José Pedraza-Chaverri**[1,*]

[1] *Chemistry School, Department of Biology, Universidad Nacional Autónoma de México (UNAM), Mexico City, Mexico*

[2] *Posgrado en Ciencias Biológicas, Universidad Nacional Autónoma de México (UNAM), Mexico City, Mexico*

Abstract: The amount of chemicals is constantly increasing, which increases the likelihood of exposure to toxic substances. The kidney is one of the organs most affected by exposure to these chemicals, medications, and environmental pollutants. Although the proximal tubules are the main target of a large majority of nephrotoxic agents, all kidney compartments can be affected by nephrotoxins, leading to one or more classic clinical renal syndromes. These include acute kidney injury, tubulopathies, proteinuric kidney disease, and chronic kidney disease. Different molecular mechanisms, such as oxidative stress, mitochondrial dysfunction, autophagy, necrosis, and apoptosis, can regulate these renal syndromes. It is important to note that the nephrotoxicity of chemicals is not always recognized due to the lack of identification of the causal link between chemicals and kidney damage; however, different clinical biomarkers have been used and discussed in recent years to determine nephrotoxicity at an early stage. This chapter provides an overview of chemical-induced kidney damage and details about relevant biomarkers for identifying nephrotoxicity. In addition, we discuss some promising therapeutic targets for the early identification of toxin nephrotoxicity.

Keywords: Acute kidney injury, Clinical markers, Chronic kidney injury, Kidney damage, Nephrotoxin, Protein disease, Tubulopathies.

INTRODUCTION

Nephrotoxicity is one of the most common kidney problems; it occurs when a drug, chemical, or toxin, which can be ingested, inhaled, injected, or a substance produced by the body, causes direct or indirect adverse effects on kidney function [1, 2]. Nephrotoxicity can affect function (e.g., acute renal failure) or structure (e.g., acute tubular necrosis). Various drugs and environmental pollutants can be included among the toxic chemical agents. Drugs that can induce nephrotoxicity

---

* **Corresponding author José Pedraza Chaverri:** Chemistry School, Department of Biology, Universidad Nacional Autónoma de México (UNAM), Mexico City, Mexico; E-mail: pedraza@unam.mx

Rafael Valdez-Ortiz, Katy Sánchez-Pozos, Ana Carolina Ariza & Enzo C. Vásquez-Jiménez (Eds.)

include cancer treatments, antibiotics, analgesics, anti-inflammatories, antineoplastics, immunosuppressants, and radiocontrast agents. Environmental pollutants include heavy metals, diglycolic acid, ethylene glycol, and hydrocarbons [3].

Additionally, toxic substances are constantly being discovered worldwide; for instance, in 1970, only 65,000 toxins were known, while by 2000, the number of toxins increased to more than 500,000, so we live in a world full of invisible molecules whose effects are poorly understood. Many of these toxins are eliminated *via* the kidneys, which could be related to several cases classified as idiopathic [4].

This is particularly relevant since the incidence of kidney disease caused by toxic substances has been increasing in recent years [5]. Additionally, the American Association of Poison Control Centers reported that over 6 years (2001-2007), there were approximately 16.8 million exposures to toxic substances, 16,444 of which showed kidney effects, while 55.2% of the subsequent exposures induced severe renal complications such as increased creatinine, oliguria/anuria, and renal failure [6].

Drug-induced nephrotoxicity is more common in hospitalized patients than in the community. In Latin America, only 2% of community-acquired acute kidney injuries are attributed to nephrotoxins in countries such as Argentina, Brazil, Colombia, Mexico, and Paraguay. On the other hand, 14% of hospital-acquired acute kidney injuries are due to nephrotoxins (13%) and radiocontrast agents (1%) in countries such as Argentina, Bolivia, Brazil, Colombia, Cuba, Mexico, Peru, Puerto Rico, and Uruguay [7]. Although community-acquired kidney injury is rare, the incidence is estimated to be 4.3% among all hospital admissions in the United Kingdom [8].

Several decades ago, in the 1970s, it was estimated that nearly four million workers in the United States were occupationally exposed to known or suspected nephrotoxins [9]. Although occupational exposure to high levels of nephrotoxins is becoming less common in industrially developed countries, it is well known that chronic exposure to low levels of nephrotoxins contributes to kidney damage and is a risk factor for developing chronic kidney disease [10]. For example, in a cohort of Native Americans (3,119 participants) exposed to low and moderate levels of arsenic through drinking water, the authors reported a positive relationship between arsenic concentration in urine and chronic kidney disease [11]. In addition, "prolonged" exposure to organic solvents, pesticides, and copper sulfate has been reported to be widely associated with renal cell cancer [12]. A relationship between kidney damage and high occupational exposure to hydrocarbons has also been observed [13]. In addition, occupational exposure and people with high environmental exposure to cadmium have been reported to have an increased risk of chronic kidney disease [14, 15].

It is important to note that the general population is exposed to several nephrotoxic substances. Although physicians prescribe the vast majority of potentially nephrotoxic drugs, numerous are available as over-the-counter preparations, increasing the probability of exposure. As mentioned above, drug-induced nephrotoxicity is more common in hospitalized patients than in the community, particularly in intensive care units (ICUs).

According to a Chinese study on patients hospitalized in ICUs, the incidence of acute kidney injury was 51%, and the majority of cases occurred on the fourth day after admission [16]. Moreover, the incidence of nephrotoxicity associated with medication is approximately 18-27% of all patients with acute kidney injury in US hospitals [17]. In general, epidemiological studies on acute kidney injury have reported that the incidence of drug-induced nephrotoxicity in adults is approximately 14% to 26%, while in hospitalized children, it is 16% [18 - 22]. The global picture of acute kidney injury describes that one in five adults and one in three children will develop acute kidney injury during hospitalization [23]. Overall mortality in critically ill patients with acute kidney injury can be over 60% [21]. Several factors can contribute to acute kidney injury and to the progression of kidney failure in hospitalized patients, including cardiovascular and liver disorders, metabolic diseases, malignancies, hypovolemia, poisoning, anemia, and vascular and surgical interventions. In addition, many of these patients require nephrotoxic iodine contrast agents for computed tomography (CT) scans and other radiological examinations [24]. Multiple studies have shown that patients with diabetic nephropathy are at high risk for contrast drug-induced acute kidney injury [25]. The mortality rate associated with acute kidney injury induced by this type of drug could be greater than 30% in patients with diabetes who receive intravenous contrast media [26]. Nephrotoxicity problems have also been found in studies on drug development. In 2014, an AstraZeneca study reported that 82% of projects failed in the preclinical phase due to safety concerns, while 8% failed due to nephrotoxicity. Likewise, 52% of the projects failed in the clinical phase due to safety reasons, and 9% failed due to kidney problems [27].

PATHOPHYSIOLOGY

High drug and toxin delivery to the kidney is due to high blood irrigation, which exposes the kidney to significant concentrations of toxins [2, 28]. In addition, the kidney is exposed to chemicals through apical contact and cell uptake or transport from the basolateral circulation through the cells with the consequent apical flow into the urine [2]. The proximal tubules are usually the main targets of several nephrotoxic agents, and tubular cells have to cope with a relatively hypoxic environment due to the high metabolic requirements associated with active solute transport driven by the ATPase Na^+-K+ [22, 29, 30]. The excessive cellular workload of these cells in this relatively hypoxic environment increases the risk of nephrotoxin-related injury [22]. However, it is essential to note that all kidney compartments can be affected by nephrotoxins, which can lead to clinical renal syndromes such as acute kidney injury, tubulopathies, proteinuric kidney disease, and chronic kidney disease [31] (Table 1). Most chemical-other factors that may influence the failure to recover kidney function are altered remodeling due to inflammation, tubular atrophy, and interstitial fibrosis [32].

Clinical Renal Syndromes

Acute Kidney Injury

Acute kidney injury is one of the most common types of damage caused by nephrotoxic agents, and it is defined as an abrupt decrease (in hours) in kidney function, which encompasses both structural injury and impaired function [33]. Traditionally, the emphasis was on the most severe acute reduction in renal function, manifested by severe prerenal azotemia, acute tubular necrosis, acute interstitial nephritis, acute glomerulonephritis, crystal nephropathy, and obstructive nephropathy [31]. Azotemia is a chemical abnormality characterized by an increase in nitrogenous products; it is attributed to the renal system's inability to filter waste products properly (decreased glomerular filtration rate [GFR]). It is a typical feature of acute and chronic kidney injury, and the main nephrotoxic agents that cause azotemia are nonsteroidal anti-inflammatory drugs [34, 35].

On the other hand, acute tubular necrosis, specifically in the tubules, is used to designate acute kidney injury. Acute tubular necrosis is the most common type of intrinsic kidney injury caused mainly by aminoglycosides and other antimicrobial agents and drugs used for cancer therapy, such as cisplatin, ifosfamide, and zoledronate radiocontrast agents [33]. Additionally, acute tubular necrosis can occur due to rhabdomyolysis, a condition in which myoglobin and serum creatine kinase are released into the bloodstream due to injury to the muscles, which depresses the filtering function in the kidneys [36]. The leading causes of rhabdomyolysis are heroin, methadone, diphenhydramine, ecstasy, baclofen methamphetamine, and statin drug abuse, as well as alcoholism [37]. Likewise, some drugs can cause inflammation in the glomeruli, tubules, and interstitium and cause fibrosis, as well as kidney scarring. This inflammatory condition, known as

Table 1. Pathophysiological effects and diagnosis of chemical nephrotoxicity.

Nephrotoxic			Doses	Physiopathology — Molecular mechanisms	Physiopathology — Renal effects	Clinic markers to diagnosis	Refs.
Therapeutic agents	Antimicrobial	Aminoglycosides (Gentamicin)	0, 20, 80, or 240 mg/kg for 14 days, a single injection of 100 mg/kg, i.p route, and 8-10 mg/kg every 8 hours, sc.	Oxidative stress; ↑ Apoptosis. ↑ Necroptosis; Mitochondrial dysfunction	**Acute kidney injury:** Acute tubular necrosis; **Tubulopathies:** Proximal RTA; Fanconi syndrome; Bartter syndrome	↑ Urea; ↑ Creatinine; ↑ Uric acid; ↓ Serum total protein; ↑ KIM-1; ↓ TFF3; ↑ NGAL	[24, 105, 128 - 130]
		Antiviral agents (Tenofovir, cidofovir, adefovir and acyclovir)	Unreported doses: clinical cases	Mitochondrial dysfunction; ↓ Mitochondrial DNA	**Acute kidney injury:** Azotemia; ↓ GFR; Acute interstitial nephritis; Crystal nephropathy **Tubulopathies:** Lactic acidosis; Proximal RTA; Fanconi syndrome; Acute tubular injury; Nephrogenic diabetes insipidus	Proteinuria; Hyperlactatemia; Renal glycosuria; Hypophosphatemia; Hypopotassemia; Crystalluria; Hematuria	[131, 132]
		Amphotericin B	Intravenous injection: 0.25, 0.5, and 1 mg/kg/d for 10 days.	Lipid peroxidation; Cell membrane damage Vasoconstriction	**Acute kidney injury:** Azotemia; ↓ GFR; Acute tubular necrosis; Tubular damage; ↓ Renal blood flow	↑ Creatinine in blood; ↑ BUN; ↓ Creatinine clearance; Hypopotassemia; Nephrocalcinosis;	[133]
		Colistin	i.p. route: 20 mg/kg/d for 7 days.	Oxidative stress; Cell cycle arrest; ↑ Autophagy; ↑ Apoptosis; Deterioration of the cell membrane; Inflammation; Cell lysis	**Acute kidney injury:** Acute tubular necrosis: Injury to the proximal tubules	↑ Serum creatinine; ↓ Creatinine clearance; Proteinuria; Cylindruria; Oliguria	[134 - 136]
		Ciprofloxacin	5-30 g in humans and 100mkd, i.p. route.	Oxidative stress; ↑ Lipid peroxidation; ↑ TNF-α; Inflammation	**Acute kidney injury:** Acute tubular necrosis; Granulomatous interstitial nephritis; Lactic acidosis	Hypovolemia; ↑ Serum creatinine; Crystalluria; ↑ NAG; ↑BUN; ↑ Nitric oxide	[137 - 139]
		Vancomycin	*In vitro*: 1–5 mM for 24 h *In vivo*: i.p. route: 443.6 mg/kg body weight on alternate days for 2 weeks (median lethal dose in rats: 2218 mg/kg body weight).	Oxidative stress; Depolarization of the mitochondrial membrane; ↑ Caspase-9 and caspase-3/7; ↑ Apoptosis	**Acute kidney injury:** Acute tubular necrosis	Hypovolemia; ↑ NAG ↑ Serum creatinine (marginal increase);	[140 - 144]
	Immunosuppressive	Cyclosporine A	Levels ranging from 150 to 200 ng/mL (trough) to 700 to 800 ng/mL (peak); 15 mg/kg, sc, and 5–6 mg/kg for 6 months. s.c. (5 ml/kg): 0, 6, 30, or 60 mkd.	↑ ROS; ↑ Peroxidation of membrane lipids; ↑Autophagy; Fibrosis Polymorphism in Pgp	**Acute kidney injury:** Effects on renal hemodynamics; Azotemia; ↓ GFR; ↓ Renal plasma flow	↑ Creatinine in blood; ↓ Creatinine clearance; ↑ Nitric oxide; ↑ OPN; ↑ NGAL	[85, 145 - 148]
		Sirolimus	Blood levels of 3 ng/ml and 30–60 ng/ml, respectively.	↑ The proliferation of tubular cells	**Acute kidney injury:** Azotemia; ↓ GFR; **Protein kidney disease:** Nephrotic syndrome; Focal segmental glomerulosclerosis; Nephritic syndrome	↑ Creatinine in blood; Proteinuria; Hypomagnesemia Hypoalbuminemia; Hyperlipidemia	[51, 149]
	Chemotherapy	Cisplatin	i.p route: (5 ml/kg): 0, 0.5, 3.5, or 7 med Single dose. 50 mg/m2 for 21 days. i.p route: 20 mg/kg (high dose) or 5 mg/kg (low dose).	Oxidative stress; DNA damage; Stress of the endoplasmic reticulum; Cell cycle arrest; ↑ Autophagy; Mitochondrial dysfunction; ↑ Apoptosis; Vasoconstriction; Inflammation; Polymorphisms in OCT2, CTR1, MATE1, MRP2	**Acute kidney injury:** Acute tubular necrosis; Azotemia; ↓ GFR; **Tubulopathies:** Proximal RTA; Fanconi syndrome; Bartter syndrome	Hypomagnesemia (dose-related and cumulative); Recurrent loss of salt; ↑ TFF3; ↑ NGAL	[59, 84, 105, 150 - 153]
		Ifosfamide	Unreported doses: clinical cases with ifosfamide as a drug.	↓ GSH; Oxidative stress; Cell cycle arrest; Inflammation; Fibrosis	**Acute kidney injury:** Azotemia; ↓ GFR; Acute tubular necrosis **Tubulopathies:** Acute tubular dysfunction; Proximal RTA; Fanconi syndrome **Chronic kidney disease**	Hyperaminoaciduria; Proteinuria	[154, 155]
		Mitomycin C	Single injection: 3000 IU/kg. i.p route: 1.7 mg/kg for 5 weeks.	Oxidative stress; DNA damage ↑ Necrosis;	**Acute kidney injury:** Crystal Nephropathy **Tubulopathies:** Tubular damage **Protein kidney disease:** Nephritic syndrome; Thrombotic microangiopathy; Nuclear atypia in glomerular and tubular cells	↑ Alanine aminopeptidase (AAP)/creatinine; Proteinuria; Hematuria	[156 - 158]
		Gemcitabine; Pemetrexed; Clofarabine	Unreported doses: clinical cases	↑ Necrosis	**Acute kidney injury:** Azotemia; ↓ GFR; Acute tubular necrosis; Acute interstitial nephritis **Tubulopathies:** RTA; Nephrogenic diabetes insipidus; **Protein kidney disease:** Nephritic syndrome; Thrombotic microangiopathy;	↑ Serum creatinine; Hypokalemia; Hypocalcemia; Hyponatremia; Hypomagnesemia; Hypernatremia; Hypophosphatemia; Proteinuria; Erythrocyturia	[49, 152]
		Methotrexate	10 mg of methotrexate for 9 years. i.p route: 20 mg/kg. Single dose.	Oxidative stress; ↑ Caspase 3; ↓ Bcl-2; ↑ Apoptosis	**Acute kidney injury:** Azotemia; ↓ GFR; Acute tubular necrosis; Crystal nephropathy	↑ Serum creatinine; ↑ Urea; ↓ Creatinine clearance	[159 - 161]
	Nonsteroidal anti-inflammatory drugs	Mefenamic acid	Oral route: 80 mg/day for 28 days. i.p route: 100 or 200 mg/kg Single dose. i.p route: 50 or 100 mg/kg for 14 days	Mitochondrial damage; Nuclear and lysosomal alterations; ↑ Autophagy; ↑ Nucleophagy; ↑ Apoptosis; Inflammation	**Acute kidney injury:** Azotemia; Glomerular necrosis; Tubular atrophy	Hematuria; ↑ BUN; ↑ Serum creatinine	[162, 163]
		Phenylbutazone	Unreported doses	↑ MDA; Inhibition of COX1 and COX2	**Acute kidney injury:** Azotemia; Acute tubular necrosis	↑ Gamma-glutamyltransferase/urinary creatinine; ↑ Glucose urinary; ↑ Urinary sodium; ↓Urea; ↑ Serum creatinine	[164]
Agents for diagnostic	Radiocontrast	Iodine contrast	Unreported doses: clinical cases	Oxidative stress; ↑ ATP hydrolysis; Vasoconstriction	↓ Blood flow in the marrow; ↑ Perivascular hydrostatic pressure; **Acute kidney injury:** Azotemia; ↓ GFR; Acute tubular necrosis; Osmotic nephrosis	↑ Serum creatinine; ↑ Nitric oxide; ↑ Adenosine	[24, 165, 166]
	Other actors	Gadolinium (in high doses)	Unreported doses: patients with percutaneous transluminal renal angioplasty with gadolinium. Doses >0.4 mmol/kg are considered high doses.	Oxidative stress; ↑ ATP hydrolysis; Vasoconstriction	**Acute kidney injury:** Azotemia; ↓ GFR	↑ Serum creatinine; ↓ Creatinine clearance; ↑ Nitric oxide	[25, 167]

(Table 1) cont.....

Nephrotoxic			Doses	Physiopathology		Clinic markers to diagnosis	Refs.
				Molecular mechanisms	Renal effects		
Environmental compounds	Heavy metals	Mercury	*In vitro:* 0, 1,25, 5 y 20 μmol/L. *In vivo:* 4 mg/kg, sc route	Oxidative stress; Mitochondrial dysfunction; Alteration in mitochondrial dynamics	**Acute kidney injury:** Acute tubular necrosis; **Protein kidney disease;** Nephrotic syndrome	↑ Serum creatinine; ↑ Urea; ↓ Creatinine clearance; Glucosuria; Hypoalbuminemia; Hyperlipidemia	[10, 168, 169]
		Lead	90 mg/kg/d for 28 days *via* gastric	↓ Acetylcholinesterase activity; Oxidative stress	**Acute kidney injury:** Azotemia; ↓GFR: Nephropathy; **Tubulopathies:** Fanconi syndrome; **Chronic kidney disease**	Glucosuria; Aminoaciduria; Phosphaturia	[10, 170]
		Cadmium	90 mkd for 28 days *via* gastric. Low body burden: β = 0.287, and high body burden: β = 0.145.	Oxidative stress; ↑ Apoptosis; Mitochondrial dysfunction; Alteration in mitochondrial dynamics	Itai-Itai disease **Acute kidney injury:** Azotemia; ↓ GFR; Acute tubular necrosis **Chronic kidney disease:** Kidney cancer	↑ Retinol binding protein; ↑ NAG; Proteinuria; ↑ KIM-1 ↑ β2 microglobulin; ↑ Metallothionein	[10, 171, 172]
		Chromium	Diet supplemented with: 5, 10, or 100 mg/kg and 15 mg/kg *via* parenteral administration.	Oxidative stress; DNA damage	**Acute kidney injury:** Acute tubular necrosis; Glomerular mesangial expansion **Chronic kidney disease**	↑ β2 microglobulin; Albuminuria; ↑ urinary 8-OHdG; ↓ Creatinine clearance;	[173, 174]
		Depleted uranium	Route i.p.: 0.5, 1, and 2 mg/kg. Single administration	Oxidative stress; ↓ The activity of complexes I and III of the CTE; ↓ Mitochondrial membrane potential	**Acute kidney injury Chronic kidney disease:**	↑ β2 microglobulin; ↑ Serum creatinine; ↑ BUN	[10, 175, 176]
		Copper	*Via* gastric: 10 and 60 mg/kg for 30 days	Oxidative stress; ↓ Autophagy; ↑Apoptosis; Inflammation	**Acute kidney injury:** Acute tubular necrosis	↑ Serum creatinine; Anuria; Oliguria; Myoglobinuria	[177, 178]
		Arsenic	Oral route: 0.5, 1, 2, 3, 4, and 5 mg/kg for 2 weeks.	Oxidative stress; ↑ Acute tubular necrosis; Apoptosis; ↓ Mitochondrial membrane potential; Polymorphisms in MRP4	**Acute kidney injury:** Azotemia; ↓ GFR; Acute tubular necrosis; **Chronic kidney disease Kidney cancer**	↑ β2 microglobulin; ↑ Serum creatinine; ↑ Cystatin C; ↑ NAG; Proteinuria; Albuminuria;	[11, 86, 179]
	Solvents	Hydrocarbons	Styrene: 300 ppm, 6 hours/day, 5 days/week for 12 weeks.	Chromosomal aberrations; Oxidative stress	**Acute kidney injury:** Glomerulonephritis **Chronic kidney disease:** Chronic glomerulopathy	↑ Serum and urinary; ↑NAG; Albuminuria; Microproteinuria	[13, 180]
	Herbicides	Glyphosate	375 mg/kg, 1/10 of the LD50, once daily *via* oral gavage for 8 weeks. Oral administration: 250, 500, 1200, and 2500 mg/kg.	Oxidative stress; ↑ Necrosis; ↑ Apoptosis	**Acute kidney injury Chronic kidney disease**	↑ NAG; ↑ Cystatin C; ↑ KIM-1	[181, 182]
		Paraquat	Unreported doses: clinical cases Rat: 15, 30, 60, and 90 mg/kg in water *via* gavage.	Oxidative stress; ↑ Necrosis	**Tubulopathies:** Dysfunction of the proximal and distal tubular cells.	↑ Sodium; ↑ Uric acid; ↑ Phosphorus; Marked amino aciduria and glucosuria.	[183-185]
	Pesticide	1,2-dibromo-3-chloropropane	i.p. route: 21-170 μmol/kg.	DNA damage	**Acute kidney injury:** Acute tubular necrosis; **Kidney cancer**	---	[186]
Alternative products	Artificial sweeteners	Aspartame	Administered orally: 40 mg/kg for 2, 4 and 6 weeks.	↑ Lipid peroxidation; Oxidative stress	**Acute kidney injury:** The glomerulus, proximal, and distal toxicity convoluted tubules	↑ Serum creatinine; ↑ Urea; ↓ Ferritin ↑ BUN; Hypokalemia; Hypocalcemia; Hypophosphatemia	[187-189]

8-OHdG: 8-hydroxydeoxyguanosine; Bcl-2: B-cell lymphoma 2; BUN, urea nitrogen in the blood; COX, cyclooxygenase; CTE: electron transport chain; CTR1: copper transporter 1; GFR: glomerular filtration rate; GSH, glutathione; *i.p.:* intraperitoneal; KIM-1: kidney damage molecule 1; MATE1: multidrug and toxin extrusion protein 1; MDA: malondialdehyde; *mkd: mg/ kg/day;* MRP2: multidrug resistance-associated protein 2; NAG: N-acetyl-β-D-glucosaminidase; OCT2: organic cation transporter 2; OPN: osteopontin; *p.o.: oral;* Pgp: P-glycoprotein; ROS: reactive oxygen species; RTA: renal tubular acidosis; *s.c.: subcutaneous;* TFF3: trefoil factor 3; TNF-α: tumor necrosis factor-alpha.

glomerulonephritis, is an idiosyncratic response and is not dose-dependent [38]. The clinical presentation of acute glomerulonephritis is often associated with acute interstitial nephritis. Acute interstitial nephritis results from an allergic response to a toxin. The chemicals bind with some kidney antigens or act as antigens themselves and settle in the interstitium, inducing an immune reaction. Examples of nephrotoxic agents that cause acute interstitial nephritis are quinolones, rifampin, and acyclovir [39].

Another manifestation of acute kidney injury is crystal nephropathy, which is caused by toxins that form insoluble crystals in the urine. These crystals precipitate, usually in the lumen of the distal convoluted tubule, obstructing the flow of urine and generating an interstitial reaction. Chemicals commonly associated with crystal production include antibiotics, antivirals, indinavir, methotrexate, and triamterene [38]. Obstructive nephropathy is a relatively common entity that can be treated and is often reversible. It is characterized by decreased reabsorption of solutes and water, inability to concentrate urine, and impaired excretion of hydrogen and potassium. In addition, renal interstitial fibrosis is a common finding in patients with long-term obstructive uropathy [40]. Chemicals that have been associated with obstructive nephropathy include some drugs, such as sulfadiazine, indinavir, atazanavir, melamine, topiramate, antipsychotics, antispasmodics, atropine, benzodiazepines, and several other medications [31, 41, 42].

Tubulopathies

Tubulopathies are a heterogeneous group of entities defined by abnormalities in renal tubular function. They are divided into simple or complex, depending on whether one or more parameters are affected, and primary or secondary, depending on their origin. The former are usually hereditary, while the latter are acquired and appear in the course of other diseases or due to the administration of toxins [43]. Tubulopathies include renal tubular acidosis (RTA)/Fanconi syndrome, sodium loss (Bartter-like syndrome), potassium loss, distal renal tubular acidosis, and nephrogenic diabetes insipidus [31]. RTAs are a group of transport defects characterized by reduced proximal tubular reabsorption of bicarbonate, distal proton secretion (hydrogen ion, H^+), or both, resulting in impaired capacity for net acid excretion and persistent hyperchloremic metabolic acidosis in the presence of a standard glomerular filtration rate. Based on pathophysiology, three main types of RTA are recognized. Type 1 (distal) RTA is secondary to impaired distal H^+ secretion, type 2 or proximal RTA is caused by impaired proximal reabsorption of filtered bicarbonate, and type 4 RTA is characterized by impaired H^+ and K^+ secretion by collecting ducts due to reduced secretion or response of aldosterone [44, 45]. The RTA 2 or proximal region is usually characterized by generalized proximal tubular dysfunction, called Fanconi syndrome. Fanconi syndrome is characterized by a generalized transport defect in the proximal tubules, which leads to renal losses of glucose, phosphate, calcium, uric acid, amino acids, bicarbonates, and other organic compounds [46]. Renal tubular acidosis and Fanconi syndrome are caused by chemicals such as tenofovir, adefovir, cidofovir, aminoglycosides, obsolete tetracycline, ifosfamide, cisplatin, heavy metals, and aristolochic acid [31].

Moreover, salt loss and Bartter syndrome are caused by aminoglycosides and cisplatin. The primary pathogenetic mechanism is a defect in sodium and chloride reabsorption in the thick ascending limb of the loop of Henle [31, 47]. Nontrogenic diabetes insipidus is a disorder of water reabsorption in the collecting tubule. It manifests as the excretion of large amounts of very dilute urine, given the inability to concentrate the urine due to the failure of the tubular response to antidiuretic hormone (ADH) or vasopressin [48]. Diabetes insipidus is induced by chemicals such as lithium, pemetrexed, tenofovir, and heavy metals [31, 49].

Protein Disease

Proteinuria is shared by a heterogeneous group of kidney diseases, including minimal change disease, focal segmental glomerulosclerosis, membranous nephropathy, and diabetic nephropathy, all of which affect millions of people worldwide, resulting in end-stage renal disease [50]. Proteinuria is a cardinal feature of kidney disease and a significant clinical finding because it is a marker for kidney disease that mediates progressive kidney dysfunction and is an independent and important risk factor for the development of cardiovascular disease [51]. Proteinuric kidney disease manifests as nephrotic and nephritic syndrome. The nephrotic syndrome includes minimal changes in glomerulonephritis, membranous glomerulonephritis, and focal segmental glomerulosclerosis [31]. Symptoms of nephrotic syndrome are severe proteinuria above 50 mg/kg/day (i.e., > 3.5 g/day in a 70 kg adult), hypoalbuminemia, edema, and hyperlipidemia (and lipiduria). Patients with edema may develop progressive edema involving the ankle, sacrum, and genitalia. Pleural effusions and ascites may also appear. Leukonychia is caused by hypoalbuminemia, and xanthelasma can also be detected [51, 52]. Among the chemicals that have been reported to induce nephrotic syndrome are nonsteroidal anti-inflammatory drugs, pamidronate, lithium, gold, penicillamine, captopril, pamidronate, sirolimus, and heroin [31]. On the other hand, nephritic syndrome comprises edema, hypertension, proteinuria with significant hematuria, a reduced glomerular filtration rate, hypersensitivity angiitis, thrombotic microangiopathy, and vasculitis. Patients have been reported to have reduced urine output and often describe their urine as having a smoky color. Ankle edema is usually present but is less marked in these patients than in those with nephrotic syndrome. Hypertension is common and can be severe. Nephritic syndrome often presents with evidence of systemic disease [31, 51, 53]. The chemicals that induce nephritic syndrome include gemcitabine, mitomycin C, antiangiogenic drugs, quinine, ticlopidine, ciprofloxacin, allopurinol, and others [31].

Chronic Kidney Disease

Chronic kidney disease is defined as functional and/or structural alterations of the kidney that persist for more than three months and may or may not be accompanied by a decrease in the glomerular filtration rate. It is classified into five categories based on the glomerular filtration measurement and microalbuminuria intensity [54]. Tubulointerstitial nephritis remains a common cause of chronic kidney disease in the developing world. It is associated with immune-mediated infiltration of the renal interstitium by inflammatory cells, which can progress to fibrosis. Patients generally do not have any symptoms, but kidney function deteriorates slowly [55]. The most common inducers of tubulointerstitial nephritis are drug-induced injuries and infections, exposure to heavy metals, and chronic obstructive nephropathy, among others [56]. Furthermore, in various ways, nephrotoxin-induced acute kidney injury might progress to chronic kidney disease.

Molecular Mechanisms Associated with Nephrotoxins

Different molecular mechanisms mediate nephrotoxin-induced damage, including oxidative stress, mitochondrial dysfunction, ATP depletion, autophagy, necrosis, and apoptosis [3]. The most common of these mechanisms is oxidative stress, a redox signaling and control disruption, including an imbalance between reactive oxygen species (ROS) and antioxidants [57]. Nephrotoxins induce oxidative stress in different ways. For instance, cisplatin induces mitochondrial dysfunction, which causes increased ROS production due to the interruption of the respiratory chain; it also depletes glutathione and antioxidant enzymes such as catalase and superoxide dismutase [58, 59]. Furthermore, cisplatin can induce ROS formation in microsomes through cytochrome P450 (CYP) enzymes [60]. Mitochondria play an essential role in the increase in ROS and, therefore, in oxidative stress. For this reason, some studies have focused on approaches to preserve mitochondrial function or improve biogenesis to protect against the nephrotoxicity of different compounds [61 - 66].

Autophagy may be essential in chemical-induced nephrotoxicity [3, 67]. Autophagy is a cellular recycling process involving self-degradation and reconstructing damaged organelles and proteins [67]. The autophagy pathway is upregulated under stress conditions, including cellular starvation, hypoxia, nutrient and growth factor deprivation, endoplasmic reticulum stress, and oxidative damage, most of which are involved in the pathogenesis of kidney injury. However, whether the activation of autophagy is a mechanism of kidney damage or a way to protect the kidneys (nephrotoxic or nephroprotective) is still debated. The study of autophagy in the kidney and its pathways may reveal potentially unique targets for therapeutic interventions for acute kidney injury, particularly mitochondrial degradation through mitophagy [68]. Recently, *in vitro* studies have shown that iodinated contrast leads to increased mitophagy, protecting the kidneys from renal tubular epithelial injury [69]. In general, multiple nephrotoxins, including various drugs for cancer therapies, antibiotics, fungal agents, and molds, alter autophagy signaling [70 - 73]. It should be noted that abnormal autophagy can cause glomerulonephritis and inflammation of the glomerulus, which are associated with chemical nephrotoxicity [3, 67].

The induction of apoptosis and necrosis are other mechanisms associated with chemical-induced nephrotoxic damage. Chemicals that induce kidney cell apoptosis include various therapies against cancer, antibiotics, fungi, molds, and heavy metals such as mercury and cadmium [74 - 76]. In addition, several compounds induce kidney necrosis and apoptosis or autophagy. The specific mechanism depends on the type of cell involved, the dose, and the duration of exposure, which is valid for all toxins. Mitochondria are also key sites for mediating cell death by releasing pro-apoptotic inducers and producing ATP, a master regulator of apoptosis, necrosis, and autophagy [77].

Transporters have also been reported to influence toxicity mechanisms induced by various nephrotoxins, including cancer treatments, antibiotics, fungal agents, and environmental pollutants such as heavy metals [78 - 82]. The transporters are distributed in both the apical and basolateral membranes of cells throughout the nephron, and they transport substances out of the kidney back to the blood (reabsorption) or substances to the cells and to the filtrate (secretion) [83]. Barnett & Cummings [3] proposed that single nucleotide polymorphisms in renal transporters could be related to the idiosyncratic responses of individuals to nephrotoxins and the variability in the patient's response to therapies directed to these transporters. This hypothesis gains strength because there are studies that report correlations between the presence of single nucleotide polymorphisms in transporters and biomarkers of kidney injury. For example, a study in Caucasians on cisplatin treatment demonstrated that the presence of single nucleotide polymorphisms in transporters such as organic cation transporter 2 (OCT2), copper transporter 1 (CTR1), multidrug and toxin extrusion protein 1 (MATE1) and multidrug resistance-associated protein 2 (MRP2) was correlated with an increase in kidney damage molecule 1 (KIM-1) [84].

Additionally, single nucleotide polymorphisms in P-glycoprotein (Pgp) have been correlated with the nephrotoxicity of cyclosporine and tacrolimus [85]. Genetic polymorphisms in renal transporters can also mediate the nephrotoxicity of environmental pollutants. For example, genetic polymorphisms in MRP4 have been shown to alter the transport of methylated arsenic metabolites *in vitro* [86].

DIAGNOSIS

The pathophysiological mechanisms mentioned above are the causes of the induction of nephrotoxicity; however, they are not always recognized due to the lack of standards for identification and the causal link between chemical and kidney damage, which can be challenging to determine and requires knowledge of the mechanism of action of the chemical [87]. Furthermore, it is known that some nephrotoxic agents can induce kidney damage without changing any established clinical marker of kidney function. For example, a study on male Sprague Dawley rats exposed to gentamicin demonstrated that proximal tubule necrosis could be significant, as shown by elevated urinary NAG levels, even before any increase in blood urea nitrogen (BUN) or serum creatinine [88]. Therefore, determining the nephrotoxicity of chemicals is a complicated process that involves a combination of different factors. The dose, exposure time, degree of aggressiveness, and the mechanism by which the kidney metabolizes and excretes the nephrotoxin are essential factors in determining chemical-induced nephrotoxicity. However, the underlying characteristics of people who increase their risk of kidney injury, such as comorbid conditions, genetic determinants of metabolism, and immune response genes, should also be taken into account [22].

Nevertheless, some biomarkers allow us to determine the relationship between toxic substances and diseases. Biomarkers determined in blood or urine are a promising approach [89]. Urine is considered an attractive and practical sample because it is noninvasive and easy to obtain in considerable quantities [90].

BUN, serum creatinine (sCr), and urine output are the most commonly used biomarkers. BUN is a protein metabolism serum product and one of the oldest prognostic biomarkers of kidney failure. Urea is formed by the liver and transported by the blood to the kidneys for excretion. Diseased or damaged kidneys cause BUN to accumulate in the blood as the GFR decreases [91]. Additionally, the serum creatinine concentration is widely interpreted as a measure of the GFR and is used as an index of renal function in clinical practice [92]. However, these biomarkers are widely debated due to their low sensitivity in detecting early kidney damage. Therefore, the discovery of initial kidney injury requires new biomarkers that are more sensitive and highly specific to provide insight into the site of the underlying kidney damage [93].

Another essential biomarker to determine the nephrotoxicity of chemicals is urinary proteins with enzymatic activity, such as alanine aminopeptidase (APN), alkaline phosphatase (ALP), α-glutathione-S-transferase (α-GST), γ-glutamyl transpeptidase (GGT), π-glutathione-S-transferase (π-GST), and N-acetyl--D-glucosaminidase (NAG). These enzymes are present in tubular epithelial cells and are shed in the urine when there is acute or chronic kidney damage [94]. Additionally, low- and high-molecular-weight proteins are known to be involved in kidney damage. Under normal conditions, filtration of the glomerulus restricts the migration of high-molecular-weight proteins from the blood to the lumen of the nephron; however, under pathological conditions, these proteins can be detected in the urine due to glomerular dysfunction [95]. Albumin (ALB), transferrin, and immunoglobulin G (IgG) are examples of high-molecular-weight proteins that can be used to diagnose nephrotoxicity [96, 97]. In turn, low molecular weight proteins can accumulate in the urine due to inadequate absorption in the glomerulus and proximal tubule, which means that there may be cell damage or overload [98]. Examples of low-molecular-weight proteins that serve as biomarkers are β2-microglobulin (B2M), α1-microglobulin (A1M), and cystatin-C (Cys C) [99 - 101]. The presence of low- and high-molecular-weight proteins is known as proteinuria.

Many more sensitive biomarkers exist besides traditional nephrotoxic biomarkers, such as BUN, serum creatinine, and proteinuria [102]. One of these biomarkers is KIM-1, a type I transmembrane glycoprotein quickly detected in urine after nephrotoxicity. KIM-1 expression has been reported to correlate with proximal tubule injury, renal tubule regeneration, and nephrotoxic immune responses [103]. Another biomarker is neutrophil gelatinase-associated lipocalin (NGAL). This protein is expressed in the epithelial cells of the proximal tubules by inflammation or tumorigenesis [104]. Urinary clover factor 3 (TFF-3) is another biomarker used; however, it is one of the least studied. TFF3, a small peptide hormone, is significantly reduced in a time- and dose-dependent manner after proximal tubular damage [105]. Finally, osteopontin (OPN) has also been included as a biomarker of kidney damage. OPN is a pleiotropic glycoprotein expressed in various cell types in animals and humans, including bone, immune, smooth muscle, epithelial, and endothelial cells. In addition, OPN is found in the kidneys (in the thick ascending limbs of the loop of Henle and the distal nephrons) and urine. Recent studies have reported elevated OPN expression in urolithiasis and acute and chronic kidney diseases [106]. Fig. (**1**) summarizes the pathophysiological effects and biological biomarkers for the diagnosis of chemical nephrotoxicity.

CURRENT AND NOVEL STUDIES (THE STATE OF THE ART)

The above information explains how mitochondria play a critical role in the pathogenesis of acute and chronic kidney injury, manifesting as significant changes in mitochondrial morphology, viability, and renal tubular epithelial cell function. This is why recent studies have focused on this organelle and its processes to find a therapeutic pathway and/or some targets. It has been established that mitochondria are involved in severe organ damage since mitochondrial damage or dysfunction has been associated with various human diseases, such as neurodegenerative diseases, metabolic diseases, and ischemia-reperfusion injury in different organs [107 - 109]. In addition, the kidney has the second-highest mitochondrial content and oxygen consumption in the human body after only the heart [110]. Therefore, maintaining mitochondrial homeostasis is crucial for kidney homeostasis.

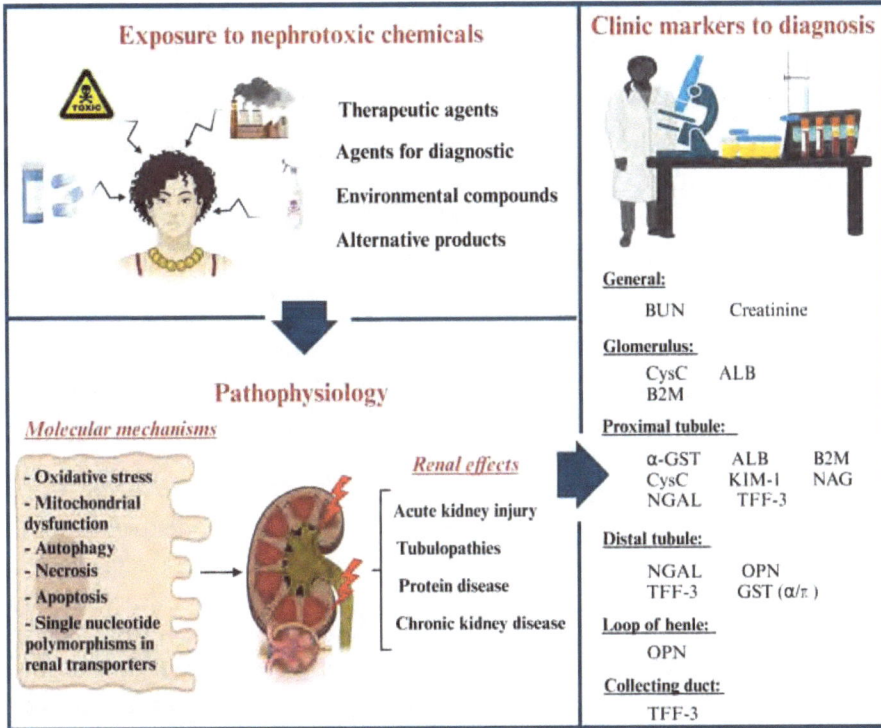

Fig. (1). Pathophysiological effects and clinic biomarkers for the diagnosis of chemical nephrotoxicity. The human body is exposed to various nephrotoxins that can induce kidney damage through various molecular mechanisms. These nephrotoxic effects cause acute kidney injury, tubulopathy, protein disease, and chronic kidney disease. So far, several biomarkers have been identified that help identify chemical nephrotoxicity. Blood urea nitrogen (BUN), cystatin-C (CysC), albumin (ALB), β2-microglobulin (B2M), α-glutathione-S-transferase (α-GST), kidney injury molecule 1 (KIM-1), N-acetyl-β-D-glucosaminidase (NAG), neutrophil gelatinase-associated lipocalin (NGAL), urinary clover factor 3 (TFF-3), osteopontin (OPN), π-glutathione-S-transferase (π-GST). Created with BioRender.

Acute or chronic kidney injury mainly affects proximal tubular cells since these cells are vulnerable to various injuries, including hypoxia and toxins, due to their high energy demands and relatively poor antioxidant ability [111]. Recent studies have shown that autophagy in the kidney is essential for renal tubular homeostasis [68, 112]. Autophagy is the primary intracellular degradation system by which cytoplasmic materials are delivered and degraded in the lysosome. Mitophagy, a type of autophagy, is the selective removal of damaged and depolarized mitochondria. Autophagy and mitophagy play important roles in acute kidney injury.

Additionally, mitochondrial damage and abnormal kidney repair play a key role after acute kidney injury. The timely elimination of damaged mitochondria in renal tubular cells represents an important quality control mechanism for cell homeostasis and survival during kidney injury and repair [113]. Indeed, *in vitro* studies have shown that increased mitophagy protects kidneys from renal tubular epithelial injury [69].

Additionally, mitochondrial damage could be detected earlier than traditional clinical markers since mitochondrial dysfunction occurs before the increase in serum creatinine [114], and mitochondrial fragmentation occurs before renal tubule cell apoptosis during ATP depletion-induced injury in cultured renal tubular cells and in a mouse model of ischemic injury [115].

Moreover, it has been shown that targeting mitochondria ameliorates renal damage. For instance, deletion of the cytosolic GTPase dynamin-related protein 1 (Drp1) (an important fission protein) accelerated renal function recovery after ischemia-reperfusion, and proximal tubular cells dramatically reduced renal fibrosis [116]. However, blocking Drp1 is not the best therapy since this protein is also needed for mitophagy. Specifically, cell culture of renal tubular cells with knockdown of Drp1 inhibited mitochondrial division and mitophagy, which is not beneficial [117]. Suppressing expression of genes PTEN induced kinase 1 (PINK1) or Parkin RBR E3 Ubiquitin Protein Ligase (Parkin) (both of which are the main proteins needed for mitophagy) increases the sensitivity of renal tubular cells to cisplatin-induced cell death or contrast-induced acute kidney injury [118, 119]. Additionally, enhancing mitophagy *via* the HIF-1α/BNIP3/BENCI signaling pathway protects against cisplatin-induced nephrotoxicity [120]. In addition, the reduction in peroxisome proliferator-activated receptor gamma coactivator 1-alpha (PGC-1α), a major transcription factor for mitochondrial biogenesis, suppresses renal recovery from acute kidney injury [121], while enhancing mitochondrial biogenesis accelerates kidney recovery after acute kidney injury [122].

Other therapies have been proposed to avoid ROS overproduction and maintain the quality of mitochondria. Thus, some mitochondrion-targeted antioxidants, including plastoquinol decylrhodamine 19 (SkQR1), Mito-Tempo, mitoquinol mesylate (MitoQ), and SS-31, have been demonstrated to attenuate acute kidney injury and accelerate kidney repair [123 - 126]. The mammalian target of the rapamycin (mTOR) signaling pathway is a master regulator of cell growth and metabolism. Deregulation of the mTOR pathway has been implicated in several human diseases, such as cancer, diabetes, obesity, neurological diseases, and genetic disorders. Rapamycin, a specific inhibitor of mTOR, helps treat certain diseases, and renal damage is not excluded. Recently, it was demonstrated that rapamycin exerts renoprotective effects against contrast-induced acute kidney injury by attenuating mitochondrial injury and oxidative stress, which might be associated with increased mitophagy due to pretreatment with rapamycin-induced overexpression of microtubule-associated protein light chain 3 I/II (LC3II/I) and Beclin-1, both of which are important proteins involved in autophagy, and that LC3-labeled autophagosomes increasingly overlap with TOMM20-labeled mitochondria [127].

CONCLUSION

Collectively, these findings provide substantial evidence that mitophagy failure results in the accumulation of abnormal mitochondria and increased ROS production, contributing to the worsening of renal function and eventual chronic kidney injury and fibrosis. Thus, mitophagy and mitochondrial biogenesis represent promising therapeutic strategies for preventing, recovering, and treating acute and chronic kidney injury.

Chemical compound-induced nephrotoxicity is a significant challenge for human health and medical treatment. Due to the fact that kidneys filter and eliminate toxins, they are especially vulnerable to toxic substances such as heavy metals, drugs, and environmental pollutants. These compounds can cause renal damage through oxidative stress, mitochondrial dysfunction, ATP depletion, autophagy, necrosis, and cellular apoptosis. Resulting renal conditions include acute kidney injury and chronic nephropathy. Identifying markers of renal damage is crucial for early and effective diagnosis. We propose focusing on the study of mitochondrial alterations, as they play a vital role in cellular bioenergetics, and their dysfunction can exacerbate renal damage. This approach can offer new perspectives for preventing nephrotoxicity and improving renal protection strategies.

ACKNOWLEDGMENTS

Research conducted for this publication was supported by grants from "Consejo Nacional de Ciencia y Tecnología" (CBF2023-2024-190), Programa de Apoyo a Proyectos de Investigación e Innovación Tecnológica (PAPIIT IN202725) of Universidad Nacional Autónoma de México (UNAM) and Programa de Apoyo a la Investigación y el Posgrado (PAIP 5000-9105) of Facultad de Química, UNAM. Hernández-Cruz is a doctoral student from Programa de Doctorado en Ciencias Biológicas from Universidad Nacional Autónoma de México (UNAM) and received fellowship 779741 from CONACyT. Medina-Reyes EI received a postdoctoral fellowship from Dirección General de Asuntos del Personal Académico (DGAPA), Universidad Nacional Autónoma de México (UNAM).

REFERENCES

[1]   Vilay AM, Wong CS, Schrader RM, Mercier RC, Seifert SA. Indicators for serious kidney complications associated with toxic exposures: an analysis of the National Poison Data System. Clin Toxicol (Phila) 2013; 51(2): 96-105.
[http://dx.doi.org/10.3109/15563650.2012.762456] [PMID: 23331216]

[2]   Perazella MA. Renal vulnerability to drug toxicity. Clin J Am Soc Nephrol 2009; 4(7): 1275-83.
        [http://dx.doi.org/10.2215/CJN.02050309] [PMID: 19520747]

[3]   Barnett LMA, Cummings BS. Nephrotoxicity and renal pathophysiology: A contemporary
        perspective. Toxicol Sci 2018; 164(2): 379-90.
        [http://dx.doi.org/10.1093/toxsci/kfy159] [PMID: 29939355]

[4]   Mendoza-Patiño N, De León-Rodríguez JA, Fernández Saavedra G, *et al.* Tóxicos renales. Revista de
        la Facultad de Medicina, UNAM 2006; 49: 34–37. Available from: https://www.medigraphic.
        com/pdfs/facmed/un-2006/un061i.pdf

[5]   Prakash J, Singh TB, Ghosh B, *et al.* Changing epidemiology of community-acquired acute kidney
        injury in developing countries: analysis of 2405 cases in 26 years from eastern India. Clin Kidney J
        2013; 6(2): 150-5.
        [http://dx.doi.org/10.1093/ckj/sfs178] [PMID: 26019843]

[6]   Bronstein AC, Spyker DA, Cantilena LR Jr, Green JL, Rumack BH, Dart RC. 2010 Annual Report of
        the American Association of Poison Control Centers' National Poison Data System (NPDS): 28th
        Annual Report. Clin Toxicol (Phila) 2011; 49(10): 910-41.
        [http://dx.doi.org/10.3109/15563650.2011.635149] [PMID: 22165864]

[7]   Chávez-Iñiguez JS, García-García G, Lombardi R. Epidemiología y desenlaces de la lesión renal
        aguda en Latinoamérica. Gac Med Mex 2023; 154(91) (Suppl. 1): S6-S14.
        [http://dx.doi.org/10.24875/GMM.M18000067] [PMID: 30074021]

[8]   Wonnacott A, Meran S, Amphlett B, Talabani B, Phillips A. Epidemiology and outcomes in
        community-acquired versus hospital-acquired AKI. Clin J Am Soc Nephrol 2014; 9(6): 1007-14.
        [http://dx.doi.org/10.2215/CJN.07920713] [PMID: 24677557]

[9]   Landrigaim PJ, Goyer RA, Clarkson TW, *et al.* The work-relatedness of renal disease. Arch Environ
        Health 1984; 39(3): 225-30.
        [http://dx.doi.org/10.1080/00039896.1984.9939529] [PMID: 6380428]

[10]   Weidemann DK, Weaver VM, Fadrowski JJ. Toxic environmental exposures and kidney health in
        children. Pediatr Nephrol 2016; 31(11): 2043-54.
        [http://dx.doi.org/10.1007/s00467-015-3222-3] [PMID: 26458883]

[11]   Zheng LY, Umans JG, Yeh F, *et al.* The association of urine arsenic with prevalent and incident
        chronic kidney disease: evidence from the Strong Heart Study. Epidemiology 2015; 26(4): 601-12.
        [http://dx.doi.org/10.1097/EDE.0000000000000313] [PMID: 25929811]

[12]   Buzio L, Tondel M, De Palma G, *et al.* Occupational risk factors for renal cell cancer. An Italian case-
        control study. Med Lav 2002; 93(4): 303-9.https://pubmed.ncbi.nlm.nih.gov/12212398/
        [PMID: 12212398]

[13]   Lacquaniti A, Fenga C, Venuti VA, *et al.* Hydrocarbons and kidney damage: potential use of
        neutrophil gelatinase-associated lipocalin and sister chromatide exchange. Am J Nephrol 2012; 35(3):
        271-8.
        [http://dx.doi.org/10.1159/000336310] [PMID: 22378219]

[14]   Li Q, Nishijo M, Nakagawa H, *et al.* Relationship between urinary cadmium and mortality in habitants
        of a cadmium-polluted area: a 22-year follow-up study in Japan. Chin Med J (Engl) 2011; 124(21):
        3504-9.https://mednexus.org/doi/pdf/10.3760/cma.j.issn.0366-6999.2011.21.013
        [PMID: 22340168]

[15]   Roels HA, Van Assche FJ, Oversteyns M, De Groof M, Lauwerys RR, Lison D. Reversibility of
        microproteinuria in cadmium workers with incipient tubular dysfunction after reduction of exposure.
        Am J Ind Med 1997; 31(5): 645-52.
        [http://dx.doi.org/10.1002/(SICI)1097-0274(199705)31:5<645::AID-AJIM21>3.0.CO;2-Y] [PMID:
        9099369]

[16]   Jiang L, Zhu Y, Luo X, *et al.* Epidemiology of acute kidney injury in intensive care units in Beijing:

the multi-center BAKIT study. BMC Nephrol 2019; 20(1): 468.
[http://dx.doi.org/10.1186/s12882-019-1660-z] [PMID: 31842787]

[17]   Taber SS, Pasko DA. The epidemiology of drug-induced disorders: the kidney. Expert Opin Drug Saf
        2008; 7(6): 679-90.
        [http://dx.doi.org/10.1517/14740330802410462] [PMID: 18983215]

[18]   Hoste EAJ, Bagshaw SM, Bellomo R, *et al.* Epidemiology of acute kidney injury in critically ill
        patients: the multinational AKI-EPI study. Intensive Care Med 2015; 41(8): 1411-23.
        [http://dx.doi.org/10.1007/s00134-015-3934-7] [PMID: 26162677]

[19]   Mehta RL, Pascual MT, Soroko S, *et al.* Spectrum of acute renal failure in the intensive care unit: The
        PICARD experience. Kidney Int 2004; 66(4): 1613-21.
        [http://dx.doi.org/10.1111/j.1523-1755.2004.00927.x] [PMID: 15458458]

[20]   Moffett BS, Goldstein SL. Acute kidney injury and increasing nephrotoxic-medication exposure in
        noncritically-ill children. Clin J Am Soc Nephrol 2011; 6(4): 856-63.
        [http://dx.doi.org/10.2215/CJN.08110910] [PMID: 21212419]

[21]   Uchino S, Kellum JA, Bellomo R, *et al.* Therapy for the Kidney (BEST Kidney) Investigators. Acute
        Renal Failure in Critically Ill Patients A Multinational, Multicenter Study. JAMA 2005; 294: 813-8.
        [http://dx.doi.org/10.1001/jama.294.7.813] [PMID: 16106006]

[22]   Perazella MA. Pharmacology behind common drug nephrotoxicities. Clin J Am Soc Nephrol 2018;
        13(12): 1897-908.
        [http://dx.doi.org/10.2215/CJN.00150118] [PMID: 29622670]

[23]   Hoe KK, Barton EN, Soyibo AK, Chávez-Iñiguez J, Garcia-Garcia G. Severity and outcomes of afro-
        caribbean patients diagnosed with community-acquired acute kidney injury at an institution in
        Jamaica. West Indian Med J 2017; 66: 141-9.
        [http://dx.doi.org/10.7727/wimj.2016.505]

[24]   Petejova N, Martinek A, Zadrazil J, *et al.* Acute Kidney Injury in Septic Patients Treated by Selected
        Nephrotoxic Antibiotic Agents—Pathophysiology and Biomarkers—A Review. Int J Mol Sci 2020;
        21(19): 7115.
        [http://dx.doi.org/10.3390/ijms21197115] [PMID: 32993185]

[25]   Calvin AD, Misra S, Pflueger A. Contrast-induced acute kidney injury and diabetic nephropathy. Nat
        Rev Nephrol 2010; 6(11): 679-88.
        [http://dx.doi.org/10.1038/nrneph.2010.116] [PMID: 20877303]

[26]   From AM, Bartholmai BJ, Williams AW, Cha SS, McDonald FS. Mortality associated with
        nephropathy after radiographic contrast exposure. Mayo Clin Proc 2008; 83(10): 1095-100.
        [http://dx.doi.org/10.4065/83.10.1095] [PMID: 18828968]

[27]   Cook D, Brown D, Alexander R, *et al.* Lessons learned from the fate of AstraZeneca's drug pipeline: a
        five-dimensional framework. Nat Rev Drug Discov 2014; 13(6): 419-31.
        [http://dx.doi.org/10.1038/nrd4309] [PMID: 24833294]

[28]   Markowitz GS, Perazella MA. Drug-induced renal failure: a focus on tubulointerstitial disease. Clin
        Chim Acta 2005; 351(1-2): 31-47.
        [http://dx.doi.org/10.1016/j.cccn.2004.09.005] [PMID: 15563870]

[29]   Perazella MA. Drug-induced acute kidney injury: Diverse mechanisms of tubular injury. Curr Opin
        Crit Care 2019; 25: 550-7.
        [http://dx.doi.org/10.1097/MCC.0000000000000653]

[30]   Cummings B, Schnellmann R. Pathophysiology of nephrotoxic cell injury. In: Schrier RW, Lippincott
        Williams & Wilkinson (eds) Diseases of the Kidney and Urogenital Tract. Philadelphia, 2001, pp.
        1071–1136. Available from: https://nephros.gr/images/books/Schriers_Diseases_of_the_Kidney_
        Vol_1_Section_5_Acute_Kidney_Injury-087-120.pdf

[31]   Kaloyanides G, Bosmans J-L, DeBroe M. Antibiotic and Immunosuppression-related renal failure. In:

Schrier RW, Lippincott Williams & Wilkinson (eds) Diseases of the Kidney and Urogenital Tract. Philadelphia, 2001, pp. 1137–1174.

[32]   Perazella MA. Toxic nephropathies: core curriculum 2010. Am J Kidney Dis 2010; 55(2): 399-409.
[http://dx.doi.org/10.1053/j.ajkd.2009.10.046] [PMID: 20042257]

[33]   Makris K, Spanou L. Acute Kidney Injury: Definition, Pathophysiology and Clinical Phenotypes. Clin Biochem Rev 2016; 37(2): 85-98. https://pmc.ncbi.nlm.nih.gov/articles/PMC5198510/
[PMID: 28303073]

[34]   Bennett WM, Henrich WL, Stoff JS. The renal effects of nonsteroidal anti-inflammatory drugs: Summary and recommendations. Am J Kidney Dis 1996; 28(1) (Suppl. 1): S56-62.
[http://dx.doi.org/10.1016/S0272-6386(96)90570-3] [PMID: 8669431]

[35]   Tyagi A, Aeddula NR. Azotemia. In: StatPearls [Internet]. 2021. Available from: https://www.ncbi.nlm.nih.gov/books/NBK538145/

[36]   Zutt R, van der Kooi AJ, Linthorst GE, Wanders RJA, de Visser M. Rhabdomyolysis: Review of the literature. Neuromuscul Disord 2014; 24(8): 651-9.
[http://dx.doi.org/10.1016/j.nmd.2014.05.005] [PMID: 24946698]

[37]   Coco TJ, Klasner AE. Drug-induced rhabdomyolysis. Curr Opin Pediatr 2004; 16(2): 206-10.
[http://dx.doi.org/10.1097/00008480-200404000-00017] [PMID: 15021204]

[38]   Naughton CA. Drug-induced nephrotoxicity. Am Fam Physician 2008; 78(6): 743-50. https://www.aafp.org/pubs/afp/issues/2008/0915/p743.html
[PMID: 18819242]

[39]   Pannu N, Nadim MK. An overview of drug-induced acute kidney injury. Crit Care Med 2008; 36(4) (Suppl.): S216-23.
[http://dx.doi.org/10.1097/CCM.0b013e318168e375] [PMID: 18382197]

[40]   Klahr S. Obstructive Nephropathy. Intern Med 2000; 39(5): 355-61.
[http://dx.doi.org/10.2169/internalmedicine.39.355] [PMID: 10830173]

[41]   Verhamme KMC, Sturkenboom MCJM, Stricker BHC, Bosch R. Drug-induced urinary retention: incidence, management and prevention. Drug Saf 2008; 31(5): 373-88.
[http://dx.doi.org/10.2165/00002018-200831050-00002] [PMID: 18422378]

[42]   Perazella MA. Drug-induced renal failure: update on new medications and unique mechanisms of nephrotoxicity. Am J Med Sci 2003; 325(6): 349-62.
[http://dx.doi.org/10.1097/00000441-200306000-00006] [PMID: 12811231]

[43]   Aguirre-Meñica M, Luis-Yanes MI. Tubulopatías. Protoc Diagn Ter Pediatr 2014; 1: 135–53. Available from: https://www.aeped.es/sites/default/files/documentos/10_tubulopatias.pdf

[44]   Bagga A, Sinha A. Renal Tubular Acidosis. Indian J Pediatr 2020; 87(9): 733-44.
[http://dx.doi.org/10.1007/s12098-020-03318-8] [PMID: 32591997]

[45]   Rodríguez Soriano J. Renal tubular acidosis: the clinical entity. J Am Soc Nephrol 2002; 13(8): 2160-70.
[http://dx.doi.org/10.1097/01.ASN.0000023430.92674.E5] [PMID: 12138150]

[46]   Cherqui S, Courtoy PJ. The renal Fanconi syndrome in cystinosis: pathogenic insights and therapeutic perspectives. Nat Rev Nephrol 2017; 13(2): 115-31.
[http://dx.doi.org/10.1038/nrneph.2016.182] [PMID: 27990015]

[47]   Gómez De la F CL, Novoa P JM, Caviedes R N. Síndrome de Bartter: una tubulopatía infrecuente de inicio antenatal. Rev Chil Pediatr 2019; 90(4): 437-42.
[http://dx.doi.org/10.32641/rchped.v90i4.932]

[48]   Bockenhauer D, Bichet DG. Nephrogenic diabetes insipidus. Curr Opin Pediatr 2017; 29(2): 199-205.
[http://dx.doi.org/10.1097/MOP.0000000000000473] [PMID: 28134709]

[49]   Vootukuru V, Liew YP, Nally JV Jr. Pemetrexed-induced acute renal failure, nephrogenic diabetes insipidus, and renal tubular acidosis in a patient with non-small cell lung cancer. Med Oncol 2006; 23(3): 419-22.
[http://dx.doi.org/10.1385/MO:23:3:419] [PMID: 17018900]

[50]   Yu CC, Fornoni A, Weins A, *et al.* Abatacept in B7-1-positive proteinuric kidney disease. N Engl J Med 2013; 369(25): 2416-23.
[http://dx.doi.org/10.1056/NEJMoa1304572] [PMID: 24206430]

[51]   Topham P. Proteinuric renal disease. Clin Med (Lond) 2009; 9(3): 284-7.
[http://dx.doi.org/10.7861/clinmedicine.9-3-284] [PMID: 19634399]

[52]   Hull RP, Goldsmith DJA. Nephrotic syndrome in adults. BMJ 2008; 336(7654): 1185-9.
[http://dx.doi.org/10.1136/bmj.39576.709711.80] [PMID: 18497417]

[53]   Yoshizawa N. Acute Glomerulonephritis. Intern Med 2000; 39(9): 687-94.
[http://dx.doi.org/10.2169/internalmedicine.39.687] [PMID: 10969898]

[54]   Clinical Practice Guideline for the Evaluation and Management of Chronic Kidney Disease. Kidney Int Suppl 2013; 3: S6-S308. https://kdigo.org/wp-content/uploads/2017/02/KDIGO_2012_CKD_GL.pdf

[55]   Joyce E, Glasner P, Ranganathan S, Swiatecka-Urban A. Tubulointerstitial nephritis: diagnosis, treatment, and monitoring. Pediatr Nephrol 2017; 32(4): 577-87.
[http://dx.doi.org/10.1007/s00467-016-3394-5] [PMID: 27155873]

[56]   Dorsainvil D, Luciano RL. Chapter 38: Chronic Tubulointerstitial Nephritis. In: Lerma E V., Rosner MH, Perazella MA (eds) CURRENT Diagnosis & Treatment: Nephrology & Hypertension, 2e. McGraw-Hill Education. 2017.

[57]   Jones DP. Redefining oxidative stress. Antioxid Redox Signal 2006; 8(9-10): 1865-79.
[http://dx.doi.org/10.1089/ars.2006.8.1865] [PMID: 16987039]

[58]   Almaghrabi OA. Molecular and biochemical investigations on the effect of quercetin on oxidative stress induced by cisplatin in rat kidney. Saudi J Biol Sci 2015; 22(2): 227-31.
[http://dx.doi.org/10.1016/j.sjbs.2014.12.008] [PMID: 25737657]

[59]   Reyes-Fermín LM, Avila-Rojas SH, Aparicio-Trejo OE, Tapia E, Rivero I, Pedraza-Chaverri J. The Protective Effect of Alpha-Mangostin against Cisplatin-Induced Cell Death in LLC-PK1 Cells is Associated to Mitochondrial Function Preservation. Antioxidants 2019; 8(5): 133.
[http://dx.doi.org/10.3390/antiox8050133] [PMID: 31096625]

[60]   Liu H, Baliga R. Cytochrome P450 2E1 null mice provide novel protection against cisplatin-induced nephrotoxicity and apoptosis. Kidney Int 2003; 63(5): 1687-96.
[http://dx.doi.org/10.1046/j.1523-1755.2003.00908.x] [PMID: 12675844]

[61]   Bhargava P, Schnellmann RG. Mitochondrial energetics in the kidney. Nat Rev Nephrol 2017; 13(10): 629-46.
[http://dx.doi.org/10.1038/nrneph.2017.107] [PMID: 28804120]

[62]   Chen J-F, Wu Q-S, Xie Y-X, *et al.* TRAP1 ameliorates renal tubulointerstitial fibrosis in mice with unilateral ureteral obstruction by protecting renal tubular epithelial cell mitochondria; TRAP1 ameliorates renal tubulointerstitial fibrosis in mice with unilateral ureteral obstruction by FASEB J 2017; 31: 4503–4514.
[http://dx.doi.org/10.1096/fj.201700283R]

[63]   Collier JB, Whitaker RM, Eblen ST, Schnellmann RG. Rapid Renal Regulation of Peroxisome Proliferator-activated Receptor γ Coactivator-1α by Extracellular Signal-Regulated Kinase 1/2 in Physiological and Pathological Conditions. J Biol Chem 2016; 291(52): 26850-9.
[http://dx.doi.org/10.1074/jbc.M116.754762] [PMID: 27875304]

[64]   Geng X, Hong Q, Wang W, *et al.* Biological Membrane-Packed Mesenchymal Stem Cells Treat Acute

Kidney Disease by Ameliorating Mitochondrial-Related Apoptosis. Sci Rep 2017; 7(1): 41136.
[http://dx.doi.org/10.1038/srep41136] [PMID: 28117405]

[65]   Ni Z, Tao L, Xiaohui X, *et al.* Polydatin impairs mitochondria fitness and ameliorates podocyte injury by suppressing Drp1 expression. J Cell Physiol 2017; 232(10): 2776-87.
[http://dx.doi.org/10.1002/jcp.25943] [PMID: 28383775]

[66]   Zhang J, Wang Q, Xu C, *et al.* MitoTEMPO Prevents Oxalate Induced Injury in NRK□52E Cells *via* Inhibiting Mitochondrial Dysfunction and Modulating Oxidative Stress. Oxid Med Cell Longev 2017; 2017(1): 7528090.
[http://dx.doi.org/10.1155/2017/7528090] [PMID: 28116040]

[67]   Lin TA, Wu VCC, Wang CY. Autophagy in Chronic Kidney Diseases. Cells 2019; 8(1): 61.
[http://dx.doi.org/10.3390/cells8010061] [PMID: 30654583]

[68]   Kaushal GP, Shah SV. Autophagy in acute kidney injury. Kidney Int 2016; 89(4): 779-91.
[http://dx.doi.org/10.1016/j.kint.2015.11.021] [PMID: 26924060]

[69]   Lei R, Zhao F, Tang CY, *et al.* Mitophagy Plays a Protective Role in Iodinated Contrast-Induced Acute Renal Tubular Epithelial Cells Injury. Cell Physiol Biochem 2018; 46(3): 975-85.
[http://dx.doi.org/10.1159/000488827] [PMID: 29680838]

[70]   Decuypere JP, Ceulemans LJ, Agostinis P, *et al.* Autophagy and the Kidney: Implications for Ischemia-Reperfusion Injury and Therapy. Am J Kidney Dis 2015; 66(4): 699-709.
[http://dx.doi.org/10.1053/j.ajkd.2015.05.021] [PMID: 26169721]

[71]   Kimura T, Isaka Y, Yoshimori T. Autophagy and kidney inflammation. Autophagy 2017; 13(6): 997-1003.
[http://dx.doi.org/10.1080/15548627.2017.1309485] [PMID: 28441075]

[72]   Kitada M, Ogura Y, Monno I, Koya D. Regulating Autophagy as a Therapeutic Target for Diabetic Nephropathy. Curr Diab Rep 2017; 17(7): 53.
[http://dx.doi.org/10.1007/s11892-017-0879-y] [PMID: 28593583]

[73]   Tang C, Han H, Yan M, *et al.* PINK1-PRKN/PARK2 pathway of mitophagy is activated to protect against renal ischemia-reperfusion injury. Autophagy 2018; 14(5): 880-97.
[http://dx.doi.org/10.1080/15548627.2017.1405880] [PMID: 29172924]

[74]   Mkaddem SB, Bens M, Vandewalle A. Differential activation of Toll-like receptor-mediated apoptosis induced by hypoxia. Oncotarget 2010; 1(8): 741-50.
[http://dx.doi.org/10.18632/oncotarget.209] [PMID: 21321383]

[75]   Rana SVS. Metals and apoptosis: Recent developments. J Trace Elem Med Biol 2008; 22(4): 262-84.
[http://dx.doi.org/10.1016/j.jtemb.2008.08.002] [PMID: 19013355]

[76]   Servais H, Ortiz A, Devuyst O, Denamur S, Tulkens PM, Mingeot-Leclercq MP. Renal cell apoptosis induced by nephrotoxic drugs: cellular and molecular mechanisms and potential approaches to modulation. Apoptosis 2008; 13(1): 11-32.
[http://dx.doi.org/10.1007/s10495-007-0151-z] [PMID: 17968659]

[77]   Linkermann A, Chen G, Dong G, Kunzendorf U, Krautwald S, Dong Z. Regulated cell death in AKI. J Am Soc Nephrol 2014; 25(12): 2689-701.
[http://dx.doi.org/10.1681/ASN.2014030262] [PMID: 24925726]

[78]   Aleo MF, Morandini F, Bettoni F, *et al.* Endogenous thiols and MRP transporters contribute to Hg2+ efflux in HgCl2-treated tubular MDCK cells. Toxicology 2005; 206(1): 137-51.
[http://dx.doi.org/10.1016/j.tox.2004.07.003] [PMID: 15590114]

[79]   George B, You D, Joy MS, Aleksunes LM. Xenobiotic transporters and kidney injury. Adv Drug Deliv Rev 2017; 116: 73-91.
[http://dx.doi.org/10.1016/j.addr.2017.01.005] [PMID: 28111348]

[80]   Lash LH, Hueni SE, Putt DA, Zalups RK. Role of organic anion and amino acid carriers in transport of

inorganic mercury in rat renal basolateral membrane vesicles: influence of compensatory renal growth. Toxicol Sci 2005; 88(2): 630-44.
[http://dx.doi.org/10.1093/toxsci/kfi328] [PMID: 16162843]

[81] Zalups RK, Ahmad S. Homocysteine and the renal epithelial transport and toxicity of inorganic mercury: role of basolateral transporter organic anion transporter 1. J Am Soc Nephrol 2004; 15(8): 2023-31.
[http://dx.doi.org/10.1097/01.ASN.0000135115.63412.A9] [PMID: 15284288]

[82] Zalups RK, Ahmad S. Handling of cysteine S-conjugates of methylmercury in MDCK cells expressing human OAT1. Kidney Int 2005; 68(4): 1684-99.
[http://dx.doi.org/10.1111/j.1523-1755.2005.00585.x] [PMID: 16164645]

[83] Breljak D, Ljubojević M, Hagos Y, *et al.* Distribution of organic anion transporters NaDC3 and OAT1-3 along the human nephron. Am J Physiol Renal Physiol 2016; 311(1): F227-38.
[http://dx.doi.org/10.1152/ajprenal.00113.2016] [PMID: 27053689]

[84] Chang C, Hu Y, Hogan S, *et al.* Pharmacogenomic Variants May Influence the Urinary Excretion of Novel Kidney Injury Biomarkers in Patients Receiving Cisplatin. Int J Mol Sci 2017; 18(7): 1333.
[http://dx.doi.org/10.3390/ijms18071333] [PMID: 28640195]

[85] Naesens M, Kuypers DRJ, Sarwal M. Calcineurin inhibitor nephrotoxicity. Clin J Am Soc Nephrol 2009; 4(2): 481-508.
[http://dx.doi.org/10.2215/CJN.04800908] [PMID: 19218475]

[86] Banerjee M, Marensi V, Conseil G, Le XC, Cole SPC, Leslie EM. Polymorphic variants of MRP4/ABCC4 differentially modulate the transport of methylated arsenic metabolites and physiological organic anions. Biochem Pharmacol 2016; 120: 72-82.
[http://dx.doi.org/10.1016/j.bcp.2016.09.016] [PMID: 27659809]

[87] Izzedine H. [Drug nephrotoxicity]. Nephrol Ther 2018; 14(3): 127-34.
[http://dx.doi.org/10.1016/j.nephro.2017.06.006] [PMID: 29540291]

[88] Zhou Y, Vaidya VS, Brown RP, *et al.* Comparison of kidney injury molecule-1 and other nephrotoxicity biomarkers in urine and kidney following acute exposure to gentamicin, mercury, and chromium. Toxicol Sci 2008; 101(1): 159-70.
[http://dx.doi.org/10.1093/toxsci/kfm260] [PMID: 17934191]

[89] Shao C, Li M, Li X, *et al.* A tool for biomarker discovery in the urinary proteome: a manually curated human and animal urine protein biomarker database. Mol Cell Proteomics 2011; 10(11): M111.010975.
[http://dx.doi.org/10.1074/mcp.M111.010975] [PMID: 21876203]

[90] Wu Y, Yang L, Su T, Wang C, Liu G, Li X. Pathological significance of a panel of urinary biomarkers in patients with drug-induced tubulointerstitial nephritis. Clin J Am Soc Nephrol 2010; 5(11): 1954-9.
[http://dx.doi.org/10.2215/CJN.02370310] [PMID: 20813857]

[91] Xue Y, Daniels LB, Maisel AS, *et al.* Cardiac Biomarkers. Reference Module in Biomedical Sciences. Elsevier 2014.
[http://dx.doi.org/10.1016/B978-0-12-801238-3.00022-2]

[92] Perrone RD, Madias NE, Levey AS. Serum creatinine as an index of renal function: new insights into old concepts. Clin Chem 1992; 38(10): 1933-53.
[http://dx.doi.org/10.1093/clinchem/38.10.1933] [PMID: 1394976]

[93] Campos MAA, de Almeida LA, Grossi MF, Tagliati CA. *In vitro* evaluation of biomarkers of nephrotoxicity through gene expression using gentamicin. J Biochem Mol Toxicol 2018; 32(9): e22189.
[http://dx.doi.org/10.1002/jbt.22189] [PMID: 29992668]

[94] Ferguson MA, Vaidya VS, Bonventre JV. Biomarkers of nephrotoxic acute kidney injury. Toxicology 2008; 245(3): 182-93.

[http://dx.doi.org/10.1016/j.tox.2007.12.024] [PMID: 18294749]

[95]   Finn W, Porter G. Urinary biomarkers and nephrotoxicity. Clinical Nephrotoxins. 2nd ed Klu. Massachusetts., 2003.
[http://dx.doi.org/10.1007/1-4020-2586-6_33]

[96]   Mogensen CE. Urinary albumin excretion in early and long-term juvenile diabetes. Scand J Clin Lab Invest 1971; 28(2): 183-93.
[http://dx.doi.org/10.3109/00365517109086899] [PMID: 5130106]

[97]   Prinsen BHCMT, De Sain-Van Der Velden MGM, Kaysen GA, *et al.* Transferrin synthesis is increased in nephrotic patients insufficiently to replace urinary losses. J Am Soc Nephrol 2001; 12(5): 1017-25.
[http://dx.doi.org/10.1681/ASN.V1251017] [PMID: 11316861]

[98]   Bernard AM, Vyskocil AA, Mahieu P, Lauwerys RR. Assessment of urinary retinol-binding protein as an index of proximal tubular injury. Clin Chem 1987; 33(6): 775-9.
[http://dx.doi.org/10.1093/clinchem/33.6.775] [PMID: 3297418]

[99]   Emeigh Hart SG. Assessment of renal injury *in vivo*. J Pharmacol Toxicol Methods 2005; 52(1): 30-45.
[http://dx.doi.org/10.1016/j.vascn.2005.04.006] [PMID: 15953738]

[100] Schaub S, Wilkins JA, Antonovici M, *et al.* Proteomic-based identification of cleaved urinary beta2-microglobulin as a potential marker for acute tubular injury in renal allografts. Am J Transplant 2005; 5(4): 729-38.
[http://dx.doi.org/10.1111/j.1600-6143.2005.00766.x] [PMID: 15760396]

[101] Conti M, Moutereau S, Zater M, *et al.* Urinary cystatin C as a specific marker of tubular dysfunction. Clin Chem Lab Med 2006; 44(3): 288-91.
[http://dx.doi.org/10.1515/CCLM.2006.050] [PMID: 16519600]

[102] Vaidya VS, Ramirez V, Ichimura T, Bobadilla NA, Bonventre JV. Urinary kidney injury molecule-1: a sensitive quantitative biomarker for early detection of kidney tubular injury. Am J Physiol Renal Physiol 2006; 290(2): F517-29.
[http://dx.doi.org/10.1152/ajprenal.00291.2005] [PMID: 16174863]

[103] Bailly V, Zhang Z, Meier W, Cate R, Sanicola M, Bonventre JV. Shedding of kidney injury molecule-1, a putative adhesion protein involved in renal regeneration. J Biol Chem 2002; 277(42): 39739-48.
[http://dx.doi.org/10.1074/jbc.M200562200] [PMID: 12138159]

[104] Nielsen BS, Borregaard N, Bundgaard JR, Timshel S, Sehested M, Kjeldsen L. Induction of NGAL synthesis in epithelial cells of human colorectal neoplasia and inflammatory bowel diseases. Gut 1996; 38(3): 414-20.
[http://dx.doi.org/10.1136/gut.38.3.414] [PMID: 8675096]

[105] Yu Y, Jin H, Holder D, *et al.* Urinary biomarkers trefoil factor 3 and albumin enable early detection of kidney tubular injury. Nat Biotechnol 2010; 28(5): 470-7.
[http://dx.doi.org/10.1038/nbt.1624] [PMID: 20458317]

[106] Kaleta B. The role of osteopontin in kidney diseases. Inflamm Res 2019; 68(2): 93-102.
[http://dx.doi.org/10.1007/s00011-018-1200-5] [PMID: 30456594]

[107] Cao R, Li L, Ying Z, *et al.* A small molecule protects mitochondrial integrity by inhibiting mTOR activity. Proc Natl Acad Sci USA 2019; 116(46): 23332-8.
[http://dx.doi.org/10.1073/pnas.1911246116] [PMID: 31653761]

[108] Chen HH, Chen YT, Yang CC, *et al.* Melatonin pretreatment enhances the therapeutic effects of exogenous mitochondria against hepatic ischemia–reperfusion injury in rats through suppression of mitochondrial permeability transition. J Pineal Res 2016; 61(1): 52-68.
[http://dx.doi.org/10.1111/jpi.12326] [PMID: 26993080]

[109] Meka DP, Müller-Rischart AK, Nidadavolu P, *et al.* Parkin cooperates with GDNF/RET signaling to

prevent dopaminergic neuron degeneration. J Clin Invest 2015; 125(5): 1873-85.
[http://dx.doi.org/10.1172/JCI79300] [PMID: 25822020]

[110] Ralto KM, Rhee EP, Parikh SM. NAD$^+$ homeostasis in renal health and disease. Nat Rev Nephrol 2020; 16(2): 99-111.
[http://dx.doi.org/10.1038/s41581-019-0216-6] [PMID: 31673160]

[111] Chevalier RL. The proximal tubule is the primary target of injury and progression of kidney disease: role of the glomerulotubular junction. Am J Physiol Renal Physiol 2016; 311(1): F145-61.
[http://dx.doi.org/10.1152/ajprenal.00164.2016] [PMID: 27194714]

[112] Mei S, Livingston M, Hao J, li L, Mei C, Dong Z. Autophagy is activated to protect against endotoxic acute kidney injury. Sci Rep 2016; 6(1): 22171.
[http://dx.doi.org/10.1038/srep22171] [PMID: 26916346]

[113] Wang Y, Cai J, Tang C, Dong Z. Mitophagy in acute kidney injury and kidney repair. Cells 2020; 9(2): 338.
[http://dx.doi.org/10.3390/cells9020338] [PMID: 32024113]

[114] Funk JA, Schnellmann RG, Schnellmann RG. Persistent disruption of mitochondrial homeostasis after acute kidney injury. Am J Physiol Renal Physiol 2012; 302(7): F853-64.
[http://dx.doi.org/10.1152/ajprenal.00035.2011] [PMID: 22160772]

[115] Brooks C, Wei Q, Cho SG, Dong Z. Regulation of mitochondrial dynamics in acute kidney injury in cell culture and rodent models. J Clin Invest 2009; 119(5): 1275-85.
[http://dx.doi.org/10.1172/JCI37829] [PMID: 19349686]

[116] Perry HM, Huang L, Wilson RJ, *et al.* Dynamin-Related Protein 1 Deficiency Promotes Recovery from AKI. J Am Soc Nephrol 2018; 29(1): 194-206.
[http://dx.doi.org/10.1681/ASN.2017060659] [PMID: 29084809]

[117] Zhao C, Chen Z, Qi J, *et al.* Drp1-dependent mitophagy protects against cisplatin-induced apoptosis of renal tubular epithelial cells by improving mitochondrial function. Oncotarget 2017; 8(13): 20988-1000.
[http://dx.doi.org/10.18632/oncotarget.15470] [PMID: 28423497]

[118] Zhou L, Zhang L, Zhang Y, *et al.* PINK1 Deficiency Ameliorates Cisplatin-Induced Acute Kidney Injury in Rats. Front Physiol 2019; 10: 1225.
[http://dx.doi.org/10.3389/fphys.2019.01225] [PMID: 31607953]

[119] Lin Q, Li S, Jiang N, *et al.* PINK1-parkin pathway of mitophagy protects against contrast-induced acute kidney injury *via* decreasing mitochondrial ROS and NLRP3 inflammasome activation. Redox Biol 2019; 26: 101254.
[http://dx.doi.org/10.1016/j.redox.2019.101254] [PMID: 31229841]

[120] Liang X, Yang Y, Huang Z, Zhou J, Li Y, Zhong X. *Panax notoginseng saponins* mitigate cisplatin induced nephrotoxicity by inducing mitophagy *via* HIF-1α. Oncotarget 2017; 8(61): 102989-3003.
[http://dx.doi.org/10.18632/oncotarget.19900] [PMID: 29262539]

[121] Tran MT, Zsengeller ZK, Berg AH, *et al.* PGC1α drives NAD biosynthesis linking oxidative metabolism to renal protection. Nature 2016; 531(7595): 528-32.
[http://dx.doi.org/10.1038/nature17184] [PMID: 26982719]

[122] Gibbs WS, Collier JB, Morris M, Beeson CC, Megyesi J, Schnellmann RG. 5-HT$_{1F}$ receptor regulates mitochondrial homeostasis and its loss potentiates acute kidney injury and impairs renal recovery. Am J Physiol Renal Physiol 2018; 315(4): F1119-28.
[http://dx.doi.org/10.1152/ajprenal.00077.2018] [PMID: 29846105]

[123] Plotnikov E, Pevzner I, Zorova L, *et al.* Mitochondrial Damage and Mitochondria-Targeted Antioxidant Protection in LPS-Induced Acute Kidney Injury. Antioxidants 2019; 8(6): 176.
[http://dx.doi.org/10.3390/antiox8060176] [PMID: 31197113]

[124] Kong MJ, Bak SH, Han KH, Kim JI, Park JW, Park KM. Fragmentation of kidney epithelial cell

primary cilia occurs by cisplatin and these cilia fragments are excreted into the urine. Redox Biol 2019; 20: 38-45.
[http://dx.doi.org/10.1016/j.redox.2018.09.017] [PMID: 30292083]

[125] Liu D, Jin F, Shu G, *et al.* Enhanced efficiency of mitochondria-targeted peptide SS-31 for acute kidney injury by pH-responsive and AKI-kidney targeted nanopolyplexes. Biomaterials 2019; 211: 57-67.
[http://dx.doi.org/10.1016/j.biomaterials.2019.04.034] [PMID: 31085359]

[126] Dutta RK, Kondeti VK, Sharma I, Chandel NS, Quaggin SE, Kanwar YS. Beneficial Effects of *Myo*-Inositol Oxygenase Deficiency in Cisplatin-Induced AKI. J Am Soc Nephrol 2017; 28(5): 1421-36.
[http://dx.doi.org/10.1681/ASN.2016070744] [PMID: 27895157]

[127] Yang X, Yan X, Yang D, Zhou J, Song J, Yang D. Rapamycin attenuates mitochondrial injury and renal tubular cell apoptosis in experimental contrast-induced acute kidney injury in rats. Biosci Rep 2018; 38(6): BSR20180876.
[http://dx.doi.org/10.1042/BSR20180876] [PMID: 30341250]

[128] Rahdar A, Hasanein P, Bilal M, Beyzaei H, Kyzas GZ. Quercetin-loaded F127 nanomicelles: Antioxidant activity and protection against renal injury induced by gentamicin in rats. Life Sci 2021; 276: 119420.
[http://dx.doi.org/10.1016/j.lfs.2021.119420] [PMID: 33785340]

[129] Wargo KA, Edwards JD. Aminoglycoside-Induced Nephrotoxicity. J Pharm Pract 2014; 27(6): 573-7.
[http://dx.doi.org/10.1177/0897190014546836] [PMID: 25199523]

[130] Palm CA, Segev G, Cowgill LD, *et al.* Urinary Neutrophil Gelatinase□associated Lipocalin as a Marker for Identification of Acute Kidney Injury and Recovery in Dogs with Gentamicin□induced Nephrotoxicity. J Vet Intern Med 2016; 30(1): 200-5.
[http://dx.doi.org/10.1111/jvim.13819] [PMID: 26725776]

[131] Atta MG, Deray G, Lucas GM. Antiretroviral Nephrotoxicities. Semin Nephrol 2008; 28(6): 563-75.
[http://dx.doi.org/10.1016/j.semnephrol.2008.08.009] [PMID: 19013327]

[132] Chan L, Asriel B, Eaton EF, Wyatt CM. Potential kidney toxicity from the antiviral drug tenofovir. Curr Opin Nephrol Hypertens 2018; 27(2): 102-12.
[http://dx.doi.org/10.1097/MNH.0000000000000392] [PMID: 29278542]

[133] Fanos V, Cataldi L. Amphotericin B-induced nephrotoxicity: a review. J Chemother 2000; 12(6): 463-70.
[http://dx.doi.org/10.1179/joc.2000.12.6.463] [PMID: 11154026]

[134] Ordooei Javan A, Shokouhi S, Sahraei Z. A review on colistin nephrotoxicity. Eur J Clin Pharmacol 2015; 71(7): 801-10.
[http://dx.doi.org/10.1007/s00228-015-1865-4] [PMID: 26008213]

[135] Zavascki AP, Nation RL. Nephrotoxicity of Polymyxins: Is There Any Difference between Colistimethate and Polymyxin B? Antimicrob Agents Chemother 2017; 61(3): e02319-16.
[http://dx.doi.org/10.1128/AAC.02319-16] [PMID: 27993859]

[136] Samodelov SL, Visentin M, Gai Z, Häusler S, Kullak-Ublick GA. Renal glycosuria as a novel early sign of colistin-induced kidney damage in mice. Antimicrob Agents Chemother 2019; 63(12): e01650-19.
[http://dx.doi.org/10.1128/AAC.01650-19] [PMID: 31591120]

[137] Raju SB, Goli R, Mukku KK, Uppin MS. Acute ciprofloxacin-induced crystal nephropathy with granulomatous interstitial nephritis. Indian J Nephrol 2017; 27(3): 231-3.
[http://dx.doi.org/10.4103/0971-4065.200522] [PMID: 28553048]

[138] Hajji M, Jebali H, Mrad A, *et al.* Nephrotoxicity of Ciprofloxacin: Five Cases and a Review of the Literature. Drug Saf Case Rep 2018; 5(1): 17.
[http://dx.doi.org/10.1007/s40800-018-0073-4] [PMID: 29671145]

[139] Shaki F, Ashari S, Ahangar N. Melatonin can attenuate ciprofloxacin induced nephrotoxicity: Involvement of nitric oxide and TNF-α. Biomed Pharmacother 2016; 84: 1172-8.
[http://dx.doi.org/10.1016/j.biopha.2016.10.053] [PMID: 27780148]

[140] Arimura Y, Yano T, Hirano M, Sakamoto Y, Egashira N, Oishi R. Mitochondrial superoxide production contributes to vancomycin-induced renal tubular cell apoptosis. Free Radic Biol Med 2012; 52(9): 1865-73.
[http://dx.doi.org/10.1016/j.freeradbiomed.2012.02.038] [PMID: 22401854]

[141] Bamgbola O. Review of vancomycin-induced renal toxicity: an update. Ther Adv Endocrinol Metab 2016; 7(3): 136-47.
[http://dx.doi.org/10.1177/2042018816638223] [PMID: 27293542]

[142] Nishino Y, Takemura S, Minamiyama Y, *et al.* Inhibition of vancomycin-induced nephrotoxicity by targeting superoxide dismutase to renal proximal tubule cells in the rat. Redox Rep 2002; 7(5): 317-9.
[http://dx.doi.org/10.1179/135100002125000884] [PMID: 12688519]

[143] Sakamoto Y, Yano T, Hanada Y, *et al.* Vancomycin induces reactive oxygen species-dependent apoptosis *via* mitochondrial cardiolipin peroxidation in renal tubular epithelial cells. Eur J Pharmacol 2017; 800: 48-56.
[http://dx.doi.org/10.1016/j.ejphar.2017.02.025] [PMID: 28216050]

[144] El Bohi KM, Abdel-Motal SM, Khalil SR, Abd-Elaal MM, Metwally MMM, ELhady WM. The efficiency of pomegranate (*Punica granatum*) peel ethanolic extract in attenuating the vancomycin-triggered liver and kidney tissues injury in rats. Environ Sci Pollut Res Int 2021; 28(6): 7134-50.
[http://dx.doi.org/10.1007/s11356-020-10999-3] [PMID: 33029776]

[145] Ragab AR, Al-Mazroua MK, Al-Dakrory SA-E. Cyclosporine toxicity and toxicokinetics profiles in renal transplant recipients. J Clin Toxicol 2013; 03: 1–8.
[http://dx.doi.org/10.4172/2161-0495.1000154]

[146] Wu Q, Wang X, Nepovimova E, Wang Y, Yang H, Kuca K. Mechanism of cyclosporine A nephrotoxicity: Oxidative stress, autophagy, and signalings. Food Chem Toxicol 2018; 118: 889-907.
[http://dx.doi.org/10.1016/j.fct.2018.06.054] [PMID: 29960018]

[147] Young BA, Burdmann EA, Johnson RJ, *et al.* Cellular proliferation and macrophage influx precede interstitial fibrosis in cyclosporine nephrotoxicity. Kidney Int 1995; 48(2): 439-48.
[http://dx.doi.org/10.1038/ki.1995.312] [PMID: 7564111]

[148] Wasilewska A, Zoch-Zwierz W, Taranta-Janusz K, Michaluk-Skutnik J. Neutrophil gelatinase-associated lipocalin (NGAL): a new marker of cyclosporine nephrotoxicity? Pediatr Nephrol 2010; 25(5): 889-97.
[http://dx.doi.org/10.1007/s00467-009-1397-1] [PMID: 20072790]

[149] Rangan GK. Sirolimus-associated proteinuria and renal dysfunction. Drug Saf 2006; 29(12): 1153-61.
[http://dx.doi.org/10.2165/00002018-200629120-00006] [PMID: 17147461]

[150] Karademir LD, Dogruel F, Kocyigit I, *et al.* The efficacy of theophylline in preventing cisplatin-related nephrotoxicity in patients with cancer. Ren Fail 2016; 38(5): 806-14.
[http://dx.doi.org/10.3109/0886022X.2016.1163154] [PMID: 27049176]

[151] Karasawa T, Steyger PS. An integrated view of cisplatin-induced nephrotoxicity and ototoxicity. Toxicol Lett 2015; 237: 219–227.
[http://dx.doi.org/10.1016/j.toxlet.2015.06.012]

[152] Małyszko J, Kozłowska K, Kozłowski L, Małyszko J. Nephrotoxicity of anticancer treatment. Nephrol Dial Transplant 2016; 32(6): gfw338.
[http://dx.doi.org/10.1093/ndt/gfw338] [PMID: 28339935]

[153] Mishra J, Mori K, Ma Q, Kelly C, Barasch J, Devarajan P. Neutrophil gelatinase-associated lipocalin: a novel early urinary biomarker for cisplatin nephrotoxicity. Am J Nephrol 2004; 24(3): 307-15.
[http://dx.doi.org/10.1159/000078452] [PMID: 15148457]

[154] Akilesh S, Juaire N, Duffield JS, Smith KD. Chronic Ifosfamide toxicity: kidney pathology and pathophysiology. Am J Kidney Dis 2014; 63(5): 843-50.
[http://dx.doi.org/10.1053/j.ajkd.2013.11.028] [PMID: 24518127]

[155] Ensergueix G, Pallet N, Joly D, *et al.* Ifosfamide nephrotoxicity in adult patients. Clin Kidney J 2020; 13(4): 660-5.
[http://dx.doi.org/10.1093/ckj/sfz183] [PMID: 32897279]

[156] Perazella MA, Moeckel GW. Nephrotoxicity from chemotherapeutic agents: clinical manifestations, pathobiology, and prevention/therapy. Semin Nephrol 2010; 30(6): 570-81.
[http://dx.doi.org/10.1016/j.semnephrol.2010.09.005] [PMID: 21146122]

[157] Rjiba-Touati K, Ayed-Boussema I, Guedri Y, Achour A, Bacha H, Abid-Essefi S. Effect of recombinant human erythropoietin on mitomycin C-induced oxidative stress and genotoxicity in rat kidney and heart tissues. Hum Exp Toxicol 2016; 35(1): 53-62.
[http://dx.doi.org/10.1177/0960327115577521] [PMID: 25733728]

[158] Verweij J, Kerpel-Fronius S, Stuurman M, *et al.* Mitomycin C-induced organ toxicity in Wistar rats: a study with special focus on the kidney. J Cancer Res Clin Oncol 1988; 114(2): 137-41.
[http://dx.doi.org/10.1007/BF00417827] [PMID: 3127399]

[159] Strang A, Pullar T. Methotrexate toxicity induced by acute renal failure. J R Soc Med 2004; 97(11): 536-7.
[http://dx.doi.org/10.1177/014107680409701106] [PMID: 15520148]

[160] Türk E, Güvenç M, Cellat M, *et al.* Zingerone protects liver and kidney tissues by preventing oxidative stress, inflammation, and apoptosis in methotrexate-treated rats. Drug Chem Toxicol 2020; 0: 1-12.
[http://dx.doi.org/10.1080/01480545.2020.1804397] [PMID: 32781857]

[161] Yang S-L, Zhao F-Y, Song H, *et al.* Clinical Study Methotrexate Associated Renal Impairment Is Related to Delayed Elimination of High-Dose Methotrexate. Scientific World Journal 2015; 2015: 8.
[http://dx.doi.org/10.1155/2015/751703]

[162] Jarrar QB, Hakim MN, Zakaria ZA, Cheema MS, Moshawih S. Renal ultrastructural alterations induced by various preparations of mefenamic acid. Ultrastruct Pathol 2020; 44(1): 130-40.
[http://dx.doi.org/10.1080/01913123.2020.1717705] [PMID: 31967489]

[163] Somchit MN, Sanat F, Hui GE, Wahab SI, Ahmad Z. Mefenamic Acid induced nephrotoxicity: an animal model. Adv Pharm Bull 2014; 4(4): 401-4.
[http://dx.doi.org/10.5681/apb.2014.059] [PMID: 25436198]

[164] El-Ashker MR, Hussein HS, El-Sebaei MG. Evaluation of urinary variables as diagnostic indicators of acute kidney injury in egyptian draft horses treated with phenylbutazone therapy. J Equine Vet Sci 2012; 32(5): 268-73.
[http://dx.doi.org/10.1016/j.jevs.2011.09.072]

[165] Barrett BJ, Parfrey PS. Clinical practice. Preventing nephropathy induced by contrast medium. N Engl J Med 2006; 354(4): 379-86.
[http://dx.doi.org/10.1056/NEJMcp050801] [PMID: 16436769]

[166] Wilhelm-Leen E, Montez-Rath ME, Chertow G. Estimating the risk of radiocontrast-associated nephropathy. J Am Soc Nephrol 2017; 28(2): 653-9.
[http://dx.doi.org/10.1681/ASN.2016010021] [PMID: 27688297]

[167] Kane GC, Stanson AW, Kalnicka D, *et al.* Comparison between gadolinium and iodine contrast for percutaneous intervention in atherosclerotic renal artery stenosis: clinical outcomes. Nephrol Dial Transplant 2007; 23(4): 1233-40.
[http://dx.doi.org/10.1093/ndt/gfm725] [PMID: 18256017]

[168] Han B, Lv Z, Han X, *et al.* Harmful Effects of Inorganic Mercury Exposure on Kidney Cells: Mitochondrial Dynamics Disorder and Excessive Oxidative Stress. Biol Trace Elem Res 2022; 200(4): 1591-7.

[http://dx.doi.org/10.1007/s12011-021-02766-3] [PMID: 34060062]

[169] Hazelhoff MH, Bulacio RP, Torres AM. Trimetazidine protects from mercury-induced kidney injury. Pharmacology 2021; 106(5-6): 332-40.
[http://dx.doi.org/10.1159/000514843] [PMID: 33849026]

[170] Baş H, Apaydın FG, Kalender S, Kalender Y. Lead nitrate and cadmium chloride induced hepatotoxicity and nephrotoxicity: Protective effects of sesamol on biochemical indices and pathological changes. J Food Biochem 2021; 45(7): e13769.
[http://dx.doi.org/10.1111/jfbc.13769] [PMID: 34021611]

[171] Gobe G, Crane D. Mitochondria, reactive oxygen species and cadmium toxicity in the kidney. Toxicol Lett 2010; 198(1): 49-55.
[http://dx.doi.org/10.1016/j.toxlet.2010.04.013] [PMID: 20417263]

[172] Satarug S. Urinary N-acetylglucosaminidase in people environmentally exposed to cadmium is minimally related to cadmium-induced nephron destruction. Toxics 2024; 12(11): 775.
[http://dx.doi.org/10.3390/toxics12110775] [PMID: 39590955]

[173] Mozaffari MS, Baban B, Abdelsayed R, *et al.* Renal and glycemic effects of high-dose chromium picolinate in db/db mice: assessment of DNA damage. J Nutr Biochem 2012; 23(8): 977-85.
[http://dx.doi.org/10.1016/j.jnutbio.2011.05.004] [PMID: 21959055]

[174] Wedeen RP, Qian LF. Chromium-induced kidney disease. Environ Health Perspect 1991; 92: 71-4.
[http://dx.doi.org/10.1289/ehp.92-1519395] [PMID: 1935854]

[175] Arzuaga X, Rieth SH, Bathija A, Cooper GS. Renal effects of exposure to natural and depleted uranium: a review of the epidemiologic and experimental data. J Toxicol Environ Health B Crit Rev 2010; 13(7-8): 527-45.
[http://dx.doi.org/10.1080/10937404.2010.509015] [PMID: 21170808]

[176] Shaki F, Hosseini MJ, Ghazi-Khansari M, Pourahmad J. Toxicity of depleted uranium on isolated rat kidney mitochondria. Biochim Biophys Acta, Gen Subj 2012; 1820(12): 1940-50.
[http://dx.doi.org/10.1016/j.bbagen.2012.08.015] [PMID: 22940002]

[177] Barceloux DG, Barceloux D. Copper. J Toxicol Clin Toxicol 1999; 37(2): 217-30.
[http://dx.doi.org/10.1081/CLT-100102421] [PMID: 10382557]

[178] Galhardi CM, Diniz YS, Faine LA, *et al.* Toxicity of copper intake: lipid profile, oxidative stress and susceptibility to renal dysfunction. Food Chem Toxicol 2004; 42(12): 2053-60.
[http://dx.doi.org/10.1016/j.fct.2004.07.020] [PMID: 15500942]

[179] Roy A, Manna P, Sil PC. Prophylactic role of taurine on arsenic mediated oxidative renal dysfunction *via* MAPKs/ NF-κ B and mitochondria dependent pathways. Free Radic Res 2009; 43(10): 995-1007.
[http://dx.doi.org/10.1080/10715760903164998] [PMID: 19672740]

[180] Mutti A, Coccini T, Alinovi R, *et al.* Exposure to hydrocarbons and renal disease: an experimental animal model. Ren Fail 1999; 21(3-4): 369-85.
[http://dx.doi.org/10.3109/08860229909085101] [PMID: 10416216]

[181] Turkmen R, Birdane YO, Demirel HH, Yavuz H, Kabu M, Ince S. Antioxidant and cytoprotective effects of N-acetylcysteine against subchronic oral glyphosate-based herbicide-induced oxidative stress in rats. Environ Sci Pollut Res Int 2019; 26(11): 11427-37.
[http://dx.doi.org/10.1007/s11356-019-04585-5] [PMID: 30805841]

[182] Wunnapuk K, Gobe G, Endre Z, *et al.* Use of a glyphosate-based herbicide-induced nephrotoxicity model to investigate a panel of kidney injury biomarkers. Toxicol Lett 2014; 225(1): 192-200.
[http://dx.doi.org/10.1016/j.toxlet.2013.12.009] [PMID: 24361898]

[183] Dinis-Oliveira RJ, Duarte JA, Sánchez-Navarro A, Remião F, Bastos ML, Carvalho F. Paraquat poisonings: mechanisms of lung toxicity, clinical features, and treatment. Crit Rev Toxicol 2008; 38(1): 13-71.
[http://dx.doi.org/10.1080/10408440701669959] [PMID: 18161502]

[184] Vaziri ND, Ness RL, Fairshter RD, Smith WR, Rosen SM. Nephrotoxicity of paraquat in man. Arch Intern Med 1979; 139(2): 172-4.
[http://dx.doi.org/10.1001/archinte.1979.03630390032014] [PMID: 434971]

[185] Wunnapuk K, Liu X, Peake P, *et al.* Renal biomarkers predict nephrotoxicity after paraquat. Toxicol Lett 2013; 222(3): 280-8.
[http://dx.doi.org/10.1016/j.toxlet.2013.08.003] [PMID: 23954200]

[186] Søderlund EJ, Låg M, Holme JA, *et al.* Species differences in kidney necrosis and DNA damage, distribution and glutathione-dependent metabolism of 1,2-dibromo-3-chloropropane (DBCP). Pharmacol Toxicol 1990; 66(4): 287-93.
[http://dx.doi.org/10.1111/j.1600-0773.1990.tb00749.x] [PMID: 2371234]

[187] Ardalan MR, Tabibi H, Ebrahimzadeh Attari V, Malek Mahdavi A. Nephrotoxic effect of aspartame as an artificial sweetener: A brief review. Iran J Kidney Dis 2017; 11(5): 339-43.
https://www.sid.ir/fileserver/je/116620170501.pdf
[PMID: 29038387]

[188] Iman I. Effect of aspartame on some oxidative stress parameters in liver and kidney of rats. Afr J Pharm Pharmacol 2011; 5(6): 678-862.
[http://dx.doi.org/10.5897/AJPP10.302]

[189] Saleh AAS. Synergistic effect of N-acetyl cysteine and folic acid against aspartame- induced nephrotoxicity in rats. Int J Adv Res (Indore) 2014; 2: 363-73. https://www.journalijar. com/article/1768/synergistic-effect-of-n-acetyl-cysteine-and-folic-acid-against-aspartame--induced-nephrotoxicity-in-rats/

CHAPTER 12

Loss of Cellular Differentiation in Renal Carcinoma

Jazmin Marlen Pérez-Rojas[1,*]

[1] *Research Division, Instituto Nacional De Cancerología, Tlalpan 14080, Mexico City, Mexico*

Abstract: Renal cell carcinoma (RCC) is a silent cancer that has increased in prevalence in the last decade, in men older than 50 years old. Clear cell RCC is the most common type of renal cancer and the most lethal urogenital cancer with a mortality rate above to 40% of frequency. More than 30% of renal cancers develop which are increasing worldwide metastatic spread. The main risk factors related with this neoplasia are smoking, hypertension, chronic kidney disease, and obesity, which are increasing worldwide. RCC has a low response to chemotherapy and radiotherapy, which has led to the investigation of new pharmaceutical strategies, such as immunotherapy and/or its combination with chemotherapy and surgery, for the treatment of this neoplasia. Unfortunately, RCC is resistant to treatment, which complicates its management.

Keywords: Cancer, Cancer therapy, Metastasis, Risk factors, Treatment resistance.

INTRODUCTION

Cancer is a major public health problem and is the second or third leading cause of death worldwide. Renal cell carcinoma (RCC) is a urinary malignancy that represents 3-4% of all types of cancers. Approximately 431,519 new RCC cases and 179,368 RCC-related deaths are registered each year worldwide, with Asia and Europe having the highest incidence. According to data from the International Agency for Research on Cancer (IARC), the mortality rate continues to increase in low- and middle-income countries, with 15,831 deaths in Latin America and the Caribbean and 10,850 deaths in Africa. RCC occurs with a high frequency in the adult population between 50 and 70 years old and with a greater prevalence in males than in females (the incidence rate is 139,216 cases compared with an incidence rate of 71,622 cases, with a 2:1 relation between men and women) [1, 2]. Similar to mortality rate is prevalence rate, it is higher in men compared to

---

[*] **Corresponding author Jazmin Marlen Pérez Rojas:** Research Division, Instituto Nacional De Cancerología, Tlalpan 14080, Mexico City, Mexico; E-mail: jazminmarlen@gmail.com.

women. RCC has a high mortality rate because it is a "silent" tumor. Only 40% of cases present one of the three common symptoms for detection: hematuria, flank pain, or a palpable abdominal mass, while 60% of cases are detected accidentally when the patient undergoes a study of abdominal imaging for nonspecific musculoskeletal or gastrointestinal complaints. RCC metastasizes in more than 25% of patients, with a median survival of 13 months once detected [3]. The main sites where metastasis occurs are the lungs, lymph nodes, liver, bone, and brain. One factor associated with the rise in the incidence of RCC is due to the increased use of diagnostic imaging techniques, such as ultrasound and computed tomography (CT) [4].

PATHOPHYSIOLOGY OF RCC

The onset of loss of cellular differentiation of renal cells egins with the gain and/or deletion of genetic material, which triggers tumorigenesis. Deletions occur frequently on chromosomes 1, 2, 3p, 5q, 6, 7, 8p, 9p, 10, 13, and 17, while gains occur on chromosomes 5q, 7, 16, 17, and 22q [5, 6]. All of these modifications cause chromatin remodeling, which leads to alterations in the genetic products of different survival pathways, such as increases in cell growth [7]. Additionally, understanding the role of altered epigenetic states in these disturbances is important for understanding RCC behavior and, therefore, carrying out pharmacological studies.

Classification

RCC shows notable heterogeneity, both histopathologically and molecularly, with a high diversity of genetic and epigenetic abnormalities, making it difficult to establish a clear line of genetic events to define the process of tumorigenesis [8]. However, it has become essential to establish an order of cellular features to choose the most appropriate and effective therapeutic strategy. The classification of RCC encompasses the histological and functional origin of the cell, the basis of molecular disturbances, the cellular morphology, and genetic alterations. Hence, the most widely accepted categorization is the TNM staging system (T, tumor size; N, lymph node involved; M, metastasis) [9]. The RCC subtypes were classified as follows:

- In clear cell renal cell carcinoma (most common), the cell of origin is in the proximal convoluted tubule of the nephron and accounts for >70%.
- Papillary renal cell carcinoma originates in the distal convoluted tubule and accounts for 15% of total renal cell carcinoma (RCC) cases.
- Chromophobic renal cell carcinoma originates in the intercalary cells of the tubule manifold and represents 5-10% of the cases.

- Collecting duct carcinoma occurs in less than 1% of cases
- Renal medulla carcinoma
- Spindle tubular cell carcinoma
- Unclassifiable renal cell carcinoma
- Papillary adenocarcinoma
- Oncocytoma is considered a benign tumor that is derived from intercalary cells and has an incidence of 7 to 10%.

The Vancouver Classification of Renal Neoplasia by the International Society of Urological Pathology [10] includes new RCC:

- Tubulocystic renal cell carcinoma
- Acquired cystic disease-associated renal cell carcinoma
- Clear cell (tubule) papillary renal cell carcinoma
- Renal cell carcinoma associated with MiT family translocation renal cell carcinoma syndrome
- Renal cell carcinoma associated with hereditary leiomyomatosis renal cell carcinoma syndrome
- Thyroid-like follicular renal cell carcinoma
- Succinic dehydrogenase B deficiency-associated renal cell carcinoma
- ALK translocation in renal cell carcinoma

Risk Factors

Two forms of RCC have been reported, the sporadic and hereditary forms, with the sporadic form being the most common [11]. Several risk factors are associated with the occurrence of sporadic RCC, including smoking [12, 13], hypertension [13, 14] and obesity [13, 15]. Other factors associated with the risk of RCC include occupational exposure to certain carcinogenic agents, such as pesticides, asbestos, benzenes, crystalline silica, sun exposure, and tobacco smoke [16]. Some medical interventions that predispose patients to sporadic RCC are dialysis and/or hemodialysis treatment and kidney transplantation [17, 18].

Hereditary forms of RCC include patients with different syndromes, such as Von Hippel–Lindau syndrome (strongly associated with mutations in chromosome 3p), papillary hereditary carcinoma, Birt-Hogg-Dubés syndrome (a hybrid carcinoma oncocytoma-chromophobic), hereditary leiomyomatosis, germ cell mutation in the B subunit of the succinate dehydrogenase enzyme-encoding gene family, hereditary nonpolyposis colorectal cancer syndrome, PTEN-associated hamartomatous tumor syndrome, and tuberous sclerosis (germline mutations in the tumor suppressor genes TSCI or TSC2). There are other nonsyndromic hereditary forms of RCC, such as the translocation of constitutional chromosome

3p (tumor suppressor gene FHIT), the nonsyndromic family of clear cell renal carcinoma, and finally, patients whose first-degree relatives are diagnosed with RCC [19].

Hypertension

Arterial hypertension is the most common disease worldwide. The relationship between hypertension and the development of RCC is not yet fully understood. Some studies have reported that hypertensive patients have a moderately increased risk for several kinds of cancer, such as RCC [13, 20]. The possible mechanisms involved are related to lipid peroxidation, renin-angiotensi--aldosterone system disturbances, inflammation, and obesity [21, 22]. Inflammation may promote hypoxia-inducing factors in the kidney, leading to cell growth dysregulation and angiogenesis [23]. In addition, hypertension may be associated with endothelial dysfunction and altered vascular remodeling, which increase the formation of reactive oxygen species [24] and consequently promote tumor development and disease progression (Fig. **1**) [25]. Christakoudi and coworkers reported positive associations of systolic and diastolic blood pressure with the development of malignant cancers; among these, RCC presented equal incidences in men and women [20].

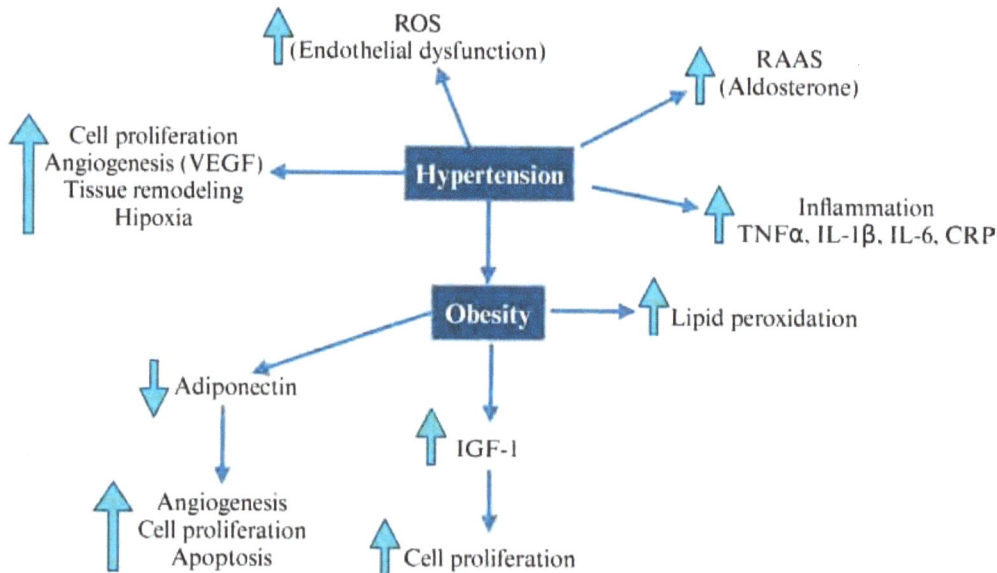

Fig. (1). Schematic diagram illustrating the relationship between hypertension and obesity. ROS, reactive oxygen species; RAAS, renin-angiotensin-aldosterone system; TNFα, tumor necrosis factor-alpha; IL-1β, interleukin-1beta; CRP, C-reactive protein; IGF-1, insulin-like growth factor 1; VEGF, vascular endothelial growth factor.

Obesity and Dyslipidemia

Currently, obesity and dyslipidemia are metabolic disturbances that are common worldwide and are frequently found in younger populations. Although the role of obesity in the development of cancer is not known, the proportion of cancer cases attributable to obesity is high. Nonetheless, several mechanisms related to the association of obesity with cancer have been proposed, including the high serum concentration of insulin-like growth factor 1 (IGF-1) in obese people; this mitogen factor has been linked to proliferation and cell cycle dysregulation [12]. Another suggested mechanism involved a decrease in the concentration of serum adiponectin. Adiponectin is involved in regulating glucose levels and fatty acid breakdown, and a decrease in adiponectin causes an increase in angiogenesis and proliferation and a decrease in apoptosis (Fig. **1**); however, additional studies to determine the participation of this hormone in RCC development are still needed [26].

There is controversy about the association between dyslipidemia and RCC. Some reports in the literature have shown that statins reduce the risk of developing RCC, while other studies have reported no association between them [27]. For this reason, investigations into the participation of this metabolic disorder in RCC development are still ongoing.

Genetics

As mentioned above, RCC has hereditary factors that influence the development of this type of neoplasia. Table **1** summarizes the main genetic alterations that occur and are associated with the different types of RCC [28, 29].

Von Hippel–Lindau (VHL) disease is an autosomal dominant disorder caused by mutations in the VHL tumor suppressor gene. Affected individuals are at high risk of developing RCC. Mutations in the VHL gene can occur at early ages, such as during adolescence [28]. The VHL gene is associated with the regulation of hypoxia-inducible factor (HIF); under normal conditions, VHL contributes to the degradation of HIF *via* the ubiquitination pathway, but when VHL is mutated or methylated, HIF accumulates in the cell and induces the transcription of genes encoding cell growth factors such as vascular endothelial growth factor (VEGF); survival genes such as transforming growth factor beta (TGFβ) and alpha (TGFα); apoptosis-inducing genes; and glucose metabolism transporters (*e.g.*, GLUT1). Genetic alterations in the different genes of the different types of RCC, whether genetic or sporadic, promote the transformation of cells into malignant cells, followed by cell invasion. However, more complex mutations occur during metastasis, allowing cancer cells to invade other organs [30].

Table 1. The most common molecular alterations corresponding to the type of RCC.

RCC Type	Genetic/Chromosomal Alterations
Clear Cell	• Deletions: 1p, 3p, 4p, 4q, 6q, 8p, 9p, 13q, 14q, Xq • Duplications: 5q, 7, 17q • Mutations or methylation of gene: VHL (chromosome 3p25), PBRM1, SETD2, KDM5C and BAP1
Papillary	• Trisomies and Tetrasomies: 7, 17 • Deletions: Chr Y • C-MET oncogene (chromosome 7q31)
Chromophobic	• Deletions: 1, 2, 6, 10, 13q, 17, 21 • BHD syndrome: BHD gene mutation (chromosome 17p11.2)
Oncocytoma	• Deletions: 1, 14, 6p, 21, Y t (5; 11) • Mitochondrial DNA

VHL, Von Hippel–Lindau; PBRM1, protein polybromo-1; SETD2, SET domain containing 2; BAP1, BRCA1-associated protein 1. BHD, Birt Hogg-Dubé. KDM5C, Lysine demethylase 5C.

In recent years, the increasing prevalence of RCC has been attributed mainly to two factors: the increase in the prevalence of risk factors associated with RCC and the development of modern diagnostic tools (computerized axial tomography and ultrasound), which have allowed the detection of tumors smaller than 4 cm. Therefore, early RCC diagnosis can increase 5-year survival. However, despite timely detection, the mortality of this neoplasia has not decreased, and some reports suggest that this is due to a change in the biology of the tumor, probably due to tobacco consumption, diet, or other carcinogenic agents [31]. Furthermore, the high prevalence of some risk factors promotes the onset of RCC; for example, arterial hypertension is present in 35% of the world population above 50 years of age, and the prevalence of obesity is detected in the adult population, with a prevalence exceeding 35%, in adults over 20 years of age, favoring neoplasia formation [32].

TREATMENT

RCC continues to be known as an intractable tumor. The first-line therapy is surgery, targeted therapy, immunotherapy, or a combination of all these treatments. Radiation and chemotherapy are not widely used due to their low efficacy and high cell resistance (Fig. **2**) [15].

Surgery

There are different surgical options for renal masses: partial nephrectomy and radical nephrectomy; the latter can be laparoscopic, which allows the patient's recovery to be faster than open surgery. Partial nephrectomy is recommended for small tumors (< 2 cm), and the advantage of this type of surgery is the preservation of kidney function. Cryotherapy is a minimally invasive ablative technique used for treating tumors smaller than 4 mm in elderly patients and/or those with compromised kidney function; it is a relatively simple surgery with a high recovery rate [15]. Radical nephrectomy is used for large tumors when the patient does not have chronic renal failure or preexisting proteinuria and when the contralateral kidney has a glomerular filtration rate above 45 mL/min/1.73 m^2 [32].

Immunotherapy

When surgery cannot be performed, either because of the characteristics of the tumor (advanced and/or metastatic carcinoma), the general conditions of the patient, or because the surgery poses a greater risk of complications, the first line of treatment is immunotherapy with monoclonal antibodies against vascular growth factor (VEGF), the most commonly used of which are sunitinib, sorafenib, and bevacizumab. In recent years, other drugs, such as monoclonal antibody-based therapies against tyrosine kinase inhibitors (mTOR), including everolimus and temsirolimus, have been used with promising results [4].

Chemotherapy and Radiotherapy

Chemotherapy is not very effective for treating RCC due to the cells' high resistance. Nevertheless, 5-fluorouracil, in combination with gemcitabine and/or capecitabine, has shown moderate efficacy. Finally, radiotherapy is rarely used in this type of carcinoma due to its modest beneficial effects and a high degree of toxicity to healthy kidney cells [15].

Other Therapies

Cytokine-based immunotherapy (interleukin-2 and interferon alpha) and developing dendritic cell vaccines with CR antigens have been used to treat RCC as alternative therapies [15]. However, no significant changes in the overall survival rate of patients have been observed, and continuing research on new therapies intended to stop and eliminate cancer cells with the least side effects and without compromising kidney function is imperative. Thus, in the last year, treatments that inhibit tumor-initiating capacity are expected to improve the treatment of RCC and promote personalized and targeted therapies [4].

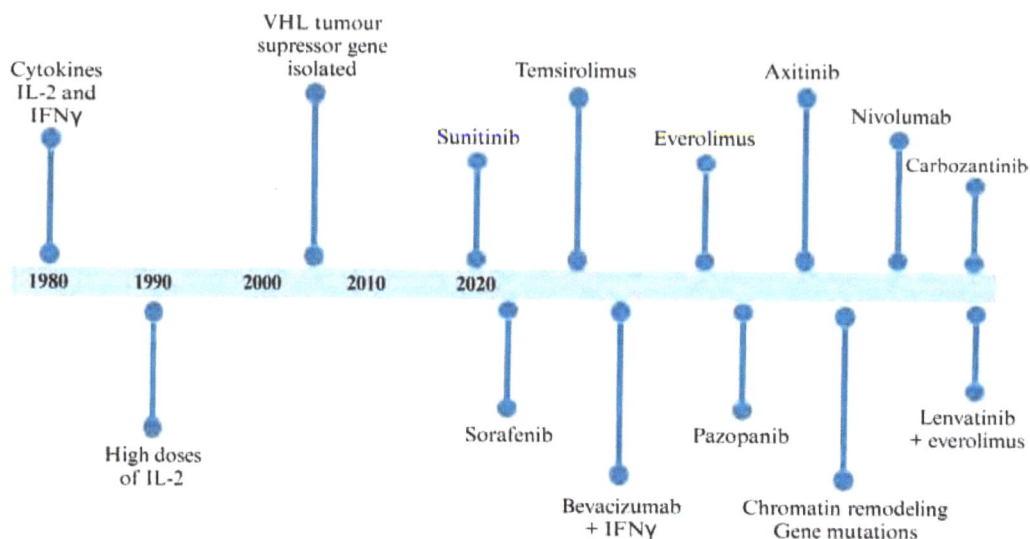

Fig. (2). Timeline of drugs approved for the treatment of RCC.

CONCLUSION

RCC is being detected more frequently around the world. The risk factors associated with this type of cancer are hypertension, obesity, tobacco use, and inherited patterns of VHL disease. For this reason, it is important to emphasize that RCC should be considered an important type of cancer in men, so screening should be mandatory in men above 50 years of age to detect tumorigenic cells in the early stages, thus improving the overall survival rate of patients. Surgical resection remains the primary therapeutic approach for treating RCC. Due to the high participation of genetic alterations that occur during the development of RCC, it is very likely that in the not-too-distant future, inhibitors of epigenetic regulators will be included as alternative therapies.

REFERENCES

[1] Bray F, Ferlay J, Soerjomataram I, Siegel RL, Torre LA, Jemal A. Global cancer statistics 2018: GLOBOCAN estimates of incidence and mortality worldwide for 36 cancers in 185 countries. CA Cancer J Clin 2018; 68(6): 394-424.
[http://dx.doi.org/10.3322/caac.21492] [PMID: 30207593]

[2] Sung H, Ferlay J, Siegel RL, *et al.* Global cancer statistics 2020: globocan estimates of incidence and mortality worldwide for 36 cancers in 185 countries. CA Cancer J Clin 2021; 71(3): 209-49.
[http://dx.doi.org/10.3322/caac.21660] [PMID: 33538338]

[3] Cairns P. Renal cell carcinoma. Cancer Biomark 2011; 9(1-6): 461-73.
[http://dx.doi.org/10.3233/CBM-2011-0176] [PMID: 22112490]

[4] Choueiri TK, Motzer RJ. Systemic therapy for metastatic renal-cell carcinoma. N Engl J Med 2017; 376(4): 354-66.
[http://dx.doi.org/10.1056/NEJMra1601333] [PMID: 28121507]

[5] Ricketts CJ, De Cubas AA, Fan H, *et al.* The cancer genome atlas comprehensive molecular

characterization of renal cell carcinoma. Cell Rep 2018; 23(12): 3698.
[http://dx.doi.org/10.1016/j.celrep.2018.06.032] [PMID: 29925010]

[6]   Kluzek K, Srebniak MI, Majer W, *et al.* Genetic characterization of Polish ccRCC patients: somatic mutation analysis of *PBRM1, BAP1* and *KDMC5*, genomic SNP array analysis in tumor biopsy and preliminary results of chromosome aberrations analysis in plasma cell free DNA. Oncotarget 2017; 8(17): 28558-74.
[http://dx.doi.org/10.18632/oncotarget.15331] [PMID: 28212566]

[7]   Roy DM, Walsh LA, Chan TA. Driver mutations of cancer epigenomes. Protein Cell 2014; 5(4): 265-96.
[http://dx.doi.org/10.1007/s13238-014-0031-6] [PMID: 24622842]

[8]   Inamura K. Major Tumor Suppressor and Oncogenic Non-Coding RNAs: Clinical Relevance in Lung Cancer. Cells 2017; 6(2): 12.
[http://dx.doi.org/10.3390/cells6020012] [PMID: 28486418]

[9]   Swami U, Nussenzveig RH, Haaland B, Agarwal N. Revisiting AJCC TNM staging for renal cell carcinoma: quest for improvement. Ann Transl Med 2019; 7(S1) (Suppl. 1): S18.
[http://dx.doi.org/10.21037/atm.2019.01.50] [PMID: 31032299]

[10]   Srigley JR, Delahunt B, Eble JN, *et al.* The International Society of Urological Pathology (ISUP) Vancouver Classification of Renal Neoplasia. Am J Surg Pathol 2013; 37(10): 1469-89.
[http://dx.doi.org/10.1097/PAS.0b013e318299f2d1] [PMID: 24025519]

[11]   Terris M, Klaassen Z, Kabaria R. Renal cell carcinoma: links and risks. Int J Nephrol Renovasc Dis 2016; 9: 45-52.
[http://dx.doi.org/10.2147/IJNRD.S75916] [PMID: 27022296]

[12]   Chow WH, Gridley G, Fraumeni JF Jr, Järvholm B. Obesity, hypertension, and the risk of kidney cancer in men. N Engl J Med 2000; 343(18): 1305-11.
[http://dx.doi.org/10.1056/NEJM200011023431804] [PMID: 11058675]

[13]   Eskelinen TJ, Kotsar A, Tammela TLJ, Murtola TJ. Components of metabolic syndrome and prognosis of renal cell cancer. Scand J Urol 2017; 51(6): 435-41.
[http://dx.doi.org/10.1080/21681805.2017.1352616] [PMID: 28743221]

[14]   Colt JS, Schwartz K, Graubard BI, *et al.* Hypertension and risk of renal cell carcinoma among white and black Americans. Epidemiology 2011; 22(6): 797-804.
[http://dx.doi.org/10.1097/EDE.0b013e3182300720] [PMID: 21881515]

[15]   Harris W, Simons J. Riñón y Uréter. In: Abeloff M, Armitage J, Niederhuber J, Eds. Oncología clínica. 2005; Vol. II.

[16]   Daniel CR, Cross AJ, Graubard BI, *et al.* Large prospective investigation of meat intake, related mutagens, and risk of renal cell carcinoma. Am J Clin Nutr 2012; 95(1): 155-62.
[http://dx.doi.org/10.3945/ajcn.111.019364] [PMID: 22170360]

[17]   Stewart JH, Vajdic CM, van Leeuwen MT, *et al.* The pattern of excess cancer in dialysis and transplantation. Nephrol Dial Transplant 2009; 24(10): 3225-31.
[http://dx.doi.org/10.1093/ndt/gfp331] [PMID: 19589786]

[18]   Dahle DO, Skauby M, Langberg CW, Brabrand K, Wessel N, Midtvedt K. Renal Cell Carcinoma and Kidney Transplantation: A Narrative Review. Transplantation 2022; 106(1): e52-63.
[http://dx.doi.org/10.1097/TP.0000000000003762] [PMID: 33741842]

[19]   Clague J, Lin J, Cassidy A, *et al.* Family history and risk of renal cell carcinoma: results from a case-control study and systematic meta-analysis. Cancer Epidemiol Biomarkers Prev 2009; 18(3): 801-7.
[http://dx.doi.org/10.1158/1055-9965.EPI-08-0601] [PMID: 19240244]

[20]   Christakoudi S, Kakourou A, Markozannes G, *et al.* Blood pressure and risk of cancer in the European Prospective Investigation into Cancer and Nutrition. Int J Cancer 2020; 146(10): 2680-93.
[http://dx.doi.org/10.1002/ijc.32576] [PMID: 31319002]

[21] Gago-Dominguez M, Castelao JE. Lipid peroxidation and renal cell carcinoma: further supportive evidence and new mechanistic insights. Free Radic Biol Med 2006; 40(4): 721-33.
[http://dx.doi.org/10.1016/j.freeradbiomed.2005.09.026] [PMID: 16458203]

[22] Gago-Dominguez M, Castelao JE, Yuan JM, Ross RK, Yu MC. Lipid peroxidation: a novel and unifying concept of the etiology of renal cell carcinoma (United States). Cancer Causes Control 2002; 13(3): 287-93.
[http://dx.doi.org/10.1023/A:1015044518505] [PMID: 12020111]

[23] Araújo WF, Naves MA, Ravanini JN, Schor N, Teixeira VPC. Renin-angiotensin system (RAS) blockade attenuates growth and metastatic potential of renal cell carcinoma in mice. Urol Oncol 2015; 33(9): 389.e1-7.
[http://dx.doi.org/10.1016/j.urolonc.2014.11.022] [PMID: 25595575]

[24] Sosa V, Moliné T, Somoza R, Paciucci R, Kondoh H, LLeonart ME. Oxidative stress and cancer: An overview. Ageing Res Rev 2013; 12(1): 376-90.
[http://dx.doi.org/10.1016/j.arr.2012.10.004] [PMID: 23123177]

[25] Miyajima A, Yazawa S, Kosaka T, *et al.* Prognostic Impact of Renin–Angiotensin System Blockade on Renal Cell Carcinoma After Surgery. Ann Surg Oncol 2015; 22(11): 3751-9.
[http://dx.doi.org/10.1245/s10434-015-4436-0] [PMID: 25691280]

[26] Rajandram R, Perumal K, Yap NY. Prognostic biomarkers in renal cell carcinoma: is there a relationship with obesity? Transl Androl Urol 2019; 8(S2) (Suppl. 2): S138-46.
[http://dx.doi.org/10.21037/tau.2018.11.10] [PMID: 31236331]

[27] Drabkin HA, Gemmill RM. Obesity, cholesterol, and clear-cell renal cell carcinoma (RCC). Adv Cancer Res 2010; 107: 39-56.
[http://dx.doi.org/10.1016/S0065-230X(10)07002-8] [PMID: 20399960]

[28] Turajlic S, Swanton C, Boshoff C. Kidney cancer: The next decade. J Exp Med 2018; 215(10): 2477-9.
[http://dx.doi.org/10.1084/jem.20181617] [PMID: 30217855]

[29] Tena Ros R, Pena Ezquerra JM. Genética molecular del cáncer renal: utilidad en pronóstico y posibilidades terapéuticas. Rev Lab Clín 2008; 1(1): 29-34.
[http://dx.doi.org/10.1016/S1888-4008(08)74952-3]

[30] Becerra MF, Reznik E, Redzematovic A, *et al.* Comparative Genomic Profiling of Matched Primary and Metastatic Tumors in Renal Cell Carcinoma. Eur Urol Focus 2018; 4(6): 986-94.
[http://dx.doi.org/10.1016/j.euf.2017.09.016] [PMID: 29066084]

[31] Hollingsworth JM, Miller DC, Daignault S, Hollenbeck BK. Rising incidence of small renal masses: a need to reassess treatment effect. J Natl Cancer Inst 2006; 98(18): 1331-4.
[http://dx.doi.org/10.1093/jnci/djj362] [PMID: 16985252]

[32] Afshin A, Forouzanfar MH, Reitsma MB, *et al.* Health Effects of Overweight and Obesity in 195 Countries over 25 Years. N Engl J Med 2017; 377(1): 13-27.
[http://dx.doi.org/10.1056/NEJMoa1614362] [PMID: 28604169]

CHAPTER 13

Epigenetics in Renal Diseases

Karina Robledo-Márquez[1], Yadira Ramírez[2] and Joyce Trujillo[3,*]

[1] *Facultad de Ingeniería, Universidad Autónoma de San Luis Potosí, San Luis Potosí, México*

[2] *División de Materiales Avanzados, Instituto Potosino de Investigación Científica y Tecnológica (IPICYT), San Luis Potosí, Mexico*

[3] *Secretaría de Ciencia, Humanidades, Tecnología e Innovación (SECIHTI) - División de Materiales Avanzados-Instituto Potosino de Investigación Científica y Tecnológica - (SECIHTI-IPICYT), San Luis Potosí, Mexico*

Abstract: AKI and CKD have been described as interconnected syndromes as CKD predisposes to AKI, and AKI, in turn, may accelerate CKD progression. Thus, they are considered as an integrated clinical syndrome. AKI and CKD remain incompletely understood. It is well known that environmental and genetic factors are involved in the process. Long-term environmental effects lead to alterations in gene expression, specifically epigenetic changes. Epigenetic mechanisms that might integrate these interactions include chromatin modification, DNA methylation and demethylation, covalent modifications of histones: methylation, acetylation, and crotonylation, and the expression of various non-coding RNAs. Recent advances in epigenetics and diagnostic tools have made the study of kidney dysfunction more efficient, as well as technological achievements that have allowed us to improve our understanding of epigenetics on the physiological and pathological state of the kidney.

Keywords: Acetylation, Chromatin, Crotonylation, Histones, Methylation.

INTRODUCTION

Acute kidney injury (AKI) and chronic kidney disease (CKD) are associated with high morbidity (13-20% of the population) and mortality in the general population. AKI is a transitory, rapid, and reversible reduction in renal function. Many risk factors, such as drugs, toxins, sepsis, ischemia-reperfusion (I/R), and COVID-19, generally cause AKI, leading to a reduced glomerular filtration rate and acute tubular damage [1 - 3] (Fig. **1**). Numerous studies have demonstrated through several different strategies [4, 5] that AKI is a leading cause of cardiovascular events and the development of CKD [6]. AKI can progress to

* **Corresponding author Joyce Trujillo:** Secretaría de Ciencia, Humanidades, Tecnología e Innovación (SECIHTI)- División de Materiales Avanzados-Instituto Potosino de Investigación Científica y Tecnológica - (SECIHTI-IPICYT), San Luis Potosí, Mexico; E-mail: daniela.trujillo@ipicyt.edu.mx.

CKD, characterized by changes in the structure and function of the kidney [7]. CKD is irreversible and progressive and is associated with chronic comorbidities such as hypertension, cardiovascular disease, diabetes, anemia, and bone diseases [8]. CKD can progress to end-stage kidney disease, which is associated with renal replacement therapy and an increased risk of premature death (Fig. **1**) [9].

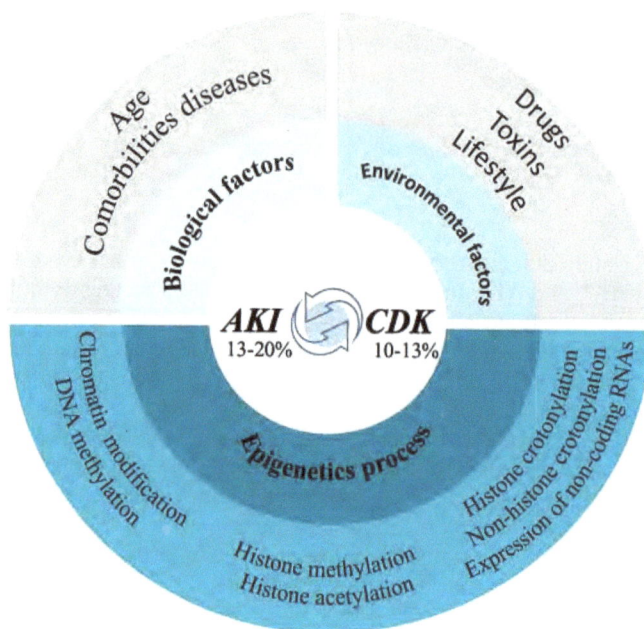

Fig. (1). Prevalence and factors involved in the development and progression of AKI and CDK. Acute kidney injury (AKI); Chronic Kidney Disease (CKD), the percentages refer to the prevalence of each pathological entity.

AKI and CKD have been described as interconnected syndromes because CKD is a risk factor for AKI, and AKI, in turn, may accelerate CKD progression; thus, they are considered integrated clinical syndromes [9]. Consequently, both entities share injury mechanisms, such as damage to vascular endothelial and/or tubular epithelial cells, cell death and proliferation, inflammation, and fibrosis [4, 10, 11]. Nonetheless, although the development and progression of AKI and CKD are incompletely understood, it is well-known that environmental and genetic factors are involved in this process (Fig. **1**) [12]. Long-term environmental effects lead to alterations in gene expression, specifically epigenetic changes [13]. Epigenetics refers to modifying and modulating gene expression without impairing the DNA sequence, which results in a modified phenotype [14]. Furthermore, epigenetics can facilitate the interconnection between genes and the environment [12]. Throughout cell division, epigenetic changes can be inherited but may be reversible and modified by age, disease, and the environment [9].

Currently, epigenetic mechanisms, including priming and tolerance, are known to be involved in all stages of AKI and CKD [11]. Therefore, this chapter aims to provide an overview of current and novel studies that explore the epigenetic mechanisms of AKI and CKD in human disease and animal models. In addition, we will discuss the implications of epigenetics in diagnosing and treating renal diseases of diverse etiologies.

PATHOPHYSIOLOGY, CURRENT AND NOVEL STUDIES

Epigenetics mechanisms include DNA methylation and demethylation, covalent modifications of histones (methylation, acetylation, and crotonylation), and the expression of various non-coding RNAs [9, 15]. There have been new efforts to investigate the contribution of epigenetic mechanisms in renal disease, concretely onset, progression, and treatment of AKI or CDK, as we will see below [14].

The principal pathological manifestations of the AKI-to-CKD transition are hypoxia and apoptosis, which are common pathways of the AKI-to-CKD transition. When renal injury is minor or short in duration (AKI), adaptive repair is initiated for renal function recovery. Nonetheless, when the injury is severe and persistent, maladaptive repair (inflammation and fibrosis) occurs to mediate CKD occurrence [15, 16]. In AKI, under hypoxic conditions, hypoxia-inducible factor 1 (HIF-1) binds to hypoxic response elements in the regulatory region of several target genes to regulate their expression under decreased oxygen conditions. These epigenetic changes have long-term effects and are called "hypoxic memory." Changes induced by hypoxia promote the expression of inflammatory and fibrotic genes, such as monocyte chemoattractant protein 1 (MCP-1), transforming growth factor-beta 1 (TGF-β1), and type III collagen, all of which aggravate hypoxia, inflammation, and fibrosis, leading to CKD [15].

DNA Methylation and Demethylation

DNA methylation is catalyzed by DNA methyltransferases, which transfer a methyl group from the donor S-adenosyl-L-methionine (SAM) to the 5'-position of cytosine residues in the DNA, specifically in the CpG dinucleotides in the promoter region of DNA, to form 5-methylcytosine. DNA methylation in the promoter region is a silencing mechanism that inhibits the binding of transcription factors or the recruitment of proteins involved in gene expression [9, 15]. Methylated DNA can be demethylated or oxidized by a demethyltransferase, and the reaction progresses from 5-methylcytosine (5mC) to 5-hydroxymethylcytosine (5hmC) to regulate gene expression [15].

In particular, Pratt *et al.* were the first group to report changes in DNA methylation, specifically the demethylation of a cytosine residue in interferon-gamma (INF-γ), in the rat kidney in an ischemia/reperfusion (I/R) model in response to cold ischemia and additional demethylation during further warm reperfusion [17]. DNA methylation was analyzed in the urine of transplant recipients, and the patients presented an increase in 5mC levels and a global decrease in 5hmC levels. In this work, the authors proposed urine epigenetics analysis as a biomarker for I/R in transplantation [18].

DNA methylation influences the inhibition of the expression of nephroprotective genes, such as Klotho, erythropoietin, and Ras GTPase-activating-like protein 1 (RASAL1), which have anti-inflammatory and antifibrotic effects in AKI, as well as in the AKI-CKD transition. In this regard, the administration of DNA methylation inhibitors, such as 5-azacytidine, 5-aza-2-deoxycytidine, and hydralazine, reduces the methylation level in murine models of AKI-CKD progression and in I/R models [15, 19, 20].

The DNMT (DNA methyltransferase) inhibitor 5-aza-2-deoxycytidine overrides UUO-induced Klotho suppression and promoter hypermethylation, thus reducing profibrotic protein expression and renal fibrosis [20]. Additionally, tubule-specific overexpression of Sirtuin-1 (SIRT1), an NAD-dependent deacetylase, prevented albuminuria by promoting hypermethylation of the Cldn1 gene. This caused the downregulation of the protein Claudin-1 in podocytes, indicating a possible interconnection between podocytes and proximal tubules mediated by epigenetic mechanisms in an animal model of streptozoticin or obese (db/db) diabetic mice [21].

In 2019, a study on renal tubular epithelial cells showed that complement activation leads to the release of the C5a component, which mediates damage; nevertheless, there is scarce information about the impact of the C5a-C5a receptor (C5aR) interaction in these cells. Nonetheless, it has been shown that C5a produces abnormal methylation, predominantly in regions implicated in cell cycle regulation, DNA damage, and Wnt4/β-catenin activation. Additionally, C5a increased the expression of proinflammatory molecules such as IL-6, MCP-1, and connective tissue growth factor and the DNA methylation of genes involved in tubular senescence [22]. Hence, understanding the epigenetic mechanisms involved in kidney damage could allow us to identify alternative therapeutic approaches.

The methylation of arginine residues by protein arginine methyltransferases is a crucial posttranslational modification for many biological processes, including DNA repair, RNA processing, and the transduction of intra- and extracellular signals. Recent studies have shown that aberrant functions of protein arginine methyltransferases and their metabolic products (symmetric dimethylarginine and asymmetric dimethylarginine) are involved in several renal pathological processes, including renal fibrosis, AKI, CKD, hypertension, and renal tumors, among others [23]. Nonetheless, the role and regulation of DNA methylation in kidney injury and repair remain largely unknown.

Chromatin Structure Modifications

Hypoxia induces changes in cellular metabolism, chromatin structure, and binding of different transcription factors, as well as an increase in the expression of proinflammatory cytokines, such as TNF-α and MCP-1, up to seven days after an AKI episode [15, 24]. These findings could be the result of epigenetic modifications associated with the activation of the multiprotein chromatin remodeling complex, which includes the SWItch/Sucrose Non-Fermentable (SWI/SNF) factor [24], which causes chromatin agglutination, increased promoter accessibility, and the upregulation of genes such as TNF-α and MCP-1 [11, 25].

Brahma-related gene 1 (BRG1) the central catalytic subunit of the SWI/SNF complex, activates the transcription of adhesion molecules and chemokines by recruiting histone-modifying enzymes and promoting macrophage adhesion and chemotaxis [26]. Additionally, BRG1 induces tubular senescence by inhibiting autophagy *via* the Wnt/β-catenin pathway, which contributes to the development of renal fibrosis [27]. Similarly, BRG1 is essential for embryonic kidney development and regulates the proliferation and differentiation of nephron progenitor cells [28]. Liu *et al.* (2019) showed that endothelial-specific deletion of BRG1 in a mouse model of obstructive nephropathy promoted the attenuation of renal inflammation associated with the downregulation of proinflammatory cytokines (interleukin (IL)-1β, TNF-α, inducible nitric oxide synthase, intercellular adhesion molecule 1, and vascular cell adhesion molecule 1, among others) and reduced the infiltration of immune cells [26].

In a study on BRG1 knockout mice subjected to I/R, BRG1 activated IL-33 transcription in endothelial cells, promoting the synthesis of profibrogenic proteins that contribute to fibrosis and, consequently, renal injury [29]. In a clinical analysis of 539 patients, Groisberg *et al.* reported the presence of abnormalities in SWI/SNF complex genes (such as BRG1) in different cancers, including renal carcinoma. BRG1 has been implicated as an oncogene and a tumor suppressor, specifically in mutations related to specific cancers [30]. In addition, BRG1 upregulation was shown to be associated with poor prognosis in patients with kidney renal clear cell carcinoma [31]. Accordingly, epigenetic regulation of endothelial function, inflammation, and fibrosis by BRG1 might contribute substantially to renal injury pathogenesis.

Histone Modifications

The importance and diversity of histone posttranslational modifications have been described in many epigenetic regulatory mechanisms. Different histone modifications may occur at the histone N-terminus, such as acetylation, methylation, ubiquitination, hydroxylation, phosphorylation, and ADP ribosylation [23]. Histone modifications are associated with activating inflammatory and fibrotic genes [32]. Specifically, histone acetylation is frequently associated with the transcriptional activation of genes [33]. In contrast, eliminating acetyl groups by histone deacetylases (HDACs) frequently suppresses gene expression [34].

Acetylation

Histone acetylation and deacetylation are catalyzed by acetyltransferase and HDAC, respectively. The acetylation and deacetylation reactions imply the addition or elimination of an acetoxy group, CH3CO [35]. These modifications have been studied in AKI and renal fibrosis. In the fibrosis model kidney, the acetylation of lysine residue 9 of histone 3 (H3K9Me) and the trimethylation of lysine residue 4 of histone 3 (H3K4Me3) is upregulated, inducing inflammatory, profibrotic, and regulatory gene transcription, which leads to CKD [36].

Marumo *et al.* (2008) demonstrated that ischemia decreases histone acetylation while reperfusion increases acetylation levels. In this way, decreased levels of HDAC5 activate a regenerative process following ischemia by inducing bone morphogenetic protein-7 (BMP-7) expression in proximal tubular cells. These findings suggest that inhibition of HDAC5 is a novel therapeutic strategy for enhancing BMP-7 expression to repair kidney injury [37].

In cisplatin-induced AKI, the overexpression of HDAC2 by cisplatin promotes tubular epithelium cell apoptosis and kidney injury. The administration of an HDAC inhibitor increased BMP-7 levels, thus suppressing epithelial cell apoptosis [38]. Class I HDACs are critical for gene expression and cell growth and differentiation in the kidney; hence, these enzymes are closely linked to the control of key developmental routes [39]. Tang *et al.* (2013) reported that MS-275-mediated inhibition of class I HDACs decreased renal proximal tubular cell proliferation and the expression of cyclin D1, the latter of which is a regulator of the cell cycle. Therefore, the inhibition of class I HDACs reduced the expression and activation of the epidermal growth factor receptor (EGFR) and reduced the phosphorylation of the activator of transcription 3 (STAT3) protein, a key element in cell proliferation. These findings suggest that class I HDACs regulate renal epithelial cell proliferation through the activation of the EGFR/STAT3 signaling pathway. Hence, inhibition of class I HDACs promotes kidney protection and functional restoration by regulating the EGFR/STAT3 signaling pathway and AKT phosphorylation, which is indispensable for renal recovery after AKI [40, 41]. Furthermore, Zhang *et al.* (2018) reported that MS-275 attenuates renal tissue injury and suppresses the generation of inflammatory cytokines and reactive oxygen species (ROS) in mice treated with lipopolysaccharide (LPS) [42]. Another study that tested romidepsin (FK228, a selective inhibitor of the enzymes HDAC1 and 2) showed a significant reduction in LPS-induced kidney injury [43].

Class II HDACs (HDAC4, HDAC5, HDAC6, HDAC7, HDAC9, and HDAC10) have been studied to understand the effect of AKI. Tubastatin A, an inhibitor of HDAC6, increases the expression of autophagy and proinflammatory cytokines, suggesting that inhibition of HDAC6 has a protective effect on cisplatin-induced AKI [44]. Additionally, Ranganathan *et al.* (2016) reported that inhibition of HDAC6 with tubastatin A, a novel anti-inflammatory and antiapoptotic protein that reduces cisplatin-induced kidney dysfunction, activates microglia/macrophage WAP domain protein expression in proximal tubular cells [45]. In some studies in which TMP195 was used as an inhibitor of HDAC4 in LPS-induced AKI, it was shown to reduce tubule injury and renal tubular cell apoptosis by reversing the increase in the expression of intermediate proteins involved in apoptosis. Furthermore, it increased the expression of BMP-7 and reduced the upregulation of proinflammatory cytokines/chemokines [23, 44]. Trichostatin A, an inhibitor of HDAC enzymes (class I/II) in cultured human renal proximal tubular cells, can prevent TGF-β1-induced epithelial-mesenchymal transition, leading to fibrosis development [46]. Valproic acid (a class I/II HDAC inhibitor) can reduce inflammatory cytokines and apoptosis/stress-related gene expression and improve regeneration through the induction of BMP-7 expression, and recent studies have shown that valproic acid can also attenuate hypertonic glycerol–induced rhabdomyolysis and AKI [38, 47, 48]. All these findings suggest that HDAC inhibitors could be an alternative therapy for cisplatin nephrotoxicity.

Methylation

In UUO-induced fibrotic and human CKD kidneys, histone H3K27Me3 and histone H3K4me3 were significantly upregulated. This increase is associated with high expression of inflammation-related genes (TNF-α), fibrosis-related genes (TGF-β1, type III collagen), and cholesterol-regulated genes (3-hydroxy-3-methylglutaryl-CoA reductase), ultimately leading to a gradual transition from AKI to CKD [15]. Histone methylation is catalyzed by specific histone methyltransferase, enhancer of zeste homolog 2 (EZH2) (H3K27me3 and H3K29me) and SET7/9 (H3K4me) [49]. Zhou *et al.* (2016) showed that EZH2 downregulation decreases the activation of renal interstitial fibroblasts and that treatment with 3-DZNeP (an EZH2 inhibitor) attenuates fibrosis in an animal model of UUO [50].

Crotonylation

Recent studies have recognized lysine crotonylation (Kcr) as a new evolutionarily conserved histone posttranslational modification observed in kidney tissue. This modification consists of an acylation that occurs on the ε-amino group of Lys, and the substrate is a donor molecule linked by a thioester to the sulfhydryl group of CoA, namely, crotonyl-CoA [51]. This type of posttranscriptional modification (PTM) is related to kidney disease. Kcr analysis of the plasma of patients with IgA nephropathy revealed 155 upregulated and 198 downregulated proteins. Gene enrichment analysis revealed proteins involved in antigen presentation and processing and complement and coagulation pathways, suggesting that these PTMs play important roles in IgA nephropathy [52]. In addition, histone lysine Kcr has been found in tubular cells from healthy murine and human kidney tissue, affecting histone crotonylation in the kidney through cells stressed by inflammatory cytokines and AKI [53]. Kcr has also been found to be very active in the plasma of ESRD patients. Proteomic analysis of plasma from hemodialysis patients revealed 1109 lysine modifications distributed on 347 proteins, including 93 and 252 crotonylated upregulated and downregulated proteins, respectively. Patients who underwent hemodialysis presented a decrease in histone protein crotonylation compared with normal controls. According to gene enrichment analysis, the pathways involved in Kcr changes were complement and coagulation cascades, cardiac muscle contraction, and hematopoietic cell lineage [54].

Among the genes regulated by Krc, PPARGC1A, a regulator of mitochondrial biogenesis, is decreased in AKI. Crotonate increased tubular cell PPARGC1A mRNA and protein levels, thus promoting the upregulation of some protective genes and the downregulation of genes involved in tissue injury in AKI. Therefore, Kcr has a very active role in kidney disease and could be directed by administering crotonate to favor nephroprotection as a therapeutic alternative.

Non-coding RNAs

miRNAs are single-stranded endogenous RNAs (20–22 nucleotides) that can control gene expression at the posttranscriptional or transcriptional level [55]. On the other hand, long non-coding RNAs (lncRNAs) are transcripts of RNA over 200 nucleotides in length that regulate gene expression by binding DNAs, RNAs, or proteins [56]. The roles of miRNAs and lncRNAs in renal diseases have been studied, and it is well known that miRNAs are important for the epigenetic regulation of diabetic nephropathy [16]. Many miRNAs are related to diabetic nephropathy. For example, phosphatase and tensin homologs are targets of miR-

22, which leads to the suppression of autophagy and the induction of the expression of profibrotic molecules such as collagen IV and α-SMA [57]. miR-23a targets the nuclear transcription corepressor Ski-related novel protein N [58], a crucial negative regulator of the TGF-β1/Smad3-mediated signaling pathway, to induce fibrosis in diabetic nephropathy [59]. As previously mentioned, SIRT1 is renoprotective; however, miR-34a-5p, miR-217, miR-133b, and miR-199b can inhibit the expression of SIRT1 under hyperglycemic conditions [60 - 62]. miR-135a targets transient receptor potential canonical 1 (TRPC1), and this interaction contributes to fibrosis in diabetic kidney injury [63]. miR-184 is expressed in tubular cells and promotes tubulointerstitial fibrosis owing to decreased expression of lipoma-preferred partner 3 [64]. miR-342 inhibits SRY-box 6 expression and suppresses the progression of diabetic nephropathy [65]. Lin *et al.* (2019) reported that miR-379 suppressed renal fibrosis by regulating mesangial cell proliferation and the deposition of extracellular matrix components in the LIN28B/let-7 metabolism pathway [66]. miR-30c, miR-98-5p, and miR- 302a-3p have protective effects *via* the modulation of renal epithelial-mesenchymal transition, a mechanism involved in fibrosis development, through the inhibition of JAK1, Snail1, high-mobility group AT-hook 2, and zinc finger E-box-binding homeobox 1, respectively [66 - 69]. miR-455–3p can inhibit renal fibrosis by inhibiting the expression of coiled-coil-containing protein kinase 2 and reversing fibrosis and inflammation [70, 71]. miR-544 ameliorated diabetic renal injury through glomerulosclerosis and inflammation suppression *via* fatty acid synthase (FASN) gene regulation [72].

For many decades, it was believed that the only function of podocytes was to ensure the normal function of the glomerular filtration barrier; however, recent literature suggests that podocytes play a role in the innate and adaptive immune systems [73]. Podocyte injury is promoted through the upregulation of miR-77-
-5p by targeting metalloproteinase-3 and Tp53-regulated inhibitor of apoptosis 1 (TRIAP1); hence, if miR770-5p is downregulated or knocked down, apoptosis and inflammation in the kidney can be reversed [74, 75]. High glucose-induced apoptosis, oxidative stress, and inflammation in podocytes are repressed by the overexpression of miR-15b-5p [76]. Overexpression of miR-34b improves inflammation and apoptosis in high glucose-induced HK-2 cells *via* the IL-6R/JAK2/STAT3 pathway [77]. There are three miRNAs related to the reduced production of proinflammatory cytokines (NADPH oxidase 4 and 5), miR-146a [78], miR-423-5p [59], and miR-485 [79], in kidney disease models. In addition, Li *et al.* (2020) reported that miR-218 regulates NF-κB-mediated inflammation and reduces the expression of the proinflammatory and profibrotic molecules TNF-α, IL-6, IL-1β, and MCP-1 [80]. Overexpression of miR-451 attenuated urinary microalbumin excretion, blood glucose, and glomerular injury [81]. miR-140-5p and miR-874 act as anti-inflammatory modulators that suppress the

expression of TNF-α, IL-6, and IL-1β in tubular epithelial cells by binding to Toll-like receptor 4 [82, 83]

LncRNAs are essential for the progression from AKI to CKD. Nuclear enriched abundant transcript 1, a psoriasis susceptibility-related RNA gene stimulated by stress, and LINC00520 mainly play a role in promoting the transition from AKI to CKD [84 - 86], while aspartyl-tRNA synthetase antisense 1 (DARS-AS1), MALAT1, and the lncRNA Miat inhibit this process [87 - 89]. Zhou *et al.* (2020) identified the lncRNA XLOC_032768 as a new target in kidney I/R injury; overexpression of XLOC_032768 ameliorated tubular epithelial cell apoptosis, protecting the kidney against injury in mice [90].

Some miRNAs and lncRNAs have been described to be associated with preventing or promoting AKI by silencing, downregulating, or upregulating different genes involved in renal pathophysiology and the transition from AKI-CKD (Fig. **2**). Nevertheless, the role and regulation of some miRNAs and lncRNAs in kidney injury and repair remain unknown; this topic continues to be a large field of study, especially for emerging pathologies such as COVID-19.

EPIGENETICS IN DIAGNOSIS

Early diagnosis of kidney function loss is an important step in preventing CKD complications. Usually, the diagnosis of CKD is based on serum creatinine (sCr) levels; however, sCr has been shown to lack high predictive value. This situation can lead to the failure to detect the early stages of AKI or CKD and, consequently, the late application of detailed diagnoses and the implementation of therapeutic interventions [91]. Due to the development of genomics, epigenetics, transcriptomics, proteomics, and metabolomics, new techniques have been introduced to identify new biomarkers for kidney diseases, aiming to provide rapid, noninvasive, and specific measurements that correlate well with kidney tissue pathology [92]. These biomarkers include asymmetric dimethylarginine and symmetric dimethylarginine biomolecules, uromodulin glycoprotein, kidney injury molecule-1, neutrophil gelatinase-associated lipocalin, proteomic and metabolomic biomarkers, and epigenetic biomarkers [91]. Identification of epigenetic changes in renal pathology is still a field under development, with great expectations of defining new therapeutic targets since these epigenetic changes are potentially reversible.

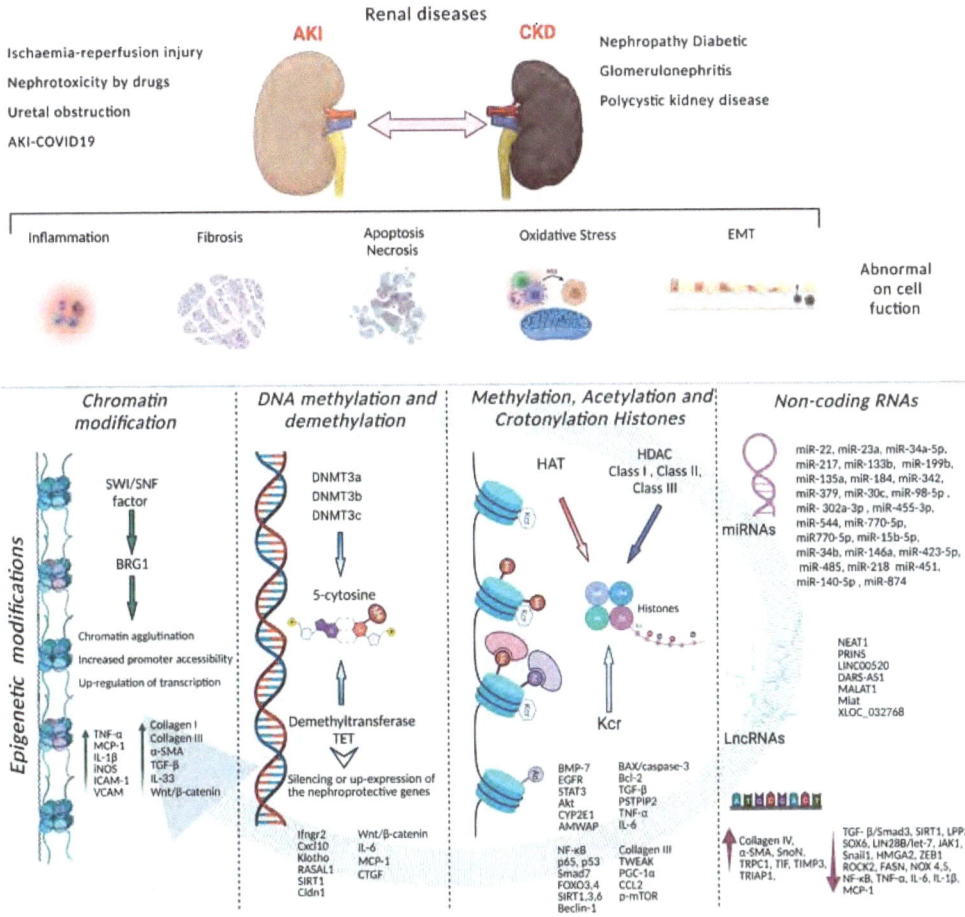

Fig. (2). Epigenetics modification in the development and progression of AKI and CDK.
The main kidney diseases and their mechanisms include epigenetic modifications (chromatin modification, DNA methylation, demethylation, covalent modifications of histones, and the expression of non-coding RNAs). They include the main epigenetic factors and the genes affected by silencing or up-regulation or down-regulation. Acute kidney injury (AKI); Chronic Kidney Disease (CKD), Coronavirus disease 2019 (COVID); Epithelial–mesenchymal transition (EMT); SWItch/Sucrose Non-Fermentable (SWI/SNF); Brahma-related gene 1 (BRG1); tumor necrosis factor (TNF-α); Monocyte Chemoattractant Protein 1 (MCP-1), Transforming Growth Factor β1 (TGF-β1), Interleukin (IL-), inducible nitric oxide synthase (iNOS); Intercellular Adhesion Molecule-1 (ICAM-1), Vascular Cell Adhesion Molecule 1 (VCAM); Smooth muscle alpha-actin (α-SMA); DNA methyltransferases (DNMT); ten–eleven translocation (TET) enzymes; Interferon gamma receptor 2 (Ifngr2); C-X-C motif chemokine ligand 10 (CXCL10); Ras GTPase-activating-like protein 1 (RASAL1); Sirtuin-1(SIRT1); Claudin 1 (Cldn1); Connective tissue growth factor (CTGF); acetyltransferase (HAT); histone deacetylase (HDAC); crotonylation (Kcr); bone morphogenetic protein-7 (BMP-7); epidermal growth factor receptor (EGRF); activators of transcription 3 (STAT3); protein kinase B (Akt); cytochrome P450 family 2 subfamily E member 1 (CYP2E1); activated microglia/macrophage WAP domain protein (AMWAP); nuclear factor -kappa B (NF-κB); Mothers against decapentaplegic homolog 7 (Smad7); Forkhead box class O 3 and 4 (FOXO3, 4); Sirtuin-3 (SIRT3); Sirtuin-6 (SIRT6); proapoptotic protein markers Bax and cleavage caspase-3 (BAX/caspase-3); antiapoptotic protein (Bcl-2); proline–serine–threonine phosphatase-interacting protein 2 (PSTPIP2); proinflammatory cytokine TWEAK;

nephroprotective gene PGC-1α; monocyte chemoattractant protein-1, MCP-1 (CCL2); mammalian target of rapamycin (p-mTOR); microRNA (miRNA); long non-coding RNA (lncRNA); nuclear enriched abundant transcript 1 (NEAT1); psoriasis susceptibility-related RNA gene induced by stress (PRINS); aspartyl-tRNA synthetase antisense 1 (DARS-AS1); Ski-related novel gene (SnoN); transient receptor potential cation channel, subfamily C, member 1 (TRPC1); Tubulointerstitial fibrosis (TIF); metalloproteinase 3 (TIMP3); Tp53 regulated inhibitor of apoptosis 1 (TRIAP1); lipid phosphate phosphatase-3 (LPP3); SRY-box 6 (SOX6); Janus kinase 1 (JAK1); Snail Family Transcriptional Repressor 1 (Snail1); high mobility group A (HMGA2); Zinc finger E-box-binding protein 1 (ZEB1); Rho-associated coiled coil-containing protein kinase 2 (ROCK2); fatty acid synthase (FASN); nicotinamide adenine dinucleotide phosphate oxidase (NOX). Created with BioRender.com

EZH2 is a component of the histone methyltransferase polycomb repressive complex 2 (PRC2) H3K27me3 [49]. Recent studies have shown that EZH2 is associated with diverse kidney diseases and pathologies. Increased EZH2 expression is related to renal tumors, AKI development [93], renal fibrosis [50], diabetic nephropathy [94], lupus nephritis [95], hyperuricemic nephropathy [96], and kidney transplantation and aging [97, 98]. Pharmacological inhibitors of EZH2, such as 3-DZNep, GSK343, EED226, and CPT-1205, can improve AKI, renal fibrosis, and lupus nephritis in animal models [49]. However, more studies are needed to confirm the benefits of these inhibitors.

Another therapeutic target is the bromodomain and extraterminal (BET) family of proteins (BRD2, BRD3, BRD4, and BRDT), which are proteins responsible for locating and linking acetylated histones and transcription factors with the transcriptional complex. This family of proteins is linked to the development of tumors, inflammation, and renal fibrosis. In a 2018 study, one of the main inhibitors of BET proteins, the compound JQ1 (thieno-triazolo-1,4-diazepine substituted at position C-6), was evaluated using *in vivo* and *in vitro* models, where it was observed that the blockage of BET proteins by this compound decreased the inflammatory response and renal fibrosis and improved renal function in a model of immune glomerulonephritis [99].

MicroRNAs (miRNAs) and non-coding RNAs (ncRNAs) are other known biomarkers. Studies on experimental models have demonstrated that different tissue expression levels of specific miRNAs (miR-145, -143, -126, -223, -155, and -125b) in plasma can be used as noninvasive markers for vascular and cardiovascular calcification and complications in CKD patients [100, 101]. Furthermore, miR-145 replacement therapy was shown to reduce atherosclerotic damage in experimental systems [102].

In patients with CKD, kidney transplantation improves survival and quality of life; therefore, kidney transplantation has become the treatment of choice for patients with ESRD [103]. According to estimates, long-term outcomes remain poor, as ~ 50% of kidney transplant patients require dialysis 10 years after surgery when developing chronic graft nephropathy. Three miRNAs (142-3p, 204, and 211) have been suggested as specific biomarkers for identifying patients with chronic graft nephropathy in the early stages; nonetheless, their usefulness should be confirmed in further studies [104, 105].

Khurana *et al.* performed an analysis of ncRNAs from CKD patients and healthy controls to identify biomarkers that may detect the presence of all stages of CKD. In their study, 211 ncRNAs showed significant differences in stage 1 CKD patients, 153 in stage 2 patients, 221 in stage 3 patients, and 117 in stage 4 patients compared to healthy controls. In addition, 16 miRNAs were identified, of which the most significant finding was miR-181a, with an exosomal abundance approximately 200 times lower in CKD patients than in healthy subjects; thus, it was proposed that ncRNA and miR-181a are potential biomarkers for the early diagnosis of CKD [106].

In another investigation of the early detection of AKI, an established rat model of I/R-induced kidney injury was used, and urine microarray analysis was performed at baseline (0 h) and 72 h after surgery to evaluate the expression profile of miRNAs. The quantitative validation of miRNAs showed that the expression of miR-30c-5p and miR-192-5p was notably elevated in urine after surgery, showing that miR-30c-5p is a better diagnostic biomarker than protein-based biomarkers such as kidney injury molecule-1 and neutrophil gelatinase-associated lipocalin. Both miR-30c-5p and miR-192-5p are potential diagnostic markers for I/R-induced AKI; nonetheless, more studies are needed to validate their diagnostic value for detecting kidney injury [107].

These are just a few of the main biomarkers currently being studied. Future studies exploiting additional models are expected to pave the way for the development of new targets and noninvasive therapeutic solutions for the early diagnosis of kidney disease.

CONCLUSION

There is no therapy that prevents kidney dysfunction or promotes total recovery from kidney dysfunction in AKI and CKD patients [108]. In addition, the high prevalence of both nephropathies indicates the need for a more in-depth understanding of the underlying molecular mechanisms, pathophysiology, and drivers of the AKI-to-CKD transition. Additionally, it is necessary to identify better diagnostic methods, prognoses, and therapies for these pathologies [12].

The complex interactions between hemodynamic, inflammatory, fibrotic, and metabolic factors drive AKI and CKD pathogenesis. Epigenetic mechanisms that might integrate these interactions include chromatin modification, DNA methylation and demethylation, covalent modifications of histones (methylation, acetylation, and Kcr), and the expression of various non-coding RNAs, as we previously discussed (Fig. **2**).

Recent advances in epigenetics and diagnostic tools have made the study of kidney dysfunction more efficient, as well as technological achievements that have improved our understanding of the effects of epigenetics on the physiological and pathological state of the kidney. In this regard, epigenetic modifications at the transcriptional and translational levels participate in various changes in several renal diseases (I/R injury, nephrotoxicity, ureteral obstruction, diabetes, glomerulonephritis, polycystic kidney disease, and COVID-19). Likewise, a few epigenetic modifications have been considered biomarkers of renal pathologies due to their high stability, simple detection techniques, and noninvasive specimen sources (blood, urine, saliva), particularly non-coding RNA analysis (in exosomes, apoptotic bodies, and extracellular vesicles), which can reduce the discomfort of sample collection, risk of complications, variability in histopathology interpretation and high costs of invasive specimen sources (tissue).

These modifications at the genetic level have potential clinical value and potential for use as biomarkers for predicting lesions. Finally, more studies on epigenetics in several pathologies, either for those with high mortality rates or those with emerging pathologies, such as COVID-19, are needed in the search for new prognostic and diagnostic biomarkers. Further improvements in computational deconvolution approaches, multiomics reference datasets, and human kidney single-cell sequencing datasets are expected.

REFERENCES

[1]   Benedetti C, Waldman M, Zaza G, Riella LV, Cravedi P. COVID-19 and the Kidneys: An Update. Front Med (Lausanne) 2020; 7: 423.
[http://dx.doi.org/10.3389/fmed.2020.00423] [PMID: 32793615]

[2]   Carlson N, Nelveg-Kristensen KE, Freese Ballegaard E, *et al.* Increased vulnerability to COVID-19 in chronic kidney disease. J Intern Med 2021; 290(1): 166-78.
[http://dx.doi.org/10.1111/joim.13239] [PMID: 33452733]

[3]   Liu Y, Xia P, Cao W, *et al.* Divergence between serum creatine and cystatin C in estimating glomerular filtration rate of critically ill COVID-19 patients. Ren Fail 2021; 43(1): 1104-14.
[http://dx.doi.org/10.1080/0886022X.2021.1948428] [PMID: 34238117]

[4]   Bao YW, Yuan Y, Chen JH, *et al.*, Kidney disease models: tools to identify mechanisms and potential therapeutic targets. Zool Res 2018; 39(2): 72-86.
[http://dx.doi.org/10.24272/j.issn.2095-8137.2017.055] [PMID: 29515089]

[5]   Yang L. Acute Kidney Injury in Asia. Kidney Dis 2016; 2(3): 95-102.
[http://dx.doi.org/10.1159/000441887] [PMID: 27921036]

[6]   Schmidt-Ott KM. [Acute kidney injury - Update 2021]. Dtsch Med Wochenschr 2021; 146(15): 988-93.
[http://dx.doi.org/10.1055/a-1198-3745] [PMID: 34344035]

[7]   Raena M. Chronic Kidney Disease: Detection and Evaluation. Osteopathic Family Physician 2020; 12(1): 14-9.
[http://dx.doi.org/10.33181/12011]

[8]   Ammirati AL. Chronic Kidney Disease. Rev Assoc Med Bras (1992); 2020; 66Suppl 1(Suppl 1): s03-s09.

[9]   Martinez-Moreno JM, Fontecha-Barriuso M, Martín-Sánchez D, *et al.* The Contribution of Histone Crotonylation to Tissue Health and Disease: Focus on Kidney Health. Front Pharmacol 2020; 11: 393.
[http://dx.doi.org/10.3389/fphar.2020.00393] [PMID: 32308622]

[10]   Andreucci M, Faga T, Serra R, De Sarro G, Michael A. Update on the renal toxicity of iodinated contrast drugs used in clinical medicine. Drug Healthc Patient Saf 2017; 9: 25-37.
[http://dx.doi.org/10.2147/DHPS.S122207] [PMID: 28579836]

[11]   Bomsztyk K, Denisenko O. Epigenetic alterations in acute kidney injury. Semin Nephrol 2013; 33(4): 327-40.
[http://dx.doi.org/10.1016/j.semnephrol.2013.05.005] [PMID: 24011575]

[12]   Kato M, Natarajan R. Epigenetics and epigenomics in diabetic kidney disease and metabolic memory. Nat Rev Nephrol 2019; 15(6): 327-45.
[http://dx.doi.org/10.1038/s41581-019-0135-6] [PMID: 30894700]

[13]   Chan K, Li X. Current Epigenetic Insights in Kidney Development. Genes (Basel) 2021; 12(8): 1281.
[http://dx.doi.org/10.3390/genes12081281] [PMID: 34440455]

[14]   Chakraborty A, Viswanathan P. Methylation-Demethylation Dynamics: Implications of Changes in Acute Kidney Injury. Anal Cell Pathol (Amst) 2018; 2018: 1-16.
[http://dx.doi.org/10.1155/2018/8764384] [PMID: 30073137]

[15]   Li Z, Li N. Epigenetic Modification Drives Acute Kidney Injury-to-Chronic Kidney Disease Progression. Nephron J 2021; 145(6): 737-47.
[http://dx.doi.org/10.1159/000517073] [PMID: 34419948]

[16]   Guo C, Dong G, Liang X, Dong Z. Epigenetic regulation in AKI and kidney repair: mechanisms and therapeutic implications. Nat Rev Nephrol 2019; 15(4): 220-39.
[http://dx.doi.org/10.1038/s41581-018-0103-6] [PMID: 30651611]

[17]   Pratt JR, Parker MD, Affleck LJ, *et al.* Ischemic epigenetics and the transplanted kidney. Transplant Proc 2006; 38(10): 3344-6.
[http://dx.doi.org/10.1016/j.transproceed.2006.10.112] [PMID: 17175268]

[18]   Mehta TK, Hoque MO, Ugarte R, *et al.* Quantitative detection of promoter hypermethylation as a biomarker of acute kidney injury during transplantation. Transplant Proc 2006; 38(10): 3420-6.
[http://dx.doi.org/10.1016/j.transproceed.2006.10.149] [PMID: 17175292]

[19]   Tampe B, Steinle U, Tampe D, *et al.* Low-dose hydralazine prevents fibrosis in a murine model of acute kidney injury–to–chronic kidney disease progression. Kidney Int 2017; 91(1): 157-76.
[http://dx.doi.org/10.1016/j.kint.2016.07.042] [PMID: 27692563]

[20]   Yin S, Zhang Q, Yang J, *et al.* TGFβ-incurred epigenetic aberrations of miRNA and DNA methyltransferase suppress Klotho and potentiate renal fibrosis. Biochim Biophys Acta Mol Cell Res 2017; 1864(7): 1207-16.
[http://dx.doi.org/10.1016/j.bbamcr.2017.03.002] [PMID: 28285987]

[21]   Hasegawa K, Wakino S, Simic P, *et al.* Renal tubular Sirt1 attenuates diabetic albuminuria by epigenetically suppressing Claudin-1 overexpression in podocytes. Nat Med 2013; 19(11): 1496-504.
[http://dx.doi.org/10.1038/nm.3363] [PMID: 24141423]

[22]   Castellano G, Franzin R, Sallustio F, *et al.* Complement component C5a induces aberrant epigenetic modifications in renal tubular epithelial cells accelerating senescence by Wnt4/βcatenin signaling after ischemia/reperfusion injury. Aging (Albany NY) 2019; 11(13): 4382-406.

[http://dx.doi.org/10.18632/aging.102059] [PMID: 31284268]

[23] Zhang W, Guan Y, Bayliss G, Zhuang S. Class IIa HDAC inhibitor TMP195 alleviates lipopolysaccharide-induced acute kidney injury. Am J Physiol Renal Physiol 2020; 319(6): F1015-26.
[http://dx.doi.org/10.1152/ajprenal.00405.2020] [PMID: 33017186]

[24] Zager RA, Johnson ACM. Renal ischemia-reperfusion injury upregulates histone-modifying enzyme systems and alters histone expression at proinflammatory/profibrotic genes. Am J Physiol Renal Physiol 2009; 296(5): F1032-41.
[http://dx.doi.org/10.1152/ajprenal.00061.2009] [PMID: 19261745]

[25] Naito M, Zager RA, Bomsztyk K. BRG1 increases transcription of proinflammatory genes in renal ischemia. J Am Soc Nephrol 2009; 20(8): 1787-96.
[http://dx.doi.org/10.1681/ASN.2009010118] [PMID: 19556365]

[26] Liu L, Mao L, Xu Y, Wu X. Endothelial-specific deletion of Brahma-related gene 1 (BRG1) assuages unilateral ureteral obstruction induced renal injury in mice. Biochem Biophys Res Commun 2019; 517(2): 244-52.
[http://dx.doi.org/10.1016/j.bbrc.2019.07.077] [PMID: 31349970]

[27] Gong W, Luo C, Peng F, *et al.* Brahma-related gene-1 promotes tubular senescence and renal fibrosis through Wnt/β-catenin/autophagy axis. Clin Sci (Lond) 2021; 135(15): 1873-95.
[http://dx.doi.org/10.1042/CS20210447] [PMID: 34318888]

[28] Basta JM, Singh AP, Robbins L, Stout L, Pherson M, Rauchman M. The core SWI/SNF catalytic subunit Brg1 regulates nephron progenitor cell proliferation and differentiation. Dev Biol 2020; 464(2): 176-87.
[http://dx.doi.org/10.1016/j.ydbio.2020.05.008] [PMID: 32504627]

[29] Liu L, Mao L, Wu X, *et al.* BRG1 regulates endothelial-derived IL-33 to promote ischemia-reperfusion induced renal injury and fibrosis in mice. Biochim Biophys Acta Mol Basis Dis 2019; 1865(9): 2551-61.
[http://dx.doi.org/10.1016/j.bbadis.2019.06.015] [PMID: 31228616]

[30] Groisberg R, Hong DS, Janku F, *et al.* SWI/SNF complex subunit aberrations in diverse cancers: Next-generation sequencing of 539 patients. J Clin Oncol 2017; 35(15_suppl): 2588.
[http://dx.doi.org/10.1200/JCO.2017.35.15_suppl.2588]

[31] Guerrero-Martínez JA, Reyes JC. High expression of SMARCA4 or SMARCA2 is frequently associated with an opposite prognosis in cancer. Sci Rep 2018; 8(1): 2043.
[http://dx.doi.org/10.1038/s41598-018-20217-3] [PMID: 29391527]

[32] Portela A, Esteller M. Epigenetic modifications and human disease. Nat Biotechnol 2010; 28(10): 1057-68.
[http://dx.doi.org/10.1038/nbt.1685] [PMID: 20944598]

[33] Sterner DE, Berger SL. Acetylation of histones and transcription-related factors. Microbiol Mol Biol Rev 2000; 64(2): 435-59.
[http://dx.doi.org/10.1128/MMBR.64.2.435-459.2000] [PMID: 10839822]

[34] Seto E, Yoshida M. Erasers of histone acetylation: the histone deacetylase enzymes. Cold Spring Harb Perspect Biol 2014; 6(4): a018713.
[http://dx.doi.org/10.1101/cshperspect.a018713] [PMID: 24691964]

[35] Allfrey VG, Mirsky AE. Structural Modifications of Histones and their Possible Role in the Regulation of RNA Synthesis. Science 1964; 144(3618): 559.
[http://dx.doi.org/10.1126/science.144.3618.559] [PMID: 17836360]

[36] Tanemoto F, Mimura I. Therapies Targeting Epigenetic Alterations in Acute Kidney Injury-to-Chronic Kidney Disease Transition. Pharmaceuticals (Basel) 2022; 15(2): 123.
[http://dx.doi.org/10.3390/ph15020123] [PMID: 35215236]

[37] Marumo T, Hishikawa K, Yoshikawa M, Fujita T. Epigenetic regulation of BMP7 in the regenerative

response to ischemia. J Am Soc Nephrol 2008; 19(7): 1311-20.
[http://dx.doi.org/10.1681/ASN.2007091040] [PMID: 18322163]

[38]   Ma T, Huang C, Xu Q, *et al*. Suppression of BMP-7 by histone deacetylase 2 promoted apoptosis of renal tubular epithelial cells in acute kidney injury. Cell Death Dis 2017; 8(10): e3139.
[http://dx.doi.org/10.1038/cddis.2017.552] [PMID: 29072686]

[39]   Chen S, Bellew C, Yao X, *et al*. Histone deacetylase (HDAC) activity is critical for embryonic kidney gene expression, growth, and differentiation. J Biol Chem 2011; 286(37): 32775-89.
[http://dx.doi.org/10.1074/jbc.M111.248278] [PMID: 21778236]

[40]   Tang J, Yan Y, Zhao TC, Bayliss G, Yan H, Zhuang S. Class I histone deacetylase activity is required for proliferation of renal epithelial cells. Am J Physiol Renal Physiol 2013; 305(3): F244-54.
[http://dx.doi.org/10.1152/ajprenal.00126.2013] [PMID: 23698124]

[41]   Tang J, Yan Y, Zhao TC, *et al*. Class I HDAC activity is required for renal protection and regeneration after acute kidney injury. Am J Physiol Renal Physiol 2014; 307(3): F303-16.
[http://dx.doi.org/10.1152/ajprenal.00102.2014] [PMID: 24808536]

[42]   Zhang H, Zhang W, Jiao F, *et al*. The Nephroprotective Effect of MS-275 on Lipopolysaccharide (LPS)-Induced Acute Kidney Injury by Inhibiting Reactive Oxygen Species (ROS)-Oxidative Stress and Endoplasmic Reticulum Stress. Med Sci Monit 2018; 24: 2620-30.
[http://dx.doi.org/10.12659/MSM.906362] [PMID: 29704392]

[43]   Cheng S, Wu T, Li Y, Huang J, Cai T. Romidepsin (FK228) in a Mouse Model of Lipopolysaccharide-Induced Acute Kidney Injury is Associated with Down-Regulation of the CYP2E1 Gene. Med Sci Monit 2020; 26: e918528.
[http://dx.doi.org/10.12659/MSM.918528] [PMID: 31954012]

[44]   Zhou X, Chen H, Shi Y, Ma X, Zhuang S, Liu N. The role and mechanism of histone deacetylases in acute kidney injury. Front Pharmacol 2021; 12: 695237.
[http://dx.doi.org/10.3389/fphar.2021.695237] [PMID: 34220520]

[45]   Ranganathan P, Hamad R, Mohamed R, Jayakumar C, Muthusamy T, Ramesh G. Histone deacetylase–mediated silencing of AMWAP expression contributes to cisplatin nephrotoxicity. Kidney Int 2016; 89(2): 317-26.
[http://dx.doi.org/10.1038/ki.2015.326] [PMID: 26509586]

[46]   Yoshikawa M, Hishikawa K, Marumo T, Fujita T. Inhibition of histone deacetylase activity suppresses epithelial-to-mesenchymal transition induced by TGF-beta1 in human renal epithelial cells. J Am Soc Nephrol 2007; 18(1): 58-65.
[http://dx.doi.org/10.1681/ASN.2005111187] [PMID: 17135397]

[47]   Hareedy MS, Abdelzaher LA, Badary DM, Mohammed Alnasser S, Abd-Eldayem AM. Valproate attenuates hypertonic glycerol-induced rhabdomyolysis and acute kidney injury. Nephrol Ther 2021; 17(3): 160-7.
[http://dx.doi.org/10.1016/j.nephro.2020.12.003] [PMID: 33781712]

[48]   Speir RW, Stallings JD, Andrews JM, Gelnett MS, Brand TC, Salgar SK. Effects of valproic acid and dexamethasone administration on early bio-markers and gene expression profile in acute kidney ischemia-reperfusion injury in the rat. PLoS One 2015; 10(5): e0126622.
[http://dx.doi.org/10.1371/journal.pone.0126622] [PMID: 25970334]

[49]   Li T, Yu C, Zhuang S. Histone methyltransferase EZH2: A potential therapeutic target for kidney diseases. Front Physiol 2021; 12: 640700.
[http://dx.doi.org/10.3389/fphys.2021.640700] [PMID: 33679454]

[50]   Zhou X, Zang X, Ponnusamy M, *et al*. Enhancer of zeste homolog 2 inhibition attenuates renal fibrosis by maintaining Smad7 and phosphatase and tensin homolog expression. J Am Soc Nephrol 2016; 27(7): 2092-108.
[http://dx.doi.org/10.1681/ASN.2015040457] [PMID: 26701983]

[51] Tan M, Luo H, Lee S, *et al.* Identification of 67 histone marks and histone lysine crotonylation as a new type of histone modification. Cell 2011; 146(6): 1016-28.
[http://dx.doi.org/10.1016/j.cell.2011.08.008] [PMID: 21925322]

[52] Lin H, Tang D, Xu Y, *et al.* Quantitative analysis of protein crotonylation identifies its association with immunoglobulin A nephropathy. Mol Med Rep 2020; 21(3): 1242-50.
[http://dx.doi.org/10.3892/mmr.2020.10931] [PMID: 32016442]

[53] Ruiz-Andres O, Sanchez-Niño MD, Moreno JA, *et al.* Downregulation of kidney protective factors by inflammation: role of transcription factors and epigenetic mechanisms. Am J Physiol Renal Physiol 2016; 311(6): F1329-40.
[http://dx.doi.org/10.1152/ajprenal.00487.2016] [PMID: 27760772]

[54] Chen W, Tang D, Xu Y, *et al.* Comprehensive analysis of lysine crotonylation in proteome of maintenance hemodialysis patients. Medicine (Baltimore) 2018; 97(37): e12035.
[http://dx.doi.org/10.1097/MD.0000000000012035] [PMID: 30212933]

[55] Wahid F, Shehzad A, Khan T, Kim YY. MicroRNAs: Synthesis, mechanism, function, and recent clinical trials. Biochim Biophys Acta Mol Cell Res 2010; 1803(11): 1231-43.
[http://dx.doi.org/10.1016/j.bbamcr.2010.06.013] [PMID: 20619301]

[56] Yao RW, Wang Y, Chen LL. Cellular functions of long noncoding RNAs. Nat Cell Biol 2019; 21(5): 542-51.
[http://dx.doi.org/10.1038/s41556-019-0311-8] [PMID: 31048766]

[57] Zhang Y, Zhao S, Wu D, *et al.* MicroRNA-22 promotes renal tubulointerstitial fibrosis by targeting PTEN and suppressing autophagy in diabetic nephropathy. J Diabetes Res 2018; 2018: 1-11.
[http://dx.doi.org/10.1155/2018/4728645] [PMID: 29850604]

[58] Tan R, Zhang J, Tan X, Zhang X, Yang J, Liu Y. Downregulation of SnoN expression in obstructive nephropathy is mediated by an enhanced ubiquitin-dependent degradation. J Am Soc Nephrol 2006; 17(10): 2781-91.
[http://dx.doi.org/10.1681/ASN.2005101055] [PMID: 16959829]

[59] Xu Y, Zhang J, Fan L, He X. miR-423-5p suppresses high-glucose-induced podocyte injury by targeting Nox4. Biochem Biophys Res Commun 2018; 505(2): 339-45.
[http://dx.doi.org/10.1016/j.bbrc.2018.09.067] [PMID: 30245133]

[60] Shao Y, Lv C, Wu C, Zhou Y, Wang Q. Mir-217 promotes inflammation and fibrosis in high glucose cultured rat glomerular mesangial cells *via* Sirt1/HIF-1α signaling pathway. Diabetes Metab Res Rev 2016; 32(6): 534-43.
[http://dx.doi.org/10.1002/dmrr.2788] [PMID: 26891083]

[61] Sun Z, Ma Y, Chen F, Wang S, Chen B, Shi J. miR-133b and miR-199b knockdown attenuate TGF-β1-induced epithelial to mesenchymal transition and renal fibrosis by targeting SIRT1 in diabetic nephropathy. Eur J Pharmacol 2018; 837: 96-104.
[http://dx.doi.org/10.1016/j.ejphar.2018.08.022] [PMID: 30125566]

[62] Xue M, Li Y, Hu F, *et al.* High glucose up-regulates microRNA-34a-5p to aggravate fibrosis by targeting SIRT1 in HK-2 cells. Biochem Biophys Res Commun 2018; 498(1): 38-44.
[http://dx.doi.org/10.1016/j.bbrc.2017.12.048] [PMID: 29371016]

[63] He F, Peng F, Xia X, *et al.* MiR-135a promotes renal fibrosis in diabetic nephropathy by regulating TRPC1. Diabetologia 2014; 57(8): 1726-36.
[http://dx.doi.org/10.1007/s00125-014-3282-0] [PMID: 24908566]

[64] Zanchi C, Macconi D, Trionfini P, *et al.* MicroRNA-184 is a downstream effector of albuminuria driving renal fibrosis in rats with diabetic nephropathy. Diabetologia 2017; 60(6): 1114-25.
[http://dx.doi.org/10.1007/s00125-017-4248-9] [PMID: 28364255]

[65] Jiang ZH, Tang YZ, Song HN, Yang M, Li B, Ni CL. miRNA-342 suppresses renal interstitial fibrosis in diabetic nephropathy by targeting SOX6. Int J Mol Med 2019; 45(1): 45-52.

[http://dx.doi.org/10.3892/ijmm.2019.4388] [PMID: 31746345]

[66]   Li N, Wang LJ, Xu WL, Liu S, Yu JY. MicroRNA-379-5p suppresses renal fibrosis by regulating the LIN28/let-7 axis in diabetic nephropathy. Int J Mol Med 2019; 44(5): 1619-28.
[http://dx.doi.org/10.3892/ijmm.2019.4325] [PMID: 31485601]

[67]   Gao B-H, Wu H, Wang X, Ji LL, Chen C. MiR-30c-5p inhibits high glucose-induced EMT and renal fibrogenesis by down-regulation of JAK1 in diabetic nephropathy. Eur Rev Med Pharmacol Sci 2020; 24(3): 1338-49.
[http://dx.doi.org/10.26355/eurrev_202002_20191] [PMID: 32096183]

[68]   Tang W, Zheng L, Yan R, *et al.* miR302a-3p may modulate renal epithelial-mesenchymal transition in diabetic kidney disease by targeting ZEB1. Nephron J 2018; 138(3): 231-42.
[http://dx.doi.org/10.1159/000481465] [PMID: 29227974]

[69]   Zhao Y, Yin Z, Li H, *et al.* MiR-30c protects diabetic nephropathy by suppressing epithelial-t--mesenchymal transition in db/db mice. Aging Cell 2017; 16(2): 387-400.
[http://dx.doi.org/10.1111/acel.12563] [PMID: 28127848]

[70]   Wu J, Liu J, Ding Y, *et al.* MiR-455-3p suppresses renal fibrosis through repression of ROCK2 expression in diabetic nephropathy. Biochem Biophys Res Commun 2018; 503(2): 977-83.
[http://dx.doi.org/10.1016/j.bbrc.2018.06.105] [PMID: 29932921]

[71]   Zhu X-J, Gong Z, Li S-J, Jia HP, Li DL. Long non-coding RNA Hottip modulates high-glucos--induced inflammation and ECM accumulation through miR-455-3p/WNT2B in mouse mesangial cells. Int J Clin Exp Pathol 2019; 12(7): 2435-45.https://pmc.ncbi.nlm.nih.gov/articles/PMC6949587/
[PMID: 31934070]

[72]   Sun T, Liu Y, Liu L, Ma F. MicroRNA-544 attenuates diabetic renal injury *via* suppressing glomerulosclerosis and inflammation by targeting FASN. Gene 2020; 723: 143986.
[http://dx.doi.org/10.1016/j.gene.2019.143986] [PMID: 31323309]

[73]   Lal MA, Patrakka J. Understanding Podocyte Biology to Develop Novel Kidney Therapeutics. Front Endocrinol (Lausanne) 2018; 9: 409.
[http://dx.doi.org/10.3389/fendo.2018.00409] [PMID: 30083135]

[74]   Wang L, Li H. MiR-770-5p facilitates podocyte apoptosis and inflammation in diabetic nephropathy by targeting TIMP3. Biosci Rep 2020; 40(4): BSR20193653.
[http://dx.doi.org/10.1042/BSR20193653] [PMID: 32309847]

[75]   Zhang S-Z, Qiu X-J, Dong S-S, *et al.* MicroRNA-770-5p is involved in the development of diabetic nephropathy through regulating podocyte apoptosis by targeting TP53 regulated inhibitor of apoptosis 1. Eur Rev Med Pharmacol Sci 2019; 23(3): 1248-56.
[http://dx.doi.org/10.26355/eurrev_201902_17018] [PMID: 30779094]

[76]   Fu Y, Wang C, Zhang D, Chu X, Zhang Y, Li J. miR-15b-5p ameliorated high glucose-induced podocyte injury through repressing apoptosis, oxidative stress, and inflammatory responses by targeting Sema3A. J Cell Physiol 2019; 234(11): 20869-78.
[http://dx.doi.org/10.1002/jcp.28691] [PMID: 31025335]

[77]   Lv N, Li C, Liu X, Qi C, Wang Z. miR-34b Alleviates High Glucose-Induced Inflammation and Apoptosis in Human HK-2 Cells *via* IL-6R/JAK2/STAT3 Signaling Pathway. Med Sci Monit 2019; 25: 8142-51.
[http://dx.doi.org/10.12659/MSM.917128] [PMID: 31665127]

[78]   Wan RJ, Li YH. MicroRNA-146a/NAPDH oxidase4 decreases reactive oxygen species generation and inflammation in a diabetic nephropathy model. Mol Med Rep 2018; 17(3): 4759-66.
[http://dx.doi.org/10.3892/mmr.2018.8407] [PMID: 29328400]

[79]   Wu J, Lu K, Zhu M, *et al.* miR-485 suppresses inflammation and proliferation of mesangial cells in an in vitro model of diabetic nephropathy by targeting NOX5. Biochem Biophys Res Commun 2020; 521(4): 984-90.

[http://dx.doi.org/10.1016/j.bbrc.2019.11.020] [PMID: 31727371]

[80]   Li M, Guo Q, Cai H, Wang H, Ma Z, Zhang X. miR-218 regulates diabetic nephropathy *via* targeting IKK-β and modulating NK-κB-mediated inflammation. J Cell Physiol 2020; 235(4): 3362-71.
       [http://dx.doi.org/10.1002/jcp.29224] [PMID: 31549412]

[81]   Sun Y, Peng R, Peng H, *et al.* miR-451 suppresses the NF-kappaB-mediated proinflammatory molecules expression through inhibiting LMP7 in diabetic nephropathy. Mol Cell Endocrinol 2016; 433: 75-86.
       [http://dx.doi.org/10.1016/j.mce.2016.06.004] [PMID: 27264074]

[82]   Su J, Ren J, Chen H, Liu B. MicroRNA-140-5p ameliorates the high glucose-induced apoptosis and inflammation through suppressing TLR4/NF-κB signaling pathway in human renal tubular epithelial cells. Biosci Rep 2020; 40(3): BSR20192384.
       [http://dx.doi.org/10.1042/BSR20192384] [PMID: 32073611]

[83]   Yao T, Zha D, Gao P, Shui H, Wu X. MiR-874 alleviates renal injury and inflammatory response in diabetic nephropathy through targeting toll-like receptor-4. J Cell Physiol 2019; 234(1): 871-9.
       [http://dx.doi.org/10.1002/jcp.26908] [PMID: 30171701]

[84]   Jiang X, Li D, Shen W, Shen X, Liu Y. LncRNA NEAT1 promotes hypoxia-induced renal tubular epithelial apoptosis through downregulating miR-27a-3p. J Cell Biochem 2019; 120(9): 16273-82.
       [http://dx.doi.org/10.1002/jcb.28909] [PMID: 31090110]

[85]   Tian X, Ji Y, Liang Y, Zhang J, Guan L, Wang C. LINC00520 targeting miR-27b-3p regulates *OSMR* expression level to promote acute kidney injury development through the PI3K/AKT signaling pathway. J Cell Physiol 2019; 234(8): 14221-33.
       [http://dx.doi.org/10.1002/jcp.28118] [PMID: 30684280]

[86]   Yu TM, Palanisamy K, Sun KT, *et al.* RANTES mediates kidney ischemia reperfusion injury through a possible role of HIF-1α and LncRNA PRINS. Sci Rep 2016; 6(1): 18424.
       [http://dx.doi.org/10.1038/srep18424] [PMID: 26725683]

[87]   Bijkerk R, Au YW, Stam W, *et al.* Long Non-coding RNAs Rian and Miat Mediate Myofibroblast Formation in Kidney Fibrosis. Front Pharmacol 2019; 10: 215.
       [http://dx.doi.org/10.3389/fphar.2019.00215] [PMID: 30914951]

[88]   Chen H, Fan Y, Jing H, Tang S, Zhou J. Emerging role of lncRNAs in renal fibrosis. Arch Biochem Biophys 2020; 692: 108530.
       [http://dx.doi.org/10.1016/j.abb.2020.108530] [PMID: 32768395]

[89]   Tian H, Wu M, Zhou P, Huang C, Ye C, Wang L. The long non-coding RNA MALAT1 is increased in renal ischemia-reperfusion injury and inhibits hypoxia-induced inflammation. Ren Fail 2018; 40(1): 527-33.
       [http://dx.doi.org/10.1080/0886022X.2018.1487863] [PMID: 30277425]

[90]   Zhou X, Li Y, Wu C, Yu W, Cheng F. Novel lncRNA XLOC_032768 protects against renal tubular epithelial cells apoptosis in renal ischemia–reperfusion injury by regulating FNDC3B/TGF-β1. Ren Fail 2020; 42(1): 994-1003.
       [http://dx.doi.org/10.1080/0886022X.2020.1818579] [PMID: 32972270]

[91]   Rysz J, Franczyk B, Ciałkowska-Rysz A, Gluba-Brzózka A. The Effect of Diet on the Survival of Patients with Chronic Kidney Disease. Nutrients 2017; 9(5): 495.
       [http://dx.doi.org/10.3390/nu9050495] [PMID: 28505087]

[92]   Kolch W, Neusüß C, Pelzing M, Mischak H. Capillary electrophoresis–mass spectrometry as a powerful tool in clinical diagnosis and biomarker discovery. Mass Spectrom Rev 2005; 24(6): 959-77.
       [http://dx.doi.org/10.1002/mas.20051] [PMID: 15747373]

[93]   Zhou X, Zang X, Guan Y, *et al.* Targeting enhancer of zeste homolog 2 protects against acute kidney injury. Cell Death Dis 2018; 9(11): 1067.
       [http://dx.doi.org/10.1038/s41419-018-1012-0] [PMID: 30341286]

[94]   Jia Y, Reddy MA, Das S, *et al.* Dysregulation of histone H3 lysine 27 trimethylation in transforming growth factor-β1–induced gene expression in mesangial cells and diabetic kidney. J Biol Chem 2019; 294(34): 12695-707.
[http://dx.doi.org/10.1074/jbc.RA119.007575] [PMID: 31266808]

[95]   Rohraff DM, He Y, Farkash EA, Schonfeld M, Tsou PS, Sawalha AH. Inhibition of EZH2 Ameliorates Lupus-Like Disease in MRL/ *lpr* Mice. Arthritis Rheumatol 2019; 71(10): 1681-90.
[http://dx.doi.org/10.1002/art.40931] [PMID: 31106974]

[96]   Shi Y, Xu L, Tao M, *et al.* Blockade of enhancer of zeste homolog 2 alleviates renal injury associated with hyperuricemia. Am J Physiol Renal Physiol 2019; 316(3): F488-505.
[http://dx.doi.org/10.1152/ajprenal.00234.2018] [PMID: 30566000]

[97]   Han X, Sun Z. Epigenetic Regulation of KL (Klotho) via H3K27me3 (Histone 3 Lysine [K] 27 Trimethylation) in Renal Tubule Cells. Hypertension 2020; 75: 1233–1241.
[http://dx.doi.org/10.1161/HYPERTENSIONAHA.120.14642]

[98]   Li L, Zhang Y, Xu M, Rong R, Wang J, Zhu T. Inhibition of histone methyltransferase EZH2 ameliorates early acute renal allograft rejection in rats. BMC Immunol 2016; 17(1): 41.
[http://dx.doi.org/10.1186/s12865-016-0179-3] [PMID: 27784285]

[99]   Morgado Pascual JL. Epigenética en la enfermedad renal: Investigación de las proteínas BET como potenciales dianas terapéuticas 2018.http://hdl.handle.net/10486/682711

[100]   Chen NX, Kiattisunthorn K, O'Neill KD, *et al.* Decreased microRNA is involved in the vascular remodeling abnormalities in chronic kidney disease (CKD). PLoS One 2013; 8(5): e64558.
[http://dx.doi.org/10.1371/journal.pone.0064558] [PMID: 23717629]

[101]   Taïbi F, Metzinger-Le Meuth V, M'Baya-Moutoula E, *et al.* Possible involvement of microRNAs in vascular damage in experimental chronic kidney disease. Biochim Biophys Acta Mol Basis Dis 2014; 1842(1): 88-98.
[http://dx.doi.org/10.1016/j.bbadis.2013.10.005] [PMID: 24140891]

[102]   Lovren F, Pan Y, Quan A, *et al.* MicroRNA-145 targeted therapy reduces atherosclerosis. Circulation 2012; 126: S81-90.
[http://dx.doi.org/10.1161/CIRCULATIONAHA.111.084186] [PMID: 22965997]

[103]   Matas AJ, Smith JM, Skeans MA, *et al.* OPTN/SRTR 2012 Annual Data Report: Kidney. Am J Transplant 2014; 14: 11-44.
[http://dx.doi.org/10.1111/ajt.12579] [PMID: 24373166]

[104]   Ben-Dov IZ, Muthukumar T, Morozov P, Mueller FB, Tuschl T, Suthanthiran M. MicroRNA sequence profiles of human kidney allografts with or without tubulointerstitial fibrosis. Transplantation 2012; 94(11): 1086-94.
[http://dx.doi.org/10.1097/TP.0b013e3182751efd] [PMID: 23131772]

[105]   Scian MJ, Maluf DG, David KG, *et al.* MicroRNA profiles in allograft tissues and paired urines associate with chronic allograft dysfunction with IF/TA. Am J Transplant 2011; 11(10): 2110-22.
[http://dx.doi.org/10.1111/j.1600-6143.2011.03666.x] [PMID: 21794090]

[106]   Khurana R, Ranches G, Schafferer S, *et al.* Identification of urinary exosomal noncoding RNAs as novel biomarkers in chronic kidney disease. RNA 2017; 23(2): 142-52.
[http://dx.doi.org/10.1261/rna.058834.116] [PMID: 27872161]

[107]   Zou YF, Wen D, Zhao Q, *et al.* Urinary MicroRNA-30c-5p and MicroRNA-192-5p as potential biomarkers of ischemia–reperfusion-induced kidney injury. Exp Biol Med (Maywood) 2017; 242(6): 657-67.
[http://dx.doi.org/10.1177/1535370216685005] [PMID: 28056546]

[108] Perez-Gomez M, Sanchez-Niño M, Sanz A, *et al.* Horizon 2020 in Diabetic Kidney Disease: The Clinical Trial Pipeline for Add-On Therapies on Top of Renin Angiotensin System Blockade. J Clin Med 2015; 4(6): 1325-47.
[http://dx.doi.org/10.3390/jcm4061325] [PMID: 26239562]

CHAPTER 14

From Stem Cells to One Functional Kidney

Ana Laura Calderón-Garcidueñas[1,*]

[1] *Neuropathology Department, Research Direction, Instituto Nacional de Neurologia y Neurocirugía, Manuel Velasco Suarez, Tlalpan 14269, Mexico City, Mexico*

Abstract: Human pluripotent stem cells (hPSCs) have self-renewal capacity and can generate cells of all three germ layers of the embryo. After division, each newly produced cell can either remain a stem cell or differentiate to form any other cell type with more defined functions, such as muscle cells, blood cells, or neural cells. There are two types of stem cells: embryonic stem cells and somatic or adult stem cells. Specifically, embryonic stem cells are pluripotential stem cells that can differentiate into all body cell types. It is possible to induce pluripotent stem cells (iPSC). These cells are somatic stem cells genetically reprogrammed to become like embryonic stem cells by inducing expressions of specific genes and other components necessary for maintaining embryonic stem cell properties. The idea that renal progenitors can give rise to a functional kidney under certain experimental conditions has encouraged hundreds of researchers to achieve this goal. Nevertheless, obtaining a fully functional organ *in vitro* is still perceived as distant. However, we can get closer to this objective as we learn more about the factors that influence cell proliferation and differentiation.

Keywords: Bioartificial, Bioengineering, Bioprinting, Chip, Organoid.

INTRODUCTION

Once the kidney is insufficient to fulfill its functions, the patient and the health system face a series of problems: the cost and availability of hemodialysis, the lack of organ availability, and the morbidity and mortality of these patients. In addition, the annual health cost per patient increases with the degree of renal failure. Hence, searching for viable alternatives to overcome this serious health problem is mandatory.

TYPES OF CELLS IN THE HUMAN BODY

According to their functions, there are three types of cells: somatic, germinal, and stem cells. Somatic cells are diploid and contain two pairs of chromosomes. They

* **Corresponding author Ana Laura Calderón Garcidueñas:** Neuropathology Department, Research Direction, Instituto Nacional de Neurologia y Neurocirugía, Manuel Velasco Suarez, Tlalpan 14269, Mexico City, Mexico; E-mail: ana.calderon@innn.edu.mx

are divided by mitosis, producing two daughter cells and constituting different organs and tissues with specific functions. Germinal cells are haploid, have a single set of 23 chromosomes, produce gametes, and are the only cells that can undergo meiosis and mitosis. The egg and the sperm are germ cells [1].

Human pluripotent stem cells (hPSCs) have self-renewal capacity and can generate cells from three embryo germ layers. Following division, newly produced cells can remain stem cells or differentiate into any other cell type with specific functions, such as muscle cells, blood cells, and neural cells. There are two types of stem cells: embryonic stem cells and somatic stem cells. Embryonic stem cells are pluripotent stem cells that can differentiate into any cell body type. On the other hand, somatic stem cells can differentiate only into different cell types present in the tissue of origin. However, it is possible to induce pluripotent stem cells (iPSCs). These cells are genetically reprogrammed to resemble embryonic stem cells through the induction of the expression of specific genes, together with other components required for maintaining embryonic cell properties. These latter cells are ideal candidates for restoring kidney function [2].

EMBRYOLOGY

The kidney has three important components: the nephron, interstitial stromal cells, and blood and lymphatic vessels. In a functional kidney, these elements are perfectly structured and coordinated. Embryologically, kidneys are formed with the participation of three types of cells: nephron progenitor cells (SIX2+), ureteric buds (GATA3+), and interstitial stromal progenitor cells (FOXD1+) [3 - 5]. The nephron is the functional unit of the kidney; it has two components: the glomerulus, which is responsible for filtering, and a system of tubules that perform selective secretion and reabsorption of numerous solutes and solvents. The kidney is a mesodermal organ that arises from the primitive streak (PS). The PS forms in the blastula and is an elongating groove at the caudal end of the embryo [6]. The mesoderm is formed from front to back by cells that migrate anteriorly from the stria. The pronephros and mesonephros form primitive nephrons in early embryogenesis to later give way to the metanephros that constitutes the functional kidney. In mice, the metanephros originate from the posterior area of the medial mesonephros [7]. Intermediate mesoderm cells also produce ureteric bud progenitor cells [8]. Feedback between both structures has been described since the metanephric mesenchyme produces fibroblast growth factor 20 (FGF20), and the ureteral buds secrete fibroblast growth factor 9 (FGF9) [9]. Finally, nephron progenitor cells (NPCs) can differentiate into functional nephron structures. However, another essential component of kidney function is the vasculature. The kidney receives 25% of the cardiac output. The embryonic vasculature originates with the constitution of a primitive vascular plexus.

Mesoderm-derived angioblasts differentiate in a process called vasculogenesis. Later, this network undergoes expansion and remodeling through angiogenesis [10].

However, it is not well known whether angioblasts arise from progenitors in the metanephros or migrate into them from the systemic circulation [11]. When the renal vesicle changes from a "coma" to an "s" shape, glomerular vascularization begins; then, a vascular cleft develops between the podocyte precursor and the proximal tubule [12]. Endothelial progenitor cells (VEGFR-2+) enter the vascular cleft under the influence of immature podocytes that produce VEGF-A (vascular endothelial growth factor, type A) and form capillary loops, which subsequently develop a lumen after excess TGF-β1-mediated "apoptotic pruning" of endothelial cells [13]. These capillary loops undergo branching and form the glomerular tuft with fenestrae [14].

VASCULAR ORGANIZATION

The renal artery, segmental artery, interlobar artery (cortex), arcuate artery (located at the border of the cortex and the medulla) (Fig. **1**), interlobular artery, afferent arteriole, glomerular hilum (which contains juxtaglomerular cells producing renin), glomerular capillary network, efferent arteriole, descending vasa recta (medullary microcirculation with continuous endothelium), and diaphragmed fenestrated ascending vasa recta constitute the complex renal vascular network [15].

Achieving this structural and functional complexity is one of the major engineering challenges of the kidney.

SIGNALING PATHWAYS AND REGENERATIVE PROCESS

The kidney's regeneration in the face of various insults involves the participation of renal progenitor cells as well as other cells, such as tubular epithelial cells, fibroblasts, and macrophages. These cells establish communication by activating several pathways, and it is important to know them.

PI3K/AKT/mTOR Pathway

HGF (hepatocyte growth factor), IGF-1 (insulin-like growth factor-1), and EGF (epidermal growth factor) contribute to the recovery of ischemic renal damage by activating phosphatidylinositol-3-kinase (PI3K), which phosphorylates phosphatidylinositol-4-5-biphosphate to yield phosphatidylinositol-3-4-5-triphosphate, which activates Akt (protein kinase B). Activated Akt stimulates the mammalian target of rapamycin (mTOR). Activated mTOR phosphorylates downstream substrates to induce cell regeneration [16].

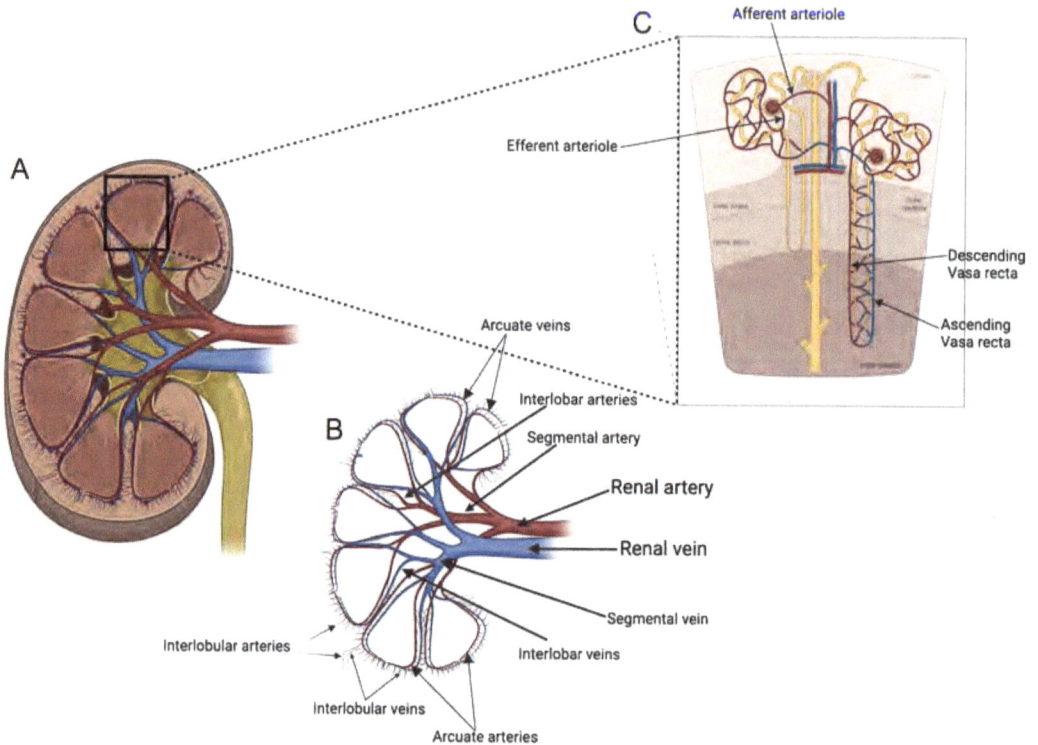

Fig. (1). Kidney structure (Panel A). Renal vascularization (Panel B). Glomerular circulation (Panel C), efferent arterioles from the outer and middle cortex constitute a peritubular plexus of capillaries. Such microvessels surround proximal and convoluted tubules; these complex microvessels-tubules function for renal reabsorption and filtrate. Efferent arterioles terminate in vasa recta, which enter the medulla as descending arterioles and exit the medulla as ascending veins (ascending vasa recta). The descending and ascending limbs of the vasa recta are connected by a thin capillary plexus. Medullary hypertonicity is preserved by countercurrent exchange through microcirculation of the vasa recta.

JAK/STAT

The JAK/STAT pathway (Janus kinases [JAKs], signal transducer, and activator of transcription proteins [STATs]) is activated when EGF binds to its receptor. Through activating the JAK/STAT pathway, erythropoiesis-stimulating proteins suppress renal tubular cell apoptosis *in vitro* and enhance renal recovery [17].

Wnt-GSK3-β-Catenin Pathway

The Wnt family (glycosylated protein ligands) can inhibit glycogen synthase kinase 3 (GSK3) *via* phosphorylation. Then, β-catenin is translocated into the nucleus and coactivates the T-cell factor/lymphoid enhancer-binding factor family of transcription factors. Wnt pathway responses are induced in the kidney following acute injury. Macrophage-derived Wnt7b, a Wnt ligand, promotes tubular epithelial cell regeneration and kidney repair [18].

MAPK/ERK Pathway

The family of mitogen-activated protein kinases (MAPKs) includes four MAPK pathways in mammalian cells: ERK1/2, c-Jun N-terminal kinase, p38MAPK, and extracellular signal-regulated kinase-5 (ERK5).

Growth factors activate ERK. *In vitro* studies have shown that ERK pathway activation enhances the survival of renal epithelial cells during oxidative injury. *In vivo*, inhibition of the ERK pathway can reduce kidney regeneration in some animal models [17].

THE LONG ROAD TO A FUNCTIONAL KIDNEY

The idea that renal progenitors can give rise to a functional kidney under certain experimental conditions has encouraged hundreds of researchers to achieve this goal. We will present the development of various techniques aimed at obtaining a functional kidney [19].

Xenotransplantation of Adult Organs or Embryonic Tissues

Cross-species transplantation, or xenotransplantation, has been attempted since the 1960s. It was initially attempted with nonhuman primate (NHP) kidneys. In 2002, an $\alpha - 1,3$-galactosyltransferase knockout (GalT-KO) pig was obtained. The deletion of a pig antigen expressed on the graft (galactose-α 1,3-galactose), together with complement-regulatory proteins and/or coagulation-regulatory proteins, has extended the life of the graft to more than a year [20].

Using CRISPR/Cas9 technology, a panel of genes vital for improving the xenograft survival rate (cytidine monophosphate-N-acetylneuraminic acid hydroxylase, B1,4 N-acetylgalactosaminyltransferase, isoglobotrihexosylceramide synthase, class I MHC, von Willebrand factor and C3) has been modified [21]. However, there is a risk of porcine infectious disease transmission to the recipient, especially porcine endogenous retroviruses (PERVs), which can be inactivated using CRISPR-Cas9 [22].

Chimeras

Chimeras are organisms composed of a mixture of cell populations from different organisms, including donor cells of embryonic, fetal, or adult origin and a host, which provides the physiological environment and life support to the donor cells.

There are two approaches in renal pathology: blastocyst complementation and targeted organ complementation [23].

Blastocyst Complementation

This procedure involves injecting embryonic stem cells (ESCs) into blastocysts and transferring the embryo to a foster mother's uterus.

Although human PSCs can be engrafted in large animal species, such as pigs and cattle, preimplantation blastocysts show limited contributions to postimplantation pig embryos [24]. This technique is in its infancy, and the problem of the vascular network is a challenge to solve.

Targeted Organ Complementation

This approach is focused on generating an organ, either by allowing PSCs to differentiate only into the organ of interest or by using committed progenitors or organ buds instead of PSCs [25]. Yamanaka *et al.* demonstrated that implantation of rat renal progenitor cells into kidney-deficient embryos led to the formation of new nephrons connected to the host uretic bud; however, there may be host-derived cells in the chimeric kidney, indicating that immunosuppressive drugs must be administered for autologous kidney transplantation [26].

Stem Cell-Based Therapies

Stem cell-based therapies for kidney disease include three basic strategies: 1) xenotransplantation of animal-derived kidneys; 2) transplantation of kidney-specific progenitor cells differentiated from PSCs; and 3) use of mesenchymal stem cells (MSCs) [27].

Whole-Kidney Grafts

Initially, 7-14-week gestation-early kidney precursors were transplanted into immunodeficient mice; a miniature kidney with functional capacity that was able to produce diluted urine was obtained. However, the mini-kidney did not integrate properly into the host and harbored cells of unwanted lineage. For this reason, more studies focused on the specific selection of precursors are needed [28].

Fetal Kidney-Derived Cells

Several experiments were performed using dissected rat fetal kidney cells. These cells produce kidney structures when injected under the renal capsule; nevertheless, nontubular cells are produced [29]. Some markers were used to select these cells. Neural cell adhesion molecule 1 (NCAM1) (CD56) is a marker previously identified for isolating stem cell populations from the kidney. NCAM1 is overexpressed in progenitor renal tissues [30]. It has been proven that human fetal kidney-derived nephron progenitors can be isolated and expanded and have the advantage of low immunogenicity [31].

Pluripotent Stem Cells

Working with embryonic and fetal human cells has ethical implications. An alternative is to generate pluripotent stem cells from fibroblasts [32]. Research has shown that by using the correct transcription factors, it is feasible to reprogram specific cells and orient them to a new phenotype [33].

Pluripotent stem cells (PSCs) are self-renewing and can differentiate into three embryonic components: the ectoderm, mesoderm, and endoderm [34]. With reprogramming technology, it is possible to generate inducible PSCs (iPSCs) from somatic cells using four factors: Oct4, Sox2, c-Myc, and Klf4 [32]. However, the direct transplant of pluripotent stem cells carries risks, such as tumor development, due to their high proliferative potential [35]. Therefore, differentiation protocols are important. Differentiation of iPSCs requires nephrogenic factors such as activin A, retinoic acid (RA), and bone morphogenetic proteins (BMPs) [36]. Self-renewing nephron progenitor cells express SIX homeobox 2 in humans (SIX2) [3].

Research on PSCs in 3D format has led to the generation of nephron-like structures (kidney organoids), similar to those of trimester 1 human kidneys, linked to a network of collecting tubules [4]. Currently, it is possible to use kidney organoids for disease modeling and, eventually, drug screening; however, we do not observe functional perfusion of vascularized kidney organoids [37]. The analysis of the different cell expansion and differentiation protocols is beyond the scope of this chapter, but there are excellent reviews in this regard [8].

Mesenchymal Stem Cells

Mesenchymal stem cells (MSCs) are self-renewing cells that can transdifferentiate and have immuno-suppressive potential [38].

MSCs are easily obtained from adipose tissue, the umbilical cord, *etc.*, and can transfer mitochondria to diseased cells by forming tubes for cell communication [39]. The transfer of mitochondria has been demonstrated in cultures of tubular epithelial cells from the kidneys of rats and of human mesenchymal cells, which opens up great possibilities in renal regenerative medicine [40].

According to the International Society for Cellular Therapy, under standard tissue culture conditions, MSCs adhere to plastic culture plates and express mesenchymal markers (CD105, CD73, and CD90) but not hematopoietic markers (CD45, CD34, CD14/CD11b, CD79a/CD19) or human leukocyte antigen (HLA-DR). MSCs can differentiate into adipocytes, skeletal tissue, osteoblasts, and chondrocytes *in vitro* [41].

MSCs have a future in kidney regeneration due to their anti-inflammatory effects. Clinical trials have already been carried out in acute renal ischemic processes and pathologies with inflammatory damage, such as lupus.

MSCs are immunomodulatory; they do not express MHC class II antigens or B7-1, B7-2, or CD40 costimulatory molecules and have low MHC class I antigens expression. Systemic administration ($\sim 10^6$-10^8 cells) of MSCs inhibits Th17 lymphocytes, augments the number and activity of regulatory T cells, and increases the expression of IL-10 [42].

MSCs can produce and release growth factors, such as epithelial growth factor (EGF), vascular endothelial growth factor (VEGF), transforming growth factor (TGF) α and β, fibroblast growth factor (FGF), and insulin-like growth factor 1 (IGF1), that stimulate the proliferation of local progenitor cells. MSCs secrete all these substances in the free state or within exosomes (spherical vesicles of endosomal origin with a diameter of 30-100 nm) or in microvesicles originating from the plasma membrane. Another advantage of these cells is that they are easily obtained from subcutaneous cellular tissue. As demonstrated by Zhang, they can be isolated from urine (2-7 cells/100 mL) [43]. Unlike MSCs, cells derived from urine (75%) exhibit telomerase activity without an increased risk of tumorigenesis. The glomerulus is the most likely origin of these MSC-like cells [44].

Renal Progenitor Cells

These cells express CD133 and CD24. In adults, RPCs can differentiate into glomerular and tubular cells. In healthy adult kidneys, glomerular progenitor cells (CD106) are located in the Bowman capsule and can differentiate toward the podocyte phenotype. Tubular progenitor cells (proximal tubules, segment S3, near the cortico-medullary junction) represent 2-6% of all tubular epithelial cells and express, in addition to CD133/CD24, vimentin, cytokeratin 6 and 9, Pax 2 and nestin. RPC has also been described in the papilla of the loop of Henle.

Unfortunately, until now, there has been no reproducible protocol to differentiate extrarenal stem cells to obtain renal progenitor cells.

The use of stem cells has vast potential in kidney regeneration, but there is still much to do.

Organ Bioengineering

Organ engineering involves combining various techniques to assemble cells, biologically relevant molecules, and scaffolds into functional organs [19].

Bioartificial Kidney

The bioartificial renal assist device (RAD) was created at the end of the 1990s as a hybrid system consisting of a multifiber bioreactor producing synthetic hollow fibers of a high-flow hemofiltration cartridge; these fibers were seeded with primary tubular epithelial cells of porcine origin [45]. The system mimicked tubular functions, providing differential reabsorption and secretion as well as metabolic and endocrine functions. At this point, RAD is the only bioartificial kidney device successfully tested in humans.

Later, the same group developed the bioartificial renal epithelial cell system (BRECS). The design included a niobium-coated carbon and cryopreserve polycarbonate seeded with human renal tubular epithelial cells originating from adult progenitor cells. It has been useful in swine models of septic shock associated with hemofilters [46].

Kidney-Derived Scaffolds

They are obtained by decellularizing or removing cellular components through detergents and enzymes without affecting the extracellular matrix. Then, the kidney is recellularized through different cell seeding strategies. Useful kidney recellularization has been achieved using epithelial cells, endothelial cells, or PSCs that can differentiate into all cell types [47]. Many important points still need to be refined before this technology can be translated to clinical trials, starting with methods for eliminating epithelial cells, preserving the vasculature, and controlling the immune response [48].

Self-Organizing Nephrons

One option for understanding renal pathophysiology and constructing assembly units is developing parts of the nephron. These parts could later be assembled to form a complete and functional organ. A brief review of renal organoids to 3D and 4D bioprinting was presented by Peired *et al.* [19].

Kidney Organoids

As mentioned earlier, kidney organoids are self-organizing 3D aggregations of relatively immature cells (embryonic kidney type from the first trimester of gestation) derived from ESCs or iPSCs. Various protocols have matured these organoids and achieved an adequate vascular network and urinary drainage. Its utility thus far has been the study of the pathophysiology of some diseases. In this context, the ability of iPSCs to form organoids from the urine of pediatric patients with several hereditary kidney diseases has been validated [49].

Kydney-on-A-Chip

Glomerulus-on-A-Chip

New drugs to model human diseases *in vitro* are needed. Microscale microfluid engineering technology has contributed to the creation of organ-on-a-chips. A model of hypertensive glomerulopathy involving the cocultivation of immortalized glomerular endothelial cells and mouse podocyte precursor cells was created *via* an organ-on-a-chip approach [50].

In 2019, a glomerulus-on-a-chip composed of human podocytes and human glomerular endothelial cells was cocultured in a three-channel version of the OrganoPlate® in the absence of an artificial membrane separating them. The authors validated the chip as a disease-modeling platform for diabetic nephropathy, genetic diseases affecting podocytes, and drug testing [51].

Tubule-on-A-Chip

Tubular cells are cultured in a three-dimensional (3D) channel, reproducing the microenvironment of the human kidney tubule and its reabsorption and secretion functions. Fluid shear stress (FSS) can be measured using microfluidic technology. The cell source in this system is frequently the immortalized human renal tubular cell line HK-2 (human kidney). Neither this cell line nor others that have been used recapitulate the primary cell phenotype, nor do they recapitulate the absorptive functions of the proximal tubules. The most useful application of this device has been to evaluate drug toxicity (cisplatin and gentamicin). Devices with multiple cell lines (liver and kidney) have even been created to understand drug metabolism and its effect on the kidney [52].

3D&4D Bioprinting

This procedure consists of depositing cells and supportive elements layer-by-layer into complex 3D functional living tissues. 3D bioprinting has been used to generate skin, cartilage, bone, and vascular tissue for transplantation in reconstructive surgery [53].

Because of the kidney's complexity and various cellular components, 3D printing technology has been principally employed to generate portions of the nephron with the intention of generating a more suitable model from an architectural and functional point of view. One research group has used 3D bioprinting technology to produce kidney organoids from cell lines efficiently [54].

4D bioprinting introduces a fourth dimension, 'time.' It utilizes a type of hydrogel responsive to physical, chemical, and biological (*e.g.*, glucose and enzymes) stimuli. The shape of the printed material can be reversibly modified to simulate physiological dynamic changes in native tissue. However, 4D bioprinting is still in the stage of proof-of-concept studies [55].

WHAT IS REQUIRED TO GENERATE A COMPLETE KIDNEY?

At least four requirements must be met to ensure an organ's functionality.

Size. The human kidney contains 200,000-2.5 million nephrons. Dialysis is needed when glomerular filtration is reduced to 10-15% of normal. On the other hand, human iPSC-derived kidney organoids are 5-7 mm in diameter and contain approximately 100 nephrons [4]. Therefore, obtaining a suitable size and number of nephrons is a limitation [56].

An appropriate structure. Structure is related to function, and this is particularly true in the kidney. For example, fluid balance regulation requires a parallel alignment of the Henle loops and the correct location of the various tubular segments in the cortex and medulla. The main challenge is to have well-vascularized nephrons that can connect to the systemic circulation [56].

Functional maturity. Cellular functional maturation has not yet been achieved with existing protocols. It is necessary to understand how the different cellular components in the kidney mature throughout the different embryonic and fetal stages, the communication signals with other cells, and the local and systemic cellular influences participating in this process. Therefore, much work is needed in this field [56].

Cellular integration. In patients with kidney damage, one theoretical alternative is to generate stem cells, the specific type of cell required to reverse the damage. However, implanting any epithelial cell that can proliferate properly requires structural support and an intact basal membrane. Therefore, more research is needed in this field [56].

CONCLUSION

Scientific and technological development can improve what already exists in a functional organ, such as optimizing treatment seeding epithelial cells of the proximal tubules in extracorporeal devices or using cells derived from iPSCs to produce erythropoietin and finishing with pharmacological dependence on this substance [56].

The ability to obtain a fully functional organ *in vitro* is still poorly understood. However, we can achieve this objective as we learn more about the factors that influence cell proliferation and differentiation.

There have been many advances in renal regenerative medicine, and the future looks promising. Moreover, a broad educational and healthcare campaign is required to prevent obstructive processes, infections, and diseases such as obesity, diabetes mellitus, and high blood pressure, which can cause irreversible damage to the kidneys.

REFERENCES

[1]   Conrad S, Azizi H, Skutella T. Single-Cell Expression Profiling and Proteomics of Primordial Germ Cells, Spermatogonial Stem Cells, Adult Germ Stem Cells, and Oocytes. Adv Exp Med Biol 2017; 1083: 77-87.
[http://dx.doi.org/10.1007/5584_2017_117] [PMID: 29299873]

[2]   Fieldès M, Ahmed E, Bourguignon C, *et al.* [Modelling the bronchial epithelium in chronic obstructive pulmonary disease using human induced pluripotential stem cells]. Rev Mal Respir 2020; 37(3): 197-200.
[http://dx.doi.org/10.1016/j.rmr.2020.02.003] [PMID: 32146059]

[3]   Kobayashi A, Valerius MT, Mugford JW, *et al.* Six2 defines and regulates a multipotent self-renewing nephron progenitor population throughout mammalian kidney development. Cell Stem Cell 2008; 3(2): 169-81.
[http://dx.doi.org/10.1016/j.stem.2008.05.020] [PMID: 18682239]

[4]   Takasato M, Er PX, Chiu HS, *et al.* Kidney organoids from human iPS cells contain multiple lineages and model human nephrogenesis. Nature 2015; 526(7574): 564-8.
[http://dx.doi.org/10.1038/nature15695] [PMID: 26444236]

[5]   Naiman N, Fujioka K, Fujino M, *et al.* Repression of interstitial identity in nephron progenitor cells by Pax2 establishes the nephron-interstitium boundary during kidney development. Dev Cell 2017; 41(4): 349-365.e3.
[http://dx.doi.org/10.1016/j.devcel.2017.04.022] [PMID: 28535371]

[6]   Mikawa T, Poh AM, Kelly KA, Ishii Y, Reese DE. Induction and patterning of the primitive streak, an organizing center of gastrulation in the amniote. Dev Dyn 2004; 229(3): 422-32.
[http://dx.doi.org/10.1002/dvdy.10458] [PMID: 14991697]

[7]   Taguchi A, Kaku Y, Ohmori T, *et al.* Redefining the in vivo origin of metanephric nephron progenitors enables generation of complex kidney structures from pluripotent stem cells. Cell Stem Cell 2014; 14(1): 53-67.
[http://dx.doi.org/10.1016/j.stem.2013.11.010] [PMID: 24332837]

[8]   Morizane R, Miyoshi T, Bonventre JV. Concise Review: Kidney Generation with Human Pluripotent

Stem Cells. Stem Cells 2017; 35(11): 2209-17.
[http://dx.doi.org/10.1002/stem.2699] [PMID: 28869686]

[9] Majumdar A, Vainio S, Kispert A, McMahon J, McMahon AP. *Wnt11* and *Ret/Gdnf* pathways cooperate in regulating ureteric branching during metanephric kidney development. Development 2003; 130(14): 3175-85.
[http://dx.doi.org/10.1242/dev.00520] [PMID: 12783789]

[10] Carmeliet P. Mechanisms of angiogenesis and arteriogenesis. Nat Med 2000; 6(4): 389-95.
[http://dx.doi.org/10.1038/74651] [PMID: 10742145]

[11] Sims-Lucas S, Schaefer C, Bushnell D, *et al.* Endothelial Progenitors Exist within the Kidney and Lung Mesenchyme. PLoS One 2013; 8(6): e65993.
[http://dx.doi.org/10.1371/journal.pone.0065993] [PMID: 23823180]

[12] Bartlett CS, Jeansson M, Quaggin SE. Vascular Growth Factors and Glomerular Disease. Annu Rev Physiol 2016; 78(1): 437-61.
[http://dx.doi.org/10.1146/annurev-physiol-021115-105412] [PMID: 26863327]

[13] Fierlbeck W, Liu A, Coyle R, Ballermann BJ. Endothelial cell apoptosis during glomerular capillary lumen formation in vivo. J Am Soc Nephrol 2003; 14(5): 1349-54.
[http://dx.doi.org/10.1097/01.ASN.0000061779.70530.06] [PMID: 12707404]

[14] Ichimura K, Stan RV, Kurihara H, Sakai T. Glomerular endothelial cells form diaphragms during development and pathologic conditions. J Am Soc Nephrol 2008; 19(8): 1463-71.
[http://dx.doi.org/10.1681/ASN.2007101138] [PMID: 18480313]

[15] Moffat DB, Fourman J. The vascular pattern of the rat kidney. J Anat 1963; 97(Pt 4): 543-53.
https://pmc.ncbi.nlm.nih.gov/articles/PMC1244518/
[PMID: 14064096]

[16] Lieberthal W, Fuhro R, Andry CC, *et al.* Rapamycin impairs recovery from acute renal failure: role of cell-cycle arrest and apoptosis of tubular cells. Am J Physiol Renal Physiol 2001; 281(4): F693-706.
[http://dx.doi.org/10.1152/ajprenal.2001.281.4.F693] [PMID: 11553517]

[17] Chou YH, Pan SY, Yang CH, Lin SL. Stem cells and kidney regeneration. J Formos Med Assoc 2014; 113(4): 201-9.
[http://dx.doi.org/10.1016/j.jfma.2013.12.001] [PMID: 24434243]

[18] Lin SL, Li B, Rao S, *et al.* Macrophage Wnt7b is critical for kidney repair and regeneration. Proc Natl Acad Sci USA 2010; 107(9): 4194-9.
[http://dx.doi.org/10.1073/pnas.0912228107] [PMID: 20160075]

[19] Peired AJ, Mazzinghi B, De Chiara L, *et al.* Bioengineering strategies for nephrologists: kidney was not built in a day. Expert Opin Biol Ther 2020; 20(5): 467-80.
[http://dx.doi.org/10.1080/14712598.2020.1709439] [PMID: 31971029]

[20] Higginbotham L, Mathews D, Breeden CA, *et al.* Pre-transplant antibody screening and anti-CD154 costimulation blockade promote long-term xenograft survival in a pig-to-primate kidney transplant model. Xenotransplantation 2015; 22(3): 221-30.
[http://dx.doi.org/10.1111/xen.12166] [PMID: 25847130]

[21] Naeimi Kararoudi M, Hejazi SS, Elmas E, *et al.* Clustered regularly interspaced short palindromic repeats/cas9 gene editing technique in xenotransplantation. Front Immunol 2018; 9: 1711.
[http://dx.doi.org/10.3389/fimmu.2018.01711] [PMID: 30233563]

[22] Niu D, Wei HJ, Lin L, *et al.* Inactivation of porcine endogenous retrovirus in pigs using CRISPR-Cas9. Science 2017; 357(6357): 1303-7.
[http://dx.doi.org/10.1126/science.aan4187] [PMID: 28798043]

[23] Wu J, Greely HT, Jaenisch R, Nakauchi H, Rossant J, Belmonte JCI. Stem cells and interspecies chimaeras. Nature 2016; 540(7631): 51-9.
[http://dx.doi.org/10.1038/nature20573] [PMID: 27905428]

[24]   Wu J, Platero-Luengo A, Sakurai M, *et al.* Interspecies chimerism with mammalian pluripotent stem cells. Cell 2017; 168(3): 473-486.e15.
[http://dx.doi.org/10.1016/j.cell.2016.12.036] [PMID: 28129541]

[25]   Li Z, Araoka T, Wu J, *et al.* 3D culture supports long-term expansion of mouse and human nephrogenic progenitors. Cell Stem Cell 2016; 19(4): 516-29.
[http://dx.doi.org/10.1016/j.stem.2016.07.016] [PMID: 27570066]

[26]   Yamanaka S, Saito Y, Fujimoto T, *et al.* Kidney regeneration in later-stage mouse embryos *via* transplanted renal progenitor cells. J Am Soc Nephrol 2019; 30(12): 2293-305.
[http://dx.doi.org/10.1681/ASN.2019020148] [PMID: 31548350]

[27]   Matsumoto T, Schäffers OJM, Yin W, *et al.* Renal Regeneration: Stem Cell-Based Therapies to Battle Kidney Disease. EMJ Nephrol 2019; 7: 54-64.

[28]   Hammerman MR. Transplantation of renal precursor cells: a new therapeutic approach. Pediatr Nephrol 2000; 14(6): 513-7.
[http://dx.doi.org/10.1007/s004670050805] [PMID: 10872196]

[29]   Kim SS, Gwak SJ, Han J, Park MH, Song KW, Kim BS. Regeneration of kidney tissue using *in vitro* cultured fetal kidney cells. Exp Mol Med 2008; 40(4): 361-9.
[http://dx.doi.org/10.3858/emm.2008.40.4.361] [PMID: 18779648]

[30]   Harari-Steinberg O, Metsuyanim S, Omer D, *et al.* Identification of human nephron progenitors capable of generation of kidney structures and functional repair of chronic renal disease. EMBO Mol Med 2013; 5(10): 1556-68.
[http://dx.doi.org/10.1002/emmm.201201584] [PMID: 23996934]

[31]   Pode-Shakked N, Gershon R, Tam G, *et al.* Evidence of *In Vitro* Preservation of Human Nephrogenesis at the Single-Cell Level. Stem Cell Reports 2017; 9(1): 279-91.
[http://dx.doi.org/10.1016/j.stemcr.2017.04.026] [PMID: 28552604]

[32]   Takahashi K, Tanabe K, Ohnuki M, *et al.* Induction of pluripotent stem cells from adult human fibroblasts by defined factors. Cell 2007; 131(5): 861-72.
[http://dx.doi.org/10.1016/j.cell.2007.11.019] [PMID: 18035408]

[33]   Slack JMW. Turning One Cell Type into Another. Curr Top Dev Biol 2016; 117: 339-58.
[http://dx.doi.org/10.1016/bs.ctdb.2015.11.017] [PMID: 26969988]

[34]   Kaminski MM, Tosic J, Pichler R, Arnold SJ, Lienkamp SS. Engineering kidney cells: reprogramming and directed differentiation to renal tissues. Cell Tissue Res 2017; 369(1): 185-97.
[http://dx.doi.org/10.1007/s00441-017-2629-5] [PMID: 28560692]

[35]   Lewandowski J, Kurpisz M. Techniques of Human Embryonic Stem Cell and Induced Pluripotent Stem Cell Derivation. Arch Immunol Ther Exp (Warsz) 2016; 64(5): 349-70.
[http://dx.doi.org/10.1007/s00005-016-0385-y] [PMID: 26939778]

[36]   Morizane R, Monkawa T, Itoh H. Differentiation of murine embryonic stem and induced pluripotent stem cells to renal lineage in vitro. Biochem Biophys Res Commun 2009; 390(4): 1334-9.
[http://dx.doi.org/10.1016/j.bbrc.2009.10.148] [PMID: 19883625]

[37]   Koning M, van den Berg CW, Rabelink TJ. Stem cell-derived kidney organoids: engineering the vasculature. Cell Mol Life Sci 2020; 77(12): 2257-73.
[http://dx.doi.org/10.1007/s00018-019-03401-0] [PMID: 31807815]

[38]   Paliwal S, Chaudhuri R, Agrawal A, Mohanty S. Regenerative abilities of mesenchymal stem cells through mitochondrial transfer. J Biomed Sci 2018; 25(1): 31.
[http://dx.doi.org/10.1186/s12929-018-0429-1] [PMID: 29602309]

[39]   Cho YM, Kim JH, Kim M, *et al.* Mesenchymal stem cells transfer mitochondria to the cells with virtually no mitochondrial function but not with pathogenic mtDNA mutations. PLoS One 2012; 7(3): e32778.

[http://dx.doi.org/10.1371/journal.pone.0032778] [PMID: 22412925]

[40]   Plotnikov EY, Khryapenkova TG, Galkina SI, Sukhikh GT, Zorov DB. Cytoplasm and organelle transfer between mesenchymal multipotent stromal cells and renal tubular cells in co-culture. Exp Cell Res 2010; 316(15): 2447-55.
[http://dx.doi.org/10.1016/j.yexcr.2010.06.009] [PMID: 20599955]

[41]   Dominici M, Le Blanc K, Mueller I, *et al.* Minimal criteria for defining multipotent mesenchymal stromal cells. The International Society for Cellular Therapy position statement. Cytotherapy 2006; 8(4): 315-7.
[http://dx.doi.org/10.1080/14653240600855905] [PMID: 16923606]

[42]   Bochon B, Kozubska M, Surygała G, *et al.* Mesenchymal Stem Cells—Potential Applications in Kidney Diseases. Int J Mol Sci 2019; 20(10): 2462.
[http://dx.doi.org/10.3390/ijms20102462] [PMID: 31109047]

[43]   Zhang Y, McNeill E, Tian H, *et al.* Urine derived cells are a potential source for urological tissue reconstruction. J Urol 2008; 180(5): 2226-33.
[http://dx.doi.org/10.1016/j.juro.2008.07.023] [PMID: 18804817]

[44]   Andrianova NV, Buyan MI, Zorova LD, *et al.* Kidney Cells Regeneration: Dedifferentiation of Tubular Epithelium, Resident Stem Cells and Possible Niches for Renal Progenitors. Int J Mol Sci 2019; 20(24): 6326.
[http://dx.doi.org/10.3390/ijms20246326] [PMID: 31847447]

[45]   Humes HD, Mackay SM, Funke AJ, Buffington DA. Tissue engineering of a bioartificial renal tubule assist device: *In vitro* transport and metabolic characteristics. Kidney Int 1999; 55(6): 2502-14.
[http://dx.doi.org/10.1046/j.1523-1755.1999.00486.x] [PMID: 10354300]

[46]   Westover AJ, Buffington DA, Johnston KA, Smith PL, Pino CJ, Humes HD. A bio-artificial renal epithelial cell system conveys survival advantage in a porcine model of septic shock. J Tissue Eng Regen Med 2017; 11(3): 649-57.
[http://dx.doi.org/10.1002/term.1961] [PMID: 25424193]

[47]   Song JJ, Guyette JP, Gilpin SE, Gonzalez G, Vacanti JP, Ott HC. Regeneration and experimental orthotopic transplantation of a bioengineered kidney. Nat Med 2013; 19(5): 646-51.
[http://dx.doi.org/10.1038/nm.3154] [PMID: 23584091]

[48]   Stahl EC, Bonvillain RW, Skillen CD, *et al.* Evaluation of the host immune response to decellularized lung scaffolds derived from α-Gal knockout pigs in a non-human primate model. Biomaterials 2018; 187: 93-104.
[http://dx.doi.org/10.1016/j.biomaterials.2018.09.038] [PMID: 30312852]

[49]   Mulder J, Sharmin S, Chow T, *et al.* Generation of infant- and pediatric-derived urinary induced pluripotent stem cells competent to form kidney organoids. Pediatr Res 2020; 87(4): 647-55.
[http://dx.doi.org/10.1038/s41390-019-0618-y] [PMID: 31629364]

[50]   Zhou M, Zhang X, Wen X, *et al.* Development of a Functional Glomerulus at the Organ Level on a Chip to Mimic Hypertensive Nephropathy. Sci Rep 2016; 6(1): 31771.
[http://dx.doi.org/10.1038/srep31771] [PMID: 27558173]

[51]   Petrosyan A, Cravedi P, Villani V, *et al.* A glomerulus-on-a-chip to recapitulate the human glomerular filtration barrier. Nat Commun 2019; 10(1): 3656.
[http://dx.doi.org/10.1038/s41467-019-11577-z] [PMID: 31409793]

[52]   Vernetti L, Gough A, Baetz N, *et al.* Functional Coupling of Human Microphysiology Systems: Intestine, Liver, Kidney Proximal Tubule, Blood-Brain Barrier and Skeletal Muscle. Sci Rep 2017; 7(1): 42296.
[http://dx.doi.org/10.1038/srep42296] [PMID: 28176881]

[53]   Cui X, Breitenkamp K, Finn MG, Lotz M, D'Lima DD. Direct human cartilage repair using three-dimensional bioprinting technology. Tissue Eng Part A 2012; 18(11-12): 1304-12.

[http://dx.doi.org/10.1089/ten.tea.2011.0543] [PMID: 22394017]

[54]   Higgins JW, Chambon A, Bishard K, *et al.* Bioprinted pluripotent stem cell-derived kidney organoids provide opportunities for high content screening. bioRxiv 2018; 505396.
[http://dx.doi.org/10.1101/505396]

[55]   Yang Q, Gao B, Xu F. Recent Advances in 4D Bioprinting. Biotechnol J 2020; 15(1): 1900086.
[http://dx.doi.org/10.1002/biot.201900086] [PMID: 31486199]

[56]   Little MH. Growing Kidney Tissue from Stem Cells: How Far from "Party Trick" to Medical Application? Cell Stem Cell 2016; 18(6): 695-8.
[http://dx.doi.org/10.1016/j.stem.2016.05.015] [PMID: 27257757]

CHAPTER 15

Pleiotropic Effects of Renal Disease Management: Role of SGLT2 Inhibitors

Iván Calderón-Lojero[1], Rafael Valdez-Ortiz[2] and Katy Sánchez-Pozos[1],*

[1] *Research Division, Hospital Juárez de México, Mexico City, Mexico*

[2] *Department of Nephrology, Hospital General de México, Mexico City, Mexico*

Abstract: Sodium-glucose cotransporter-2 inhibitors (SGLT2i), also called gliflozins, are a group of drugs to lower blood glucose in adults with type 2 diabetes (T2D) by inhibiting the reabsorption of glucose in the proximal tubules of the kidney and increasing glucose excretion in urine. Furthermore, some studies have demonstrated that SGLT2i increases insulin sensitivity and incretin-stimulated insulin secretion and reduces blood pressure, plasma lipids, and risk of cardiovascular events. SGLT2i have a low risk of hypoglycemia or serious events and have demonstrated other advantages. In general, SGLT2i, besides reducing glucotoxicity by decreasing glucose reabsorption in tubules, can reduce inflammation, oxidative stress, body weight, visceral adiposity, and arterial stiffness. Its beneficial effects go beyond glycemic control. Also, it is important to mention that the beneficial effects of SGLT2i are independent of ethnic origin, kidney function, doses, and age, which allows clinicians to expand their use. Furthermore, the SGLT2i provides a wide margin of safety.

Keywords: Adverse events, Beta cell, Glycemic control, Hyperglycemia, Insulin resistance, Renoprotection.

INTRODUCTION

As mentioned in previous chapters, the kidney contributes to glucose homeostasis through gluconeogenesis and renal glucose reabsorption. In this process, sodium-glucose cotransporters (SGLTs) play a crucial role. Specifically, SGLTs are responsible for the transport of glucose from the tubular lumen to epithelial cells by means of sodium electrochemical potential gradients sustained by sodium- and potassium-activated adenosine 5′-triphosphatase (Na+/K+-ATPase) [1]. There are two main isoforms of SGLT cotransporters: SGLT1 and SLGT2. SGLT1 is localized on the luminal side of the proximal tubular S1/S2 segments, while

---

*** Corresponding author Katy Sánchez Pozos:** Research Division, Hospital Juárez de México, Mexico City, Mexico;
E-mail: katypozos@gmail.com

Rafael Valdez-Ortiz, Katy Sánchez-Pozos, Ana Carolina Ariza & Enzo C. Vásquez-Jiménez (Eds.)

SGLT2 is localized on the luminal side of the proximal tubular S3 segment [2]. Specifically, SGLT2 is responsible for 90% of glucose reabsorption in proximal tubules [3].

Sodium-glucose cotransporter-2 inhibitors (SGLT2is), also called gliflozins, are a group of drugs used to lower blood glucose in adults with type 2 diabetes (T2D) by inhibiting the reabsorption of glucose in the proximal tubules of the kidney and increasing glucose excretion in the urine [4, 5]. The FDA has approved SGLT2, which includes canagliflozin, dapagliflozin, and empagliflozin. Among the benefits of SGLT2 therapeutic management are reduced insulin resistance and improved pancreatic b-cell function, cell mass, and function [6, 7]. Furthermore, some studies have demonstrated that SGLT2i increases insulin sensitivity and incretin-stimulated insulin secretion and reduces blood pressure, plasma lipids, and the risk of cardiovascular events [8, 9]. In addition, SGLT2i impacts pancreatic a-cells, increasing glucagon and gluconeogenesis [10]. Current therapies for glycemic control improve the majority of risk factors; however, CV mortality is not decreased, in addition to adverse effects such as hypoglycemia and body weight alterations. Thus, glycemic control is not enough to ameliorate cardiovascular disease [11]. SGLT2i have been proposed as a good alternative to diminish these adverse effects, although they are accompanied by other metabolic responses, such as increased lipolysis, endogenous glucose, and ketone body production [6, 12, 13]. Nevertheless, SGLT2i are associated with a low risk of hypoglycemia or serious adverse events and have other advantages, as we will see below.

CARDIOPROTECTIVE EFFECTS

Cardiovascular disease is the leading cause of mortality among patients affected with end-stage renal disease (ESRD) [14]. Eighty-seven percent of adult patients aged 45 years or older with chronic kidney disease (CKD) reported cardiovascular disease at the time of ESRD [15]. There are well-known risk factors for cardiovascular disease, such as age, smoking status, hyperglycemia, hypertension, dyslipidemia, and obesity [16]. One decade ago, several studies revealed cardioprotection in patients with diabetes treated with SGLT2i therapy. Randomized clinical trials have shown that SGLT2i therapy reduces hospitalizations for heart failure and deaths, independent of glycemic control [17 - 19]. In the phase III placebo-controlled trial, 4,744 patients with class II, III, or IV heart failure and an ejection fraction of 40% were randomly assigned to receive 10 mg/day dapagliflozin or placebo. Patients treated with dapagliflozin presented a lower risk of worsening heart failure or death from cardiovascular causes than patients who received a placebo [20]. In the DEFENCE study, dapagliflozin add-on therapy improved endothelial function compared with metformin, as assessed by the change in flow-mediated dilation.

Additionally, in the urine, the level of the biomarker of oxidative stress, 8-hydroxy-2'-deoxyguanosine, was significantly lower in the dapagliflozin group. The authors suggested that endothelial function improvement results from reduced oxidative stress [21]. The mechanisms underlying such cardioprotection are still not clear, but some theories have been proposed [22 - 24]. Another meta-analysis carried out by Yeong *et al.* showed that SGLT2i, compared with metformin and Glucagon-like peptide-1 receptor agonists (GLP1-RA) was superior in improving the left ventricular ejection fraction in diabetic patients and improving maximal oxygen consumption and serum N-terminal prohormone of brain natriuretic peptide (NT-proBNP) levels in non-diabetic patients. The investigators proposed that the benefits observed are mediated by increased hematocrit and positive effects on cardiac and renal metabolism [25, 26].

Despite numerous studies on SGLT2i effects in model animals and humans, the mechanisms involved in cardiovascular protection are still under investigation. These studies revealed that the cardioprotective effects include natriuretic, diuretic, and antihypertensive effects, as well as the regulation of plasma and interstitial fluid volume. The excretion of glucose in urine has an impact on osmotic diuresis and natriuresis, which in turn could be favorable for heart failure [17]. This latter is one of the main theories for the cardiovascular benefits of SGLT2i. The administration of SGLT2i resulted in plasma volume contraction and, in turn, volume reduction [27, 28].

Furthermore, high levels of serum uric acid have been associated with cardiovascular diseases [29, 30]. Hyperuricemia increases the risk of heart failure by 65% and 20% for every 1 mg/mL increase in serum uric acid [31]. Elevated serum uric acid levels stimulate smooth cell proliferation and release proinflammatory cytokines [32]. In addition, patients with heart failure and high levels of uric acid present impaired ventricular function, ventricular filling pressures and volumes, and limited functional capacity [33, 34]. SGLT2i reduce serum uric acid levels independently of therapy for regulating uric acid and independent of diabetes [35]. SGLT2i may influence uric acid levels through sirtuin 1 (SIRT1). As mentioned in previous chapters, sirtuins are deacetylases involved in many biological processes, including the regulation of cellular homeostasis, metabolism, inflammation, oxidative stress, and aging [36 - 39]. SIRT1 has been shown to ameliorate hyperuricemia in animal models [40 - 42]. Hence, SGLT2i promotes the activity of SIRT1, which in turn reduces oxidative stress and xanthine oxidase activity and, consequently, the formation of uric acid

[43]. Thus, restoring serum uric acid levels protects against heart failure by reducing oxidative stress and improving endothelial function [44].

Blood Pressure

One of the possible causes of hypertension in diabetes patients could be excessive sodium and water reabsorption due to the enhanced activity of SGLT. SGLT2i reduce blood pressure through the diuretic effect of glycosuria and increase sodium excretion through the inhibition of Na+ reabsorption, the latter of which is coupled to glucose transport [45]. In a model of diabetic rats fed a high-salt diet, the animals developed hyperglycemia and high blood pressure. The administration of phlorizin prevented the increase in SGLT2 RNAm and urinary glucose compared with those in rats that did not receive phlorizin. In addition, SGLT2 blockade resulted in blood pressure restoration. Thus, the authors concluded that SGLT2 inhibition prevents hyperglycemia and hypertension associated with increased SGLT2 activity [46]. In support of these findings, Li *et al.* determined the effect of SGLT2i on blood pressure in patients with heart failure in a recent systemic review and meta-analysis. The administration of SGLT2i in patients with heart failure was associated with a reduction in systolic blood pressure compared to controls [47].

Other mechanisms that contribute to hypertension in diabetes patients are increased arterial stiffness through the suppression of nitric oxide production by hyperglycemia, excess free fatty acids, and insulin resistance [48]. A post hoc analysis from a phase III trial in patients with T2D and hypertension showed that the administration of empagliflozin produced a reduction in blood pressure in participants. The findings suggest that the mechanisms involved in these improvements were related to favorable effects on markers of arterial stiffness and vascular resistance as well as on a marker of myocardial workload, preventing endothelial dysfunction [49].

PANCREATIC PROTECTIVE EFFECTS

Loss of pancreatic beta cell mass and function is a classic characteristic of diabetes [50]. Elevated concentrations of glucose during diabetes induce β-cell hyperexcitability, persistently increased intracellular calcium concentrations, and insulin hypersecretion, all of which contribute to the loss of β-cell mass [51, 52]. In addition, chronic hyperglycemia induces oxidative and endoplasmic reticulum stress, causing β-cell depletion [53]. Studies on*db/db* and *ob/ob* mouse models of hyperglycemia and obesity showed that animals treated with SGLT2i presented an increase in β-cell mass and β-cell replication and an increase in the conversion of a to β-cells, together with a decrease in β-cells [54 - 58]. In recent decades, insulin hypersecretion has been hypothesized to drive β-cell failure; however, a recent study on a model of neonatal diabetes mellitus (NMD) and SGLT2i showed that not insulin secretion but rather hyperglycemia *per se* causes β-cell malfunction. Hence, the recovery of β-cell function in animals treated with SGLT2i was mediated through a reduction in oxidative and endoplasmic reticulum stress. Interestingly, SGLT2i has been shown to prevent β-cell failure in the early stages of diabetes but not in the absence of β-cells [59]. Thus, these findings suggest that SGLT2i protect against B-cell failure by reducing oxidative stress.

In prediabetic Sprague–Dawley rats that received empagliflozin, the increase in the size of Langerhans islets was restored to the size of those in the control group. In addition, the disequilibrium in the proportions of b-cells and a-cells observed in prediabetic animals was corrected [60]. According to a study on T2D in humans, dapagliflozin may increase plasma glucagon and endogenous glucose production. Remarkably, the authors showed that the *SLC5A2* gene, which encodes SGLT2 in glucagon-secreting alpha cells, is subexpressed. In contrast, the *GCG* gene, which encodes glucagon, is overexpressed in T2D subjects compared to non-diabetic subjects. Hereafter, Bonner *et al.* proposed SGLT2 and dapagliflozin as secretagogues of alpha cells in the pancreas [10]. In contrast, a recent study by Chae *et al.* suggested that the increase in plasma glucagon induced by SGLT2i is not due to direct effects on islet cells. Therefore, an increase in plasma glucagon is secondary to insulin-independent glucose-lowering effects [61]. Thus, this latter study suggested that SGLT2is are not secretagogues of alpha cells and that their effect on glucagon production is indirect.

HEPATOPROTECTIVE EFFECTS

Non-alcoholic fatty liver disease (NAFLD) has become a worldwide health problem. The increasing prevalence of T2D has led to an increase in NAFLD incidence, and it has been calculated that up to 55% of patients affected with T2D present with NAFLD [62, 63]. To date, there is no specific therapy for NAFLD; however, some antihyperglycemic drugs, such as pioglitazone, metformin, glucagon-like peptide 1 analog drugs, and recently SGLT2i, have shown hepatoprotection effects [64 - 67].

There are various reports indicating that the SGLT1 and SGLT2 genes are expressed in the hepatic tissues of rats and mice [68 - 70]. The first studies that showed the protective effects of SGLT2i on the liver were performed in animals. Several studies have focused on liver functionality, and other studies have explored the effect of SGLT2i in the advanced stages of liver disease, which involves hepatic fibrosis and steatosis. In a study on rats fed a choline-deficient l-amino acid-defined diet, a model of liver steatosis, treatment with ipragliflozin, an SGLT2i, prevented hepatic triglyceride accumulation and the formation of large lipid droplets. Additionally, ipragliflozin decreases the fibrosis score in these animals [71]. Another study on a model of obese T2D mice (CD1 mice treated with monosodium glutamate for the first 5 days of life) showed that phlorizin administration restored insulinemia, triglyceride levels, and hepatic inflammation markers. More importantly, phlorizin ameliorated NAFLD in mice by reversing hepatic steatosis and hepatocyte ballooning [72]. Briefly, the amelioration of intracellular fatty acid, total cholesterol, and triglyceride accumulation is the result of SGLT2i regulation of lipogenesis, lipolysis, and β-oxidation in hepatocytes through the regulation of gene expression [68, 73 - 75]. Although the mechanisms underlying the hepatoprotective effects of SGLT2i have not yet been elucidated, early studies have shown that the beneficial effects of this therapy are due to its anti-inflammatory and antifibrotic properties.

Moreover, the beneficial effects of SGLT2i on liver function have been observed in humans. In the majority of studies, SGLT2i therapy has improved the serum levels of liver enzymes and hepatic steatosis [76 - 78]. In a prospective randomized, double-blind, placebo-controlled trial that evaluated the efficacy of empagliflozin in patients with NAFLD and T2D, the authors associated the administration of empagliflozin for 24 weeks with improvements in liver steatosis and fibrosis compared with patients who received pioglitazone [79]. A meta-analysis that included 12 randomized controlled trials testing the efficacy of SGLT2i for treating NAFLD during a median period of 24 weeks in 850 middle-aged overweight or obese individuals showed that treatment with SGLT2i significantly decreased the serum alanine aminotransferase and gamma-glutamyltransferase levels and the absolute percentage of liver fat content. Hence, these findings suggest that these compounds are good options for NAFLD treatment [80]. Another meta-analysis conducted to evaluate the effect of SGLT2is on T2D patients with NAFLD revealed that the administration of SGLT2is significantly decreased alanine transaminase and aspartate transaminase levels, visceral fat mass area, and subcutaneous fat area [81]. Therefore, SGLT2i, in addition to their antihyperglycemic effects, can protect the liver mainly through fatty acid utilization, as suggested by findings in animal models and clinical trials.

NEUROPROTECTIVE EFFECTS

It is well known that neurodegenerative diseases are associated with metabolic disorders, although the connection between cognitive dysfunction and metabolic disturbances has not been elucidated [82 - 85]. There are few studies on animal models that have demonstrated the neuroprotective effect of SGLT2i administration, specifically in a Parkinson's disease rat model, Alzheimer's disease, peripheral neuropathy, neuroinflammation, and cerebral ischemia/reperfusion injury murine models [86 - 90]. The proposed neuro-protective effects of SGLT2i are attributed to antioxidant, anti-inflammatory, and antiapoptotic properties [90].

Alzheimer's disease constitutes approximately two-thirds of dementia cases [91]. The main mechanism involved in Alzheimer's disease development is the accumulation of plaques built of beta-amyloid peptide and neurofibrillary tangle aggregates of tau protein, which promotes neuron and synapse loss and, consequently, a gradual decline in cognitive function [92]. Hierro-Bujalance *et al.* demonstrated that treatment with 10 mg/kg empagliflozin reduced neuronal loss, hemorrhage, and microglial burdens and that the number of senile plaques was low in a mixed murine model of Alzheimer's disease and T2D [93].

On the other hand, Parkinson's disease is characterized by the progressive loss of dopaminergic neurons, accompanied by the accumulation of cytoplasmic protein aggregates called Lewy bodies, which encompass α-synuclein protein fibrils [94]. In a rotenone-induced Parkinson's disease rat model, the administration of dapagliflozin improved motor dysfunction, reduced histopathological alterations and α-synuclein expression, and increased tyrosine hydroxylase and dopamine levels. These results were attributed to diminished lipoperoxidation, neuronal oxidative stress, and apoptosis. Interestingly, glial cell line-derived neurotrophic factor (GDNF) was increased in the same study. GDNF is a potent factor that promotes the survival and differentiation of dopaminergic neurons and is considered a protector factor for neuronal survival [86].

Diabetes has been linked to cognitive impairment and neurodegenerative diseases [95 - 98]. In this context, several investigations have focused on structural changes in diabetic *db/db mice*. These authors described ultrastructural remodeling within the neurovascular unit of cerebral cortical gray matter and transitional subcortical white matter in diabetic mice compared with non-diabetic mice [98]. One of the first studies in animals in which the administration of empagliflozin improved cognitive function and ameliorated oxidative stress in the brains of 17-week-old *db/db* mice was the study by Lin *et al.* They suggested that SGLT2i therapy could prevent the progression of macrovascular diseases and cognitive impairment in diabetes [99].

In addition, treatment of diabetic animals with dapagliflozin and empagliflozin prevented characteristic structural changes in the brain of hyperglycemic animals, as well as memory and cognition impairments; therefore, SGLT2i has neuroprotective effects on diabetic brains [100, 101].

Four studies explored the neuroprotective effects of SGLT2i in humans [102 - 105]. Two studies were performed to investigate the impact of SGLT2i on frailty [102, 104]. Frailty is a condition in older adults and is defined as a syndrome that involves functional decline, disability, and cognitive impairment [106, 107]. The administration of empagliflozin in older adults with T2D and hypertension reduced frailty, as determined by the Montreal Cognitive Assessment (MoCA) score, and the treatment also had beneficial effects on physical impairment [102, 104]. Mone *et al.* showed that these improvements were due to decreased oxidative stress in the mitochondria of endothelial cells [104]. In a recent randomized trial that included patients with T2D, the administration of dapagliflozin did not restore cognitive impairment or brain activation compared with diabetic patients who received liraglutide [105]. These findings suggest that more clinical trials evaluating the impact of SGLT2i on cognitive impairment in humans are needed to assess the neuroprotective effects of these drugs in humans in the real world.

RENOPROTECTIVE EFFECTS

Since the introduction of SGLT2i to the market, multiple studies evaluating renal function have been conducted. These reports have suggested that therapy with SGLT2i is renoprotective for both type 1 and T2D patients; in fact, these trials revealed up to a 40% reduction in the risk of progression of kidney disease. Five important trials have evaluated the renoprotective effects of SGLT2i in T2D patients: EMPA-REG OUTCOME (empagliflozin) [19]; CANVAS and CANVAS-R (canagliflozin) [18]; DECLARE-TIMI 58 (dapagliflozin) [108]; and VERTIS CV (ertugliflozin) [109]. These studies revealed that patients receiving SGLT2i had preserved kidney function, as determined by a delay in progression to macroalbuminuria and renal replacement therapy [18, 19, 108 - 110]. The first clinical trial that investigated the efficacy of SGLT2is in the CKD population was the CREDENCE trial (Canagliflozin and Renal Outcomes in Type 2 Diabetes and Nephropathy). Compared with the placebo group, the group treated with canagliflozin presented a 30% reduction in kidney failure and a lower risk of CV death and myocardial infarction or stroke [111]. After this first study, the DAPA-CKD (Dapagliflozin in Patients with Chronic Kidney Disease) trial and the EMPA-KIDNEY (Empagliflozin in Patients with Chronic Kidney Disease) appeared. Like in the CREDENCE trial, the progression and hospitalization rates decreased in these latter studies [112, 113]. In addition, the EMPA-KIDNEY trial results showed a 23% reduced risk of acute kidney injury and a 23% reduced risk of CV death or hospitalization for heart failure [113]. Briefly, these two studies showed that therapy with SGLT2i reduces the risk of worsening CKD. Additionally, the beneficial effects of SGLT2i on renal outcomes are independent of dose, as demonstrated through a systematic review and meta-analysis by Hedge *et al.* The authors included 43,434 references in this investigation, with 48,067 patients mentioning the flozin dose and eGFR as endpoints. The authors found that renoprotective efficacy was independent of dose; they suggested that low doses of SGLT2i are enough to improve kidney function [114].

A previous study by Lin *et al.* in 2019 showed that SGLT2i therapy reduced hospitalization due to acute kidney injury by more than 40% in the year after beginning treatment [115]. Furthermore, SGLT2i reduces the risk of dialysis, transplantation, or death due to kidney disease [116].

Notably, the renoprotective effect of SGLT2i is irrespective of the patient's baseline kidney function. In support of these findings, a study in Taiwan that included 13,666 matched pairs of patients receiving SGLT-2i and glucose-lowering drugs grouped into eGFR ≤ 60, $60 < $ eGFR ≤ 90, and eGFR > 90 subgroups showed that groups receiving SGLT2i independent of the eGFR decreased the eGFR in the first three months, but then this parameter improved and was maintained until the end of the study. Therefore, the use of SGLT2i was significantly associated with a reduction in the eGFR independent of the kidney function stage [117]. Hence, the decrease in the eGFR has a duration of 2-4 weeks, even in patients with CKD, after which the renal benefit of SGLT2i appears and remains stable [118]. Some authors have explained the biphasic change in the eGFR after SGLT2i treatment as a result of reduced hyperfiltration in viable nephrons. Additionally, a hemodynamic improvement through reduced reabsorption of sodium in the proximal tubule has been proposed to alleviate glomerular hypertension and hyperfiltration (Table **1**) [119, 120].

Table 1. Mechanisms proposed for the renoprotective effects of SGLT2i.

Mechanism	-	Model	References
Hemodynamic improvement	Enhanced natriuresis	Wistar rat with streptozotocin	[120]
	Decrease of glomerular hyperfiltration		
	Increase sodium delivery to distal nephron segments, leading to vasoconstriction of the afferent arterioles.		
	Reduced intraglomerular pressure and subsequent glomerular injury		
	Adenosine-dependent restoration of tubuloglomerular feedback		
	Decrease in extracellular fluid and plasma volume.		
	Decrease in proximal tubular sodium and water reabsorption.		

Mechanism	-	Model	References
Metabolic mechanisms	Attenuation of neutral lipid deposition	Diabetic mice	[133]
	Improve insulin resistance and islet damage.	Zucker diabetic fatty rats	[134]
	Facilitates lipolysis and ketogenesis	Obese mice	[135]
	Augmented β-cell glucose sensitivity and decreased tissue glucose disposal	T2D patients	[6]
Oxidative stress and inflammation	Lowering inflammatory mediators that can result in tissue injury	Report of a Scientific Workshop Sponsored by the National Kidney Foundation	[136]
	Reducing oxidative stress and workload of the proximal tubular cells	Type 1 and T2D patients	[137]
	Reduction of nitric oxide		
Decrease in serum uric acid levels.	Prevention of formation of uric acid crystals and reduction of glomerular hypertension	T2D patients and rats	[121]

Interestingly, a systemic review reported a reduction in serum uric acid levels with SGLT2i compared with placebo (Table **1**) [121]. This latter could be another important renoprotective mechanism because some studies have reported that uric acid-lowering agents abrogate increases in serum creatinine, decrease albuminuria, improve the decline in eGFR, and reduce the risk of renal failure [122 - 125]. The probable benefits of reducing serum uric acid levels are preventing the formation and adherence of uric acid crystals to renal epithelial cells and, in turn, preventing inflammation [126]. Additionally, hyperuricemia can induce arteriolopathy and glomerular hypertension in rats; hence, decreases in hyperuricemia could prevent glomerular hypertension [127, 128].

Renoprotective effects of SGLT2is have also been observed in non-diabetic kidney disease patients. Several systemic reviews and meta-analyses have demonstrated that SGLT2i reduce the urine albumin/creatinine ratio, prevent the progression to macroalbuminuria, diminish the decrease in the eGFR, increase the serum creatinine level, and increase the incidence of acute kidney injury [129 - 131].

The favorable effects of SGLT2is are not limited to one population. Forbes et al.'s study involved 34 studies across 15 countries. In this study, SGLT2i was associated with a 46% lower risk of kidney failure than other glucose-lowering drugs [132].

Several mechanisms have been proposed to explain the mentioned renoprotective effects (Table **1**).

ADVERSE EVENTS OF SGLT2I

Several adverse effects of SGLT2is have been reported, as shown in Table **2**. Despite a decrease of approximately 10% in the eGFR at the beginning of therapy with SGLT2i, specifically with empagliflozin treatment, the efficacy of empagliflozin remains, and a decrease in the eGFR does not impact the beneficial effects of empagliflozin [138]. Similar results were obtained with dapagliflozin [139].

Table 2. Adverse effects reported for SGLT2i treatment.

Adverse Effect	OR/RR (95% CI)	References
Acute drop of GFR	2.36-2.70 (2.07 - 3.00)	[138, 139]
Hypoglycemia	0.89 (0.80 - 0.98)	[141]
Euglycemic DKA	2.12 (1.49 - 3.04)	[141]
Genital Mycotic Infections	3.57 (3.14 - 4.06)	[141]
Urinary Tract Infections	2.11 (1.20 – 3.79)	[142]
Lower-Limb Amputation	1.97 (1.41 - 2.75)	[18, 141]

One of SGLT2i's beneficial effects is its low risk of hypoglycemia, in addition to protecting organs. In support of these findings, no significant hypoglycemia events were registered in large clinical randomized trials [140, 141].

CONCLUSION

In general, SGLT2i, in addition to reducing glucotoxicity by decreasing glucose reabsorption in tubules, can reduce inflammation, oxidative stress, body weight, visceral adiposity, and arterial stiffness. Its beneficial effects go beyond glycemic control. Notably, the beneficial effects of SGLT2i are independent of ethnic origin, kidney function, dose, and age, which allows clinicians to expand their use of SGLT2i. Furthermore, SGLT2i provide a wide margin of safety.

REFERENCES

[1]   DeFronzo RA, Davidson JA, Del Prato S. The role of the kidneys in glucose homeostasis: a new path towards normalizing glycaemia. Diabetes Obes Metab 2012; 14(1): 5-14.
[http://dx.doi.org/10.1111/j.1463-1326.2011.01511.x] [PMID: 21955459]

[2]   Vrhovac I, Balen Eror D, Klessen D, *et al.* Localizations of Na+-d-glucose cotransporters SGLT1 and SGLT2 in human kidney and of SGLT1 in human small intestine, liver, lung, and heart. Pflugers Arch 2015; 467(9): 1881-98.
[http://dx.doi.org/10.1007/s00424-014-1619-7] [PMID: 25304002]

[3]   Chao EC. SGLT-2 Inhibitors: A New Mechanism for Glycemic Control. Clin Diabetes 2014; 32(1): 4-11.
[http://dx.doi.org/10.2337/diaclin.32.1.4] [PMID: 26246672]

[4]   Abdul-Ghani MA, DeFronzo RA. Inhibition of renal glucose reabsorption: a novel strategy for achieving glucose control in type 2 diabetes mellitus. Endocr Pract 2008; 14(6): 782-90.
        [http://dx.doi.org/10.4158/EP.14.6.782] [PMID: 18996802]

[5]   Plosker GL. Canagliflozin: a review of its use in patients with type 2 diabetes mellitus. Drugs 2014; 74(7): 807-24.
        [http://dx.doi.org/10.1007/s40265-014-0225-5] [PMID: 24831734]

[6]   Ferrannini E, Muscelli E, Frascerra S, *et al.* Metabolic response to sodium-glucose cotransporter 2 inhibition in type 2 diabetic patients. J Clin Invest 2014; 124(2): 499-508.
        [http://dx.doi.org/10.1172/JCI72227] [PMID: 24463454]

[7]   Merovci A, Mari A, Solis C, *et al.* Dapagliflozin lowers plasma glucose concentration and improves β-cell function. J Clin Endocrinol Metab 2015; 100(5): 1927-32.
        [http://dx.doi.org/10.1210/jc.2014-3472] [PMID: 25710563]

[8]   Kaneto H, Obata A, Kimura T, *et al.* Beneficial effects of sodium–glucose cotransporter 2 inhibitors for preservation of pancreatic β-cell function and reduction of insulin resistance. J Diabetes 2017; 9(3): 219-25.
        [http://dx.doi.org/10.1111/1753-0407.12494] [PMID: 27754601]

[9]   Ahn CH, Oh TJ, Kwak SH, Cho YM. Sodium-glucose cotransporter-2 inhibition improves incretin sensitivity of pancreatic β-cells in people with type 2 diabetes. Diabetes Obes Metab 2018; 20(2): 370-7.
        [http://dx.doi.org/10.1111/dom.13081] [PMID: 28786557]

[10]   Bonner C, Kerr-Conte J, Gmyr V, *et al.* Inhibition of the glucose transporter SGLT2 with dapagliflozin in pancreatic alpha cells triggers glucagon secretion. Nat Med 2015; 21(5): 512-7.
        [http://dx.doi.org/10.1038/nm.3828] [PMID: 25894829]

[11]   Kelly TN, Bazzano LA, Fonseca VA, Thethi TK, Reynolds K, He J. Systematic review: glucose control and cardiovascular disease in type 2 diabetes. Ann Intern Med 2009; 151(6): 394-403.
        [http://dx.doi.org/10.7326/0003-4819-151-6-200909150-00137] [PMID: 19620144]

[12]   Merovci A, Solis-Herrera C, Daniele G, *et al.* Dapagliflozin improves muscle insulin sensitivity but enhances endogenous glucose production. J Clin Invest 2014; 124(2): 509-14.
        [http://dx.doi.org/10.1172/JCI70704] [PMID: 24463448]

[13]   Ferrannini E. Sodium-Glucose Co-transporters and Their Inhibition: Clinical Physiology. Cell Metab 2017; 26(1): 27-38.
        [http://dx.doi.org/10.1016/j.cmet.2017.04.011] [PMID: 28506519]

[14]   Foley RN, Parfrey PS, Sarnak MJ. Clinical epidemiology of cardiovascular disease in chronic renal disease. Am J Kidney Dis 1998; 32(5) (Suppl. 3): S112-9.
        [http://dx.doi.org/10.1053/ajkd.1998.v32.pm9820470] [PMID: 9820470]

[15]   Modi ZJ, Lu Y, Ji N, *et al.* Risk of Cardiovascular Disease and Mortality in Young Adults With End-stage Renal Disease. JAMA Cardiol 2019; 4(4): 353-62.
        [http://dx.doi.org/10.1001/jamacardio.2019.0375] [PMID: 30892557]

[16]   Mok Y, Ballew SH, Matsushita K. Chronic kidney disease measures for cardiovascular risk prediction. Atherosclerosis 2021; 335: 110-8.
        [http://dx.doi.org/10.1016/j.atherosclerosis.2021.09.007] [PMID: 34556333]

[17]   Inzucchi SE, Zinman B, Wanner C, *et al.* SGLT-2 inhibitors and cardiovascular risk: Proposed pathways and review of ongoing outcome trials. Diab Vasc Dis Res 2015; 12(2): 90-100.
        [http://dx.doi.org/10.1177/1479164114559852] [PMID: 25589482]

[18]   Neal B, Perkovic V, Mahaffey KW, *et al.* Canagliflozin and Cardiovascular and Renal Events in Type 2 Diabetes. N Engl J Med 2017; 377(7): 644-57.
        [http://dx.doi.org/10.1056/NEJMoa1611925] [PMID: 29166232]

[19]   Zinman B, Wanner C, Lachin JM, *et al.* Empagliflozin, Cardiovascular Outcomes, and Mortality in Type 2 Diabetes. N Engl J Med 2015; 373(22): 2117-28.
[http://dx.doi.org/10.1056/NEJMoa1504720] [PMID: 26378978]

[20]   McMurray JJV, Solomon SD, Inzucchi SE, *et al.* Dapagliflozin in Patients with Heart Failure and Reduced Ejection Fraction. N Engl J Med 2019; 381(21): 1995-2008.
[http://dx.doi.org/10.1056/NEJMoa1911303] [PMID: 31535829]

[21]   Shigiyama F, Kumashiro N, Miyagi M, *et al.* Effectiveness of dapagliflozin on vascular endothelial function and glycemic control in patients with early-stage type 2 diabetes mellitus: DEFENCE study. Cardiovasc Diabetol 2017; 16(1): 84.
[http://dx.doi.org/10.1186/s12933-017-0564-0] [PMID: 28683796]

[22]   Fuchs Andersen C, Omar M, Glenthøj A, *et al.* Effects of empagliflozin on erythropoiesis in heart failure: data from the Empire HF trial. Eur J Heart Fail 2023; 25(2): 226-34.
[http://dx.doi.org/10.1002/ejhf.2735] [PMID: 36377106]

[23]   Zinman B, Inzucchi SE, Lachin JM, *et al.* Rationale, design, and baseline characteristics of a randomized, placebo-controlled cardiovascular outcome trial of empagliflozin (EMPA-REG OUTCOME™). Cardiovasc Diabetol 2014; 13(1): 102.
[http://dx.doi.org/10.1186/1475-2840-13-102] [PMID: 24943000]

[24]   Hiruma S, Shigiyama F, Hisatake S, *et al.* A prospective randomized study comparing effects of empagliflozin to sitagliptin on cardiac fat accumulation, cardiac function, and cardiac metabolism in patients with early-stage type 2 diabetes: the ASSET study. Cardiovasc Diabetol 2021; 20(1): 32.
[http://dx.doi.org/10.1186/s12933-021-01228-3] [PMID: 33530982]

[25]   Yeong T, Mai AS, Lim OZH, *et al.* Can glucose-lowering medications improve outcomes in non-diabetic heart failure patients? A Bayesian network meta-analysis. ESC Heart Fail 2022; 9(2): 1338-50.
[http://dx.doi.org/10.1002/ehf2.13822] [PMID: 35092176]

[26]   Inzucchi SE, Zinman B, Fitchett D, *et al.* How Does Empagliflozin Reduce Cardiovascular Mortality? Insights From a Mediation Analysis of the EMPA-REG OUTCOME Trial. Diabetes Care 2018; 41(2): 356-63.
[http://dx.doi.org/10.2337/dc17-1096] [PMID: 29203583]

[27]   Heise T, Jordan J, Wanner C, *et al.* Pharmacodynamic Effects of Single and Multiple Doses of Empagliflozin in Patients With Type 2 Diabetes. Clin Ther 2016; 38(10): 2265-76.
[http://dx.doi.org/10.1016/j.clinthera.2016.09.001] [PMID: 27692976]

[28]   Rajasekeran H, Lytvyn Y, Cherney DZI. Sodium–glucose cotransporter 2 inhibition and cardiovascular risk reduction in patients with type 2 diabetes: the emerging role of natriuresis. Kidney Int 2016; 89(3): 524-6.
[http://dx.doi.org/10.1016/j.kint.2015.12.038] [PMID: 26880444]

[29]   Wang X, Hou Y, Wang X, *et al.* Relationship between serum uric acid levels and different types of atrial fibrillation: An updated meta-analysis. Nutr Metab Cardiovasc Dis 2021; 31(10): 2756-65.
[http://dx.doi.org/10.1016/j.numecd.2021.05.034] [PMID: 34348878]

[30]   Deng X, Yi H, Xiao J, *et al.* Serum uric acid: A risk factor for right ventricular dysfunction and prognosis in heart failure with preserved ejection fraction. Front Endocrinol (Lausanne) 2023; 14: 1143458.
[http://dx.doi.org/10.3389/fendo.2023.1143458] [PMID: 36950688]

[31]   Huang H, Huang B, Li Y, *et al.* Uric acid and risk of heart failure: a systematic review and meta-analysis. Eur J Heart Fail 2014; 16(1): 15-24.
[http://dx.doi.org/10.1093/eurjhf/hft132] [PMID: 23933579]

[32]   Bjornstad P, Lanaspa MA, Ishimoto T, *et al.* Fructose and uric acid in diabetic nephropathy. Diabetologia 2015; 58(9): 1993-2002.

[http://dx.doi.org/10.1007/s00125-015-3650-4] [PMID: 26049401]

[33]   Oki Y, Kawai M, Minai K, *et al.* High Serum Uric Acid is Highly Associated with a Reduced Left Ventricular Ejection Fraction Rather than Increased Plasma B-type Natriuretic Peptide in Patients with Cardiovascular Diseases. Sci Rep 2019; 9(1): 682.
[http://dx.doi.org/10.1038/s41598-018-37053-0] [PMID: 30679647]

[34]   Sakai H, Tsutamoto T, Tsutsui T, Tanaka T, Ishikawa C, Horie M. Serum level of uric acid, partly secreted from the failing heart, is a prognostic marker in patients with congestive heart failure. Circ J 2006; 70(8): 1006-11.
[http://dx.doi.org/10.1253/circj.70.1006] [PMID: 16864933]

[35]   Zhao Y, Xu L, Tian D, *et al.* Effects of sodium-glucose co-transporter 2 (SGLT2) inhibitors on serum uric acid level: A meta-analysis of randomized controlled trials. Diabetes Obes Metab 2018; 20(2): 458-62.
[http://dx.doi.org/10.1111/dom.13101] [PMID: 28846182]

[36]   Houtkooper RH, Pirinen E, Auwerx J. Sirtuins as regulators of metabolism and healthspan. Nat Rev Mol Cell Biol 2012; 13(4): 225-38.
[http://dx.doi.org/10.1038/nrm3293] [PMID: 22395773]

[37]   Haigis MC, Sinclair DA. Mammalian sirtuins: biological insights and disease relevance. Annu Rev Pathol 2010; 5(1): 253-95.
[http://dx.doi.org/10.1146/annurev.pathol.4.110807.092250] [PMID: 20078221]

[38]   Santos L, Escande C, Denicola A. Potential Modulation of Sirtuins by Oxidative Stress. Oxid Med Cell Longev 2016; 2016(1): 9831825.
[http://dx.doi.org/10.1155/2016/9831825] [PMID: 26788256]

[39]   Sack MN, Finkel T. Mitochondrial metabolism, sirtuins, and aging. Cold Spring Harb Perspect Biol 2012; 4(12): a013102.
[http://dx.doi.org/10.1101/cshperspect.a013102] [PMID: 23209156]

[40]   Wang J, Zhu XX, Liu L, Xue Y, Yang X, Zou HJ. SIRT1 prevents hyperuricemia *via* the PGC-1α/PPARγ-ABCG2 pathway. Endocrine 2016; 53(2): 443-52.
[http://dx.doi.org/10.1007/s12020-016-0896-7] [PMID: 27022940]

[41]   Lu C, Zhao H, Liu Y, *et al.* Novel Role of the SIRT1 in Endocrine and Metabolic Diseases. Int J Biol Sci 2023; 19(2): 484-501.
[http://dx.doi.org/10.7150/ijbs.78654] [PMID: 36632457]

[42]   Chen H, Zheng S, Wang Y, *et al.* The effect of resveratrol on the recurrent attacks of gouty arthritis. Clin Rheumatol 2016; 35(5): 1189-95.
[http://dx.doi.org/10.1007/s10067-014-2836-3] [PMID: 25451618]

[43]   Huang XF, Li HQ, Shi L, Xue JY, Ruan BF, Zhu HL. Synthesis of resveratrol analogues, and evaluation of their cytotoxic and xanthine oxidase inhibitory activities. Chem Biodivers 2008; 5(4): 636-42.
[http://dx.doi.org/10.1002/cbdv.200890059] [PMID: 18421756]

[44]   Packer M. Uric Acid Is a Biomarker of Oxidative Stress in the Failing Heart: Lessons Learned from Trials With Allopurinol and SGLT2 Inhibitors. J Card Fail 2020; 26(11): 977-84.
[http://dx.doi.org/10.1016/j.cardfail.2020.08.015] [PMID: 32890737]

[45]   Ferrannini E, Solini A. SGLT2 inhibition in diabetes mellitus: rationale and clinical prospects. Nat Rev Endocrinol 2012; 8(8): 495-502.
[http://dx.doi.org/10.1038/nrendo.2011.243] [PMID: 22310849]

[46]   Osorio H, Bautista R, Rios A, *et al.* Effect of phlorizin on SGLT2 expression in the kidney of diabetic rats. J Nephrol 2010; 23(5): 541-6. https://pubmed.ncbi.nlm.nih.gov/20349407/
[PMID: 20349407]

[47]   Li M, Yi T, Fan F, *et al.* Effect of sodium-glucose cotransporter-2 inhibitors on blood pressure in

patients with heart failure: a systematic review and meta-analysis. Cardiovasc Diabetol 2022; 21(1): 139.
[http://dx.doi.org/10.1186/s12933-022-01574-w] [PMID: 35879763]

[48]   Lastra G, Syed S, Kurukulasuriya LR, Manrique C, Sowers JR. Type 2 diabetes mellitus and hypertension: an update. Endocrinol Metab Clin North Am 2014; 43(1): 103-22.
[http://dx.doi.org/10.1016/j.ecl.2013.09.005] [PMID: 24582094]

[49]   Chilton R, Tikkanen I, Cannon CP, *et al.* Effects of empagliflozin on blood pressure and markers of arterial stiffness and vascular resistance in patients with type 2 diabetes. Diabetes Obes Metab 2015; 17(12): 1180-93.
[http://dx.doi.org/10.1111/dom.12572] [PMID: 26343814]

[50]   Cnop M, Welsh N, Jonas JC, Jörns A, Lenzen S, Eizirik DL. Mechanisms of pancreatic beta-cell death in type 1 and type 2 diabetes: many differences, few similarities. Diabetes 2005; 54 (Suppl. 2): S97-S107.
[http://dx.doi.org/10.2337/diabetes.54.suppl_2.S97] [PMID: 16306347]

[51]   Syeda K, Mohammed AM, Arora DK, Kowluru A. Glucotoxic conditions induce endoplasmic reticulum stress to cause caspase 3 mediated lamin B degradation in pancreatic β-cells: Protection by nifedipine. Biochem Pharmacol 2013; 86(9): 1338-46.
[http://dx.doi.org/10.1016/j.bcp.2013.08.023] [PMID: 23994168]

[52]   Rorsman P, Ashcroft FM. Pancreatic β-Cell Electrical Activity and Insulin Secretion: Of Mice and Men. Physiol Rev 2018; 98(1): 117-214.
[http://dx.doi.org/10.1152/physrev.00008.2017] [PMID: 29212789]

[53]   Chan JY, Luzuriaga J, Maxwell EL, West PK, Bensellam M, Laybutt DR. The balance between adaptive and apoptotic unfolded protein responses regulates β-cell death under ER stress conditions through XBP1, CHOP and JNK. Mol Cell Endocrinol 2015; 413: 189-201.
[http://dx.doi.org/10.1016/j.mce.2015.06.025] [PMID: 26135354]

[54]   Kimura T, Obata A, Shimoda M, *et al.* Protective effects of the SGLT2 inhibitor luseogliflozin on pancreatic β-cells in *db/db* mice: The earlier and longer, the better. Diabetes Obes Metab 2018; 20(10): 2442-57.
[http://dx.doi.org/10.1111/dom.13400] [PMID: 29873444]

[55]   Takahashi K, Nakamura A, Miyoshi H, *et al.* Effect of the sodium–glucose cotransporter 2 inhibitor luseogliflozin on pancreatic beta cell mass in db/db mice of different ages. Sci Rep 2018; 8(1): 6864.
[http://dx.doi.org/10.1038/s41598-018-25126-z] [PMID: 29717223]

[56]   Kanno A, Asahara S, Kawamura M, *et al.* Early administration of dapagliflozin preserves pancreatic β-cell mass through a legacy effect in a mouse model of type 2 diabetes. J Diabetes Investig 2019; 10(3): 577-90.
[http://dx.doi.org/10.1111/jdi.12945] [PMID: 30290061]

[57]   Wei R, Cui X, Feng J, *et al.* Dapagliflozin promotes beta cell regeneration by inducing pancreatic endocrine cell phenotype conversion in type 2 diabetic mice. Metabolism 2020; 111: 154324.
[http://dx.doi.org/10.1016/j.metabol.2020.154324] [PMID: 32712220]

[58]   Jurczak MJ, Saini S, Ioja S, *et al.* SGLT2 knockout prevents hyperglycemia and is associated with reduced pancreatic β-cell death in genetically obese mice. Islets 2018; 10(5): 181-9.
[http://dx.doi.org/10.1080/19382014.2018.1503027] [PMID: 30118626]

[59]   Shyr ZA, Yan Z, Ustione A, Egan EM, Remedi MS. SGLT2 inhibitors therapy protects glucotoxicity-induced β-cell failure in a mouse model of human KATP-induced diabetes through mitigation of oxidative and ER stress. PLoS One 2022; 17(2): e0258054.
[http://dx.doi.org/10.1371/journal.pone.0258054] [PMID: 35180212]

[60]   Abdel-Hamid AAM, Firgany AEDL. Modulatory effect of empagliflozin on cellular parameters of endocrine pancreas in experimental pre-diabetes. Ann Anat 2019; 224: 153-60.
[http://dx.doi.org/10.1016/j.aanat.2019.05.002] [PMID: 31108190]

[61]   Chae H, Augustin R, Gatineau E, *et al.* SGLT2 is not expressed in pancreatic α- and β-cells, and its inhibition does not directly affect glucagon and insulin secretion in rodents and humans. Mol Metab 2020; 42: 101071.
[http://dx.doi.org/10.1016/j.molmet.2020.101071] [PMID: 32896668]

[62]   Younossi ZM, Koenig AB, Abdelatif D, Fazel Y, Henry L, Wymer M. Global epidemiology of nonalcoholic fatty liver disease—Meta-analytic assessment of prevalence, incidence, and outcomes. Hepatology 2016; 64(1): 73-84.
[http://dx.doi.org/10.1002/hep.28431] [PMID: 26707365]

[63]   Younossi ZM, Golabi P, de Avila L, *et al.* The global epidemiology of NAFLD and NASH in patients with type 2 diabetes: A systematic review and meta-analysis. J Hepatol 2019; 71(4): 793-801.
[http://dx.doi.org/10.1016/j.jhep.2019.06.021] [PMID: 31279902]

[64]   Handzlik G, Holecki M, Kozaczka J, *et al.* Evaluation of metformin therapy using controlled attenuation parameter and transient elastography in patients with non-alcoholic fatty liver disease. Pharmacol Rep 2019; 71(2): 183-8.
[http://dx.doi.org/10.1016/j.pharep.2018.10.013] [PMID: 30780126]

[65]   Kamolvisit S, Chirnaksorn S, Nimitphong H, Sungkanuparph S. Pioglitazone for the Treatment of Metabolic-Associated Fatty Liver Disease in People Living With HIV and Prediabetes. Cureus 2021; 13(10): e19046.
[http://dx.doi.org/10.7759/cureus.19046] [PMID: 34858740]

[66]   Dwinata M, Putera D, Hasan I, Raharjo M. SGLT2 inhibitors for improving hepatic fibrosis and steatosis in non-alcoholic fatty liver disease complicated with type 2 diabetes mellitus: a systematic review. Clin Exp Hepatol 2020; 6(4): 339-46.
[http://dx.doi.org/10.5114/ceh.2020.102173] [PMID: 33511282]

[67]   Mantovani A, Byrne CD, Targher G. Efficacy of peroxisome proliferator-activated receptor agonists, glucagon-like peptide-1 receptor agonists, or sodium-glucose cotransporter-2 inhibitors for treatment of non-alcoholic fatty liver disease: a systematic review. Lancet Gastroenterol Hepatol 2022; 7(4): 367-78.
[http://dx.doi.org/10.1016/S2468-1253(21)00261-2] [PMID: 35030323]

[68]   Nasiri-Ansari N, Nikolopoulou C, Papoutsi K, *et al.* Empagliflozin Attenuates Non-Alcoholic Fatty Liver Disease (NAFLD) in High Fat Diet Fed ApoE$^{(-/-)}$ Mice by Activating Autophagy and Reducing ER Stress and Apoptosis. Int J Mol Sci 2021; 22(2): 818.
[http://dx.doi.org/10.3390/ijms22020818] [PMID: 33467546]

[69]   Jojima T, Wakamatsu S, Kase M, *et al.* The SGLT2 Inhibitor Canagliflozin Prevents Carcinogenesis in a Mouse Model of Diabetes and Non-Alcoholic Steatohepatitis-Related Hepatocarcinogenesis: Association with SGLT2 Expression in Hepatocellular Carcinoma. Int J Mol Sci 2019; 20(20): 5237.
[http://dx.doi.org/10.3390/ijms20205237] [PMID: 31652578]

[70]   Li L, Li Q, Huang W, *et al.* Dapagliflozin Alleviates Hepatic Steatosis by Restoring Autophagy *via* the AMPK-mTOR Pathway. Front Pharmacol 2021; 12: 589273.
[http://dx.doi.org/10.3389/fphar.2021.589273] [PMID: 34093169]

[71]   Hayashizaki-Someya Y, Kurosaki E, Takasu T, *et al.* Ipragliflozin, an SGLT2 inhibitor, exhibits a prophylactic effect on hepatic steatosis and fibrosis induced by choline-deficient l-amino acid-defined diet in rats. Eur J Pharmacol 2015; 754: 19-24.
[http://dx.doi.org/10.1016/j.ejphar.2015.02.009] [PMID: 25701721]

[72]   David-Silva A, Esteves JV, Morais MRPT, *et al.* Dual SGLT1/SGLT2 Inhibitor Phlorizin Ameliorates Non-Alcoholic Fatty Liver Disease and Hepatic Glucose Production in Type 2 Diabetic Mice. Diabetes Metab Syndr Obes 2020; 13: 739-51.
[http://dx.doi.org/10.2147/DMSO.S242282] [PMID: 32231437]

[73]   Petito-da-Silva TI, Souza-Mello V, Barbosa-da-Silva S. Empaglifozin mitigates NAFLD in high-fa--fed mice by alleviating insulin resistance, lipogenesis and ER stress. Mol Cell Endocrinol 2019; 498:

110539.
[http://dx.doi.org/10.1016/j.mce.2019.110539] [PMID: 31419466]

[74]   Hüttl M, Markova I, Miklankova D, *et al.* In a Prediabetic Model, Empagliflozin Improves Hepatic Lipid Metabolism Independently of Obesity and before Onset of Hyperglycemia. Int J Mol Sci 2021; 22(21): 11513.
[http://dx.doi.org/10.3390/ijms222111513] [PMID: 34768942]

[75]   Luo J, Sun P, Wang Y, *et al.* Dapagliflozin attenuates steatosis in livers of high-fat diet-induced mice and oleic acid-treated L02 cells *via* regulating AMPK/mTOR pathway. Eur J Pharmacol 2021; 907: 174304.
[http://dx.doi.org/10.1016/j.ejphar.2021.174304] [PMID: 34224699]

[76]   Sinha B, Datta D, Ghosal S. Meta-analysis of the effects of sodium glucose cotransporter 2 inhibitors in non-alcoholic fatty liver disease patients with type 2 diabetes. JGH Open 2021; 5(2): 219-27.
[http://dx.doi.org/10.1002/jgh3.12473] [PMID: 33553659]

[77]   Mo M, Huang Z, Liang Y, Liao Y, Xia N. The safety and efficacy evaluation of sodium-glucose co-transporter 2 inhibitors for patients with non-alcoholic fatty liver disease: An updated meta-analysis. Dig Liver Dis 2022; 54(4): 461-8.
[http://dx.doi.org/10.1016/j.dld.2021.08.017] [PMID: 34507895]

[78]   Wong C, Yaow CYL, Ng CH, *et al.* Sodium-Glucose Co-Transporter 2 Inhibitors for Non-Alcoholic Fatty Liver Disease in Asian Patients With Type 2 Diabetes: A Meta-Analysis. Front Endocrinol (Lausanne) 2021; 11: 609135.
[http://dx.doi.org/10.3389/fendo.2020.609135] [PMID: 33643221]

[79]   Chehrehgosha H, Sohrabi MR, Ismail-Beigi F, *et al.* Empagliflozin Improves Liver Steatosis and Fibrosis in Patients with Non-Alcoholic Fatty Liver Disease and Type 2 Diabetes: A Randomized, Double-Blind, Placebo-Controlled Clinical Trial. Diabetes Ther 2021; 12(3): 843-61.
[http://dx.doi.org/10.1007/s13300-021-01011-3] [PMID: 33586120]

[80]   Mantovani A, Petracca G, Csermely A, Beatrice G, Targher G. Sodium-Glucose Cotransporter-2 Inhibitors for Treatment of Nonalcoholic Fatty Liver Disease: A Meta-Analysis of Randomized Controlled Trials. Metabolites 2020; 11(1): 22.
[http://dx.doi.org/10.3390/metabo11010022] [PMID: 33396949]

[81]   Wei Q, Xu X, Guo L, Li J, Li L. Effect of SGLT2 Inhibitors on Type 2 Diabetes Mellitus With Non-Alcoholic Fatty Liver Disease: A Meta-Analysis of Randomized Controlled Trials. Front Endocrinol (Lausanne) 2021; 12: 635556.
[http://dx.doi.org/10.3389/fendo.2021.635556] [PMID: 34220701]

[82]   Li Y, Shang S, Fei Y, *et al.* Interactive relations of type 2 diabetes and abdominal obesity to cognitive impairment: A cross-sectional study in rural area of Xi'an in China. J Diabetes Complications 2018; 32(1): 48-55.
[http://dx.doi.org/10.1016/j.jdiacomp.2017.09.006] [PMID: 29056468]

[83]   Sánchez-Alegría K, Arias C. Functional consequences of brain exposure to saturated fatty acids: From energy metabolism and insulin resistance to neuronal damage. Endocrinol Diabetes Metab 2023; 6(1): e386.
[http://dx.doi.org/10.1002/edm2.386] [PMID: 36321333]

[84]   Ghetti S, Kuppermann N, Rewers A, *et al.* Cognitive function following diabetic ketoacidosis in young children with type 1 diabetes. Endocrinol Diabetes Metab 2023; 6(3): e412.
[http://dx.doi.org/10.1002/edm2.412] [PMID: 36788736]

[85]   Biessels GJ, Despa F. Cognitive decline and dementia in diabetes mellitus: mechanisms and clinical implications. Nat Rev Endocrinol 2018; 14(10): 591-604.
[http://dx.doi.org/10.1038/s41574-018-0048-7] [PMID: 30022099]

[86]   Arab HH, Safar MM, Shahin NN. Targeting ROS-Dependent AKT/GSK-3β/NF-κB and DJ-1/Nrf2 Pathways by Dapagliflozin Attenuates Neuronal Injury and Motor Dysfunction in Rotenone-Induced

Parkinson's Disease Rat Model. ACS Chem Neurosci 2021; 12(4): 689-703.
[http://dx.doi.org/10.1021/acschemneuro.0c00722] [PMID: 33543924]

[87] Heimke M, Lenz F, Rickert U, Lucius R, Cossais F. Anti-Inflammatory Properties of the SGLT2 Inhibitor Empagliflozin in Activated Primary Microglia. Cells 2022; 11(19): 3107.
[http://dx.doi.org/10.3390/cells11193107] [PMID: 36231069]

[88] Ibrahim WW, Kamel AS, Wahid A, Abdelkader NF. Dapagliflozin as an autophagic enhancer *via* LKB1/AMPK/SIRT1 pathway in ovariectomized/d-galactose Alzheimer's rat model. Inflammopharmacology 2022; 30(6): 2505-20.
[http://dx.doi.org/10.1007/s10787-022-00973-5] [PMID: 35364737]

[89] Abdelsameea AA, Kabil SL. Mitigation of cisplatin-induced peripheral neuropathy by canagliflozin in rats. Naunyn Schmiedebergs Arch Pharmacol 2018; 391(9): 945-52.
[http://dx.doi.org/10.1007/s00210-018-1521-5] [PMID: 29862426]

[90] Amin EF, Rifaai RA, Abdel-latif RG. Empagliflozin attenuates transient cerebral ischemia/reperfusion injury in hyperglycemic rats *via* repressing oxidative–inflammatory–apoptotic pathway. Fundam Clin Pharmacol 2020; 34(5): 548-58.
[http://dx.doi.org/10.1111/fcp.12548] [PMID: 32068294]

[91] Kumar A, Sidhu J, Goyal A, *et al.* Alzheimer Disease 2023. https://pubmed.ncbi.nlm.nih.gov/29763097/

[92] Murphy MP, LeVine H III. Alzheimer's disease and the amyloid-beta peptide. J Alzheimers Dis 2010; 19(1): 311-23.
[http://dx.doi.org/10.3233/JAD-2010-1221] [PMID: 20061647]

[93] Hierro-Bujalance C, Infante-Garcia C, del Marco A, *et al.* Empagliflozin reduces vascular damage and cognitive impairment in a mixed murine model of Alzheimer's disease and type 2 diabetes. Alzheimers Res Ther 2020; 12(1): 40.
[http://dx.doi.org/10.1186/s13195-020-00607-4] [PMID: 32264944]

[94] Schneider SA, Obeso JA. Clinical and pathological features of Parkinson's disease. Curr Top Behav Neurosci 2014; 22: 205-20.
[http://dx.doi.org/10.1007/7854_2014_317] [PMID: 24850081]

[95] Hayden MR, Banks WA, Shah GN, Gu Z, Sowers JR. Cardiorenal metabolic syndrome and diabetic cognopathy. Cardiorenal Med 2013; 3(4): 265-82.
[http://dx.doi.org/10.1159/000357113] [PMID: 24474955]

[96] Ott A, Stolk RP, van Harskamp F, Pols HAP, Hofman A, Breteler MMB. Diabetes mellitus and the risk of dementia. Neurology 1999; 53(9): 1937-42.
[http://dx.doi.org/10.1212/WNL.53.9.1937] [PMID: 10599761]

[97] Leibson CL, Rocca WA, Hanson VA, *et al.* Risk of dementia among persons with diabetes mellitus: a population-based cohort study. Am J Epidemiol 1997; 145(4): 301-8.
[http://dx.doi.org/10.1093/oxfordjournals.aje.a009106] [PMID: 9054233]

[98] Hayden M, Grant D, Aroor A, DeMarco V. Ultrastructural Remodeling of the Neurovascular Unit in the Female Diabetic db/db Model—Part III: Oligodendrocyte and Myelin. Neuroglia 2018; 1(2): 351-64.
[http://dx.doi.org/10.3390/neuroglia1020024]

[99] Lin B, Koibuchi N, Hasegawa Y, *et al.* Glycemic control with empagliflozin, a novel selective SGLT2 inhibitor, ameliorates cardiovascular injury and cognitive dysfunction in obese and type 2 diabetic mice. Cardiovasc Diabetol 2014; 13(1): 148.
[http://dx.doi.org/10.1186/s12933-014-0148-1] [PMID: 25344694]

[100] Hayden M, Grant D, Aroor A, DeMarco V. Empagliflozin Ameliorates Type 2 Diabetes-Induced Ultrastructural Remodeling of the Neurovascular Unit and Neuroglia in the Female *db/db* Mouse. Brain Sci 2019; 9(3): 57.

[http://dx.doi.org/10.3390/brainsci9030057] [PMID: 30866531]

[101] El-Safty H, Ismail A, Abdelsalam RM, El-Sahar AE, Saad MA. Dapagliflozin diminishes memory and cognition impairment in Streptozotocin induced diabetes through its effect on Wnt/β-Catenin and CREB pathway. Brain Res Bull 2022; 181: 109-20.
[http://dx.doi.org/10.1016/j.brainresbull.2022.01.017] [PMID: 35093471]

[102] Mone P, Lombardi A, Gambardella J, *et al.* Empagliflozin Improves Cognitive Impairment in Frail Older Adults With Type 2 Diabetes and Heart Failure With Preserved Ejection Fraction. Diabetes Care 2022; 45(5): 1247-51.
[http://dx.doi.org/10.2337/dc21-2434] [PMID: 35287171]

[103] Bhanu C, Nimmons D, Petersen I, *et al.* Drug-induced orthostatic hypotension: A systematic review and meta-analysis of randomised controlled trials. PLoS Med 2021; 18(11): e1003821.
[http://dx.doi.org/10.1371/journal.pmed.1003821] [PMID: 34752479]

[104] Mone P, Varzideh F, Jankauskas SS, et al. SGLT2 Inhibition via Empagliflozin Improves Endothelial Function and Reduces Mitochondrial Oxidative Stress: Insights From Frail Hypertensive and Diabetic Patients. Hypertension (Dallas, Tex : 1979) 2022; 79: 1633–1643.
[http://dx.doi.org/10.1161/HYPERTENSIONAHA.122.19586]

[105] Cheng H, Zhang Z, Zhang B, *et al.* Enhancement of Impaired Olfactory Neural Activation and Cognitive Capacity by Liraglutide, but Not Dapagliflozin or Acarbose, in Patients With Type 2 Diabetes: A 16-Week Randomized Parallel Comparative Study. Diabetes Care 2022; 45(5): 1201-10.
[http://dx.doi.org/10.2337/dc21-2064] [PMID: 35263425]

[106] Xue QL. The frailty syndrome: definition and natural history. Clin Geriatr Med 2011; 27(1): 1-15.
[http://dx.doi.org/10.1016/j.cger.2010.08.009] [PMID: 21093718]

[107] Satake S, Arai H. Chapter 1 Frailty: Definition, diagnosis, epidemiology. Geriatr Gerontol Int 2020; 20(S1) (Suppl. 1): 7-13.
[http://dx.doi.org/10.1111/ggi.13830] [PMID: 32050303]

[108] Wiviott SD, Raz I, Bonaca MP, *et al.* Dapagliflozin and Cardiovascular Outcomes in Type 2 Diabetes. N Engl J Med 2019; 380(4): 347-57.
[http://dx.doi.org/10.1056/NEJMoa1812389] [PMID: 30415602]

[109] Cannon CP, Pratley R, Dagogo-Jack S, *et al.* Cardiovascular Outcomes with Ertugliflozin in Type 2 Diabetes. N Engl J Med 2020; 383(15): 1425-35.
[http://dx.doi.org/10.1056/NEJMoa2004967] [PMID: 32966714]

[110] Wanner C, Inzucchi SE, Lachin JM, *et al.* Empagliflozin and Progression of Kidney Disease in Type 2 Diabetes. N Engl J Med 2016; 375(4): 323-34.
[http://dx.doi.org/10.1056/NEJMoa1515920] [PMID: 27806236]

[111] Perkovic V, Jardine MJ, Neal B, *et al.* Canagliflozin and Renal Outcomes in Type 2 Diabetes and Nephropathy. N Engl J Med 2019; 380(24): 2295-306.
[http://dx.doi.org/10.1056/NEJMoa1811744] [PMID: 30990260]

[112] Heerspink HJL, Stefánsson BV, Correa-Rotter R, *et al.* Dapagliflozin in Patients with Chronic Kidney Disease. N Engl J Med 2020; 383(15): 1436-46.
[http://dx.doi.org/10.1056/NEJMoa2024816] [PMID: 32970396]

[113] Herrington WG, Wanner C, Green JB, *et al.* Design, recruitment, and baseline characteristics of the EMPA-KIDNEY trial. Nephrol Dial Transplant 2022; 37(7): 1317-29.
[http://dx.doi.org/10.1093/ndt/gfac040] [PMID: 35238940]

[114] Hegde NC, Kumar A, Patil AN, *et al.* Dose-dependent renoprotection efficacy of sglt2 inhibitors in type 2 diabetes: systematic review and network meta-analysis. Acta Diabetol 2023; 60(10): 1311-31.
[http://dx.doi.org/10.1007/s00592-023-02126-8] [PMID: 37322184]

[115] Lin YH, Huang YY, Hsieh SH, Sun JH, Chen ST, Lin CH. Renal and Glucose-Lowering Effects of Empagliflozin and Dapagliflozin in Different Chronic Kidney Disease Stages. Front Endocrinol

(Lausanne) 2019; 10: 820.
[http://dx.doi.org/10.3389/fendo.2019.00820] [PMID: 31824432]

[116]   Neuen BL, Young T, Heerspink HJL, *et al.* SGLT2 inhibitors for the prevention of kidney failure in patients with type 2 diabetes: a systematic review and meta-analysis. Lancet Diabetes Endocrinol 2019; 7(11): 845-54.
[http://dx.doi.org/10.1016/S2213-8587(19)30256-6] [PMID: 31495651]

[117]   Lin FJ, Wang CC, Hsu CN, Yang CY, Wang CY, Ou HT. Renoprotective effect of SGLT-2 inhibitors among type 2 diabetes patients with different baseline kidney function: a multi-center study. Cardiovasc Diabetol 2021; 20(1): 203.
[http://dx.doi.org/10.1186/s12933-021-01396-2] [PMID: 34620182]

[118]   Duo Y, Gao J, Yuan T, Zhao W. Effect of sodium-glucose cotransporter 2 inhibitors on the rate of decline in kidney function: A systematic review and meta-analysis. J Diabetes 2023; 15(1): 58-70.
[http://dx.doi.org/10.1111/1753-0407.13348] [PMID: 36610036]

[119]   De Nicola L, Gabbai FB, Garofalo C, Conte G, Minutolo R. Nephroprotection by SGLT2 Inhibition: Back to the Future? J Clin Med 2020; 9(7): 2243.
[http://dx.doi.org/10.3390/jcm9072243] [PMID: 32679744]

[120]   Thomson SC, Rieg T, Miracle C, *et al.* Acute and chronic effects of SGLT2 blockade on glomerular and tubular function in the early diabetic rat. Am J Physiol Regul Integr Comp Physiol 2012; 302(1): R75-83.
[http://dx.doi.org/10.1152/ajpregu.00357.2011] [PMID: 21940401]

[121]   Xin Y, Guo Y, Li Y, Ma Y, Li L, Jiang H. Effects of sodium glucose cotransporter-2 inhibitors on serum uric acid in type 2 diabetes mellitus: A systematic review with an indirect comparison meta-analysis. Saudi J Biol Sci 2019; 26(2): 421-6.
[http://dx.doi.org/10.1016/j.sjbs.2018.11.013] [PMID: 31485187]

[122]   Bose B, Badve SV, Hiremath SS, *et al.* Effects of uric acid-lowering therapy on renal outcomes: a systematic review and meta-analysis. Nephrol Dial Transplant 2014; 29(2): 406-13.
[http://dx.doi.org/10.1093/ndt/gft378] [PMID: 24042021]

[123]   Kim S, Kim HJ, Ahn HS, *et al.* Renoprotective effects of febuxostat compared with allopurinol in patients with hyperuricemia: A systematic review and meta-analysis. Kidney Res Clin Pract 2017; 36(3): 274-81.
[http://dx.doi.org/10.23876/j.krcp.2017.36.3.274] [PMID: 28904879]

[124]   Su X, Xu B, Yan B, Qiao X, Wang L. Effects of uric acid-lowering therapy in patients with chronic kidney disease: A meta-analysis. PLoS One 2017; 12(11): e0187550.
[http://dx.doi.org/10.1371/journal.pone.0187550] [PMID: 29095953]

[125]   Wada T, Hosoya T, Honda D, *et al.* Uric acid-lowering and renoprotective effects of topiroxostat, a selective xanthine oxidoreductase inhibitor, in patients with diabetic nephropathy and hyperuricemia: a randomized, double-blind, placebo-controlled, parallel-group study (UPWARD study). Clin Exp Nephrol 2018; 22(4): 860-70.
[http://dx.doi.org/10.1007/s10157-018-1530-1] [PMID: 29372470]

[126]   Khan SR. Crystal-induced inflammation of the kidneys: results from human studies, animal models, and tissue-culture studies. Clin Exp Nephrol 2004; 8(2): 75-88.
[http://dx.doi.org/10.1007/s10157-004-0292-0] [PMID: 15235923]

[127]   Mazzali M, Kanellis J, Han L, *et al.* Hyperuricemia induces a primary renal arteriolopathy in rats by a blood pressure-independent mechanism. Am J Physiol Renal Physiol 2002; 282(6): F991-7.
[http://dx.doi.org/10.1152/ajprenal.00283.2001] [PMID: 11997315]

[128]   Sánchez-Lozada LG, Tapia E, Avila-Casado C, *et al.* Mild hyperuricemia induces glomerular hypertension in normal rats. Am J Physiol Renal Physiol 2002; 283(5): F1105-10.
[http://dx.doi.org/10.1152/ajprenal.00170.2002] [PMID: 12372787]

[129] Zhou T, Yao K, Xie Y, Lin Y, Wang J, Chen X. Renal Protection and Safety of Sodium-glucose Cotransporter-2 Inhibitors in Chronic Kidney Disease. Curr Pharm Des 2023; 29(21): 1659-70.
[http://dx.doi.org/10.2174/1381612829666230804103643] [PMID: 37537933]

[130] Ma C, Li X, Li W, Li Y, Shui F, Zhu P. The efficacy and safety of SGLT2 inhibitors in patients with non-diabetic chronic kidney disease: a systematic review and meta-analysis. Int Urol Nephrol 2023; 55(12): 3167-74.
[http://dx.doi.org/10.1007/s11255-023-03586-1] [PMID: 37046125]

[131] Shiau CH, Tsau LY, Kao CC, *et al.* Efficacy and safety of sodium-glucose cotransporter-2 inhibitors in patients with chronic kidney disease: a systematic review and meta-analysis. Int Urol Nephrol 2023; 56(4): 1359-81.
[http://dx.doi.org/10.1007/s11255-023-03789-6] [PMID: 37752340]

[132] Forbes AK, Suckling RJ, Hinton W, *et al.* Sodium-glucose cotransporter-2 inhibitors and kidney outcomes in real-world type 2 diabetes populations: A systematic review and meta-analysis of observational studies. Diabetes Obes Metab 2023; 25(8): 2310-30.
[http://dx.doi.org/10.1111/dom.15111] [PMID: 37202870]

[133] Wang XX, Levi J, Luo Y, *et al.* SGLT2 Protein Expression Is Increased in Human Diabetic Nephropathy: SGLT2 protein inhibition decreases renal lipid accumulation, inflammation, and the development of nephropathy in diabetic mice. J Biol Chem 2017; 292(13): 5335-48.
[http://dx.doi.org/10.1074/jbc.M117.779520] [PMID: 28196866]

[134] Kuriyama C, Xu JZ, Lee SP, *et al.* Analysis of the effect of canagliflozin on renal glucose reabsorption and progression of hyperglycemia in zucker diabetic Fatty rats. J Pharmacol Exp Ther 2014; 351(2): 423-31.
[http://dx.doi.org/10.1124/jpet.114.217992] [PMID: 25216746]

[135] Osataphan S, Macchi C, Singhal G, *et al.* SGLT2 inhibition reprograms systemic metabolism *via* FGF21-dependent and -independent mechanisms. JCI Insight 2019; 4(5): e123130.
[http://dx.doi.org/10.1172/jci.insight.123130] [PMID: 30843877]

[136] Tuttle KR, Brosius FC III, Cavender MA, *et al.* SGLT2 Inhibition for CKD and Cardiovascular Disease in Type 2 Diabetes: Report of a Scientific Workshop Sponsored by the National Kidney Foundation. Am J Kidney Dis 2021; 77(1): 94-109.
[http://dx.doi.org/10.1053/j.ajkd.2020.08.003] [PMID: 33121838]

[137] Lytvyn Y, Kimura K, Peter N, *et al.* Renal and Vascular Effects of Combined SGLT2 and Angiotensin-Converting Enzyme Inhibition. Circulation 2022; 146(6): 450-62.
[http://dx.doi.org/10.1161/CIRCULATIONAHA.122.059150] [PMID: 35862082]

[138] Kraus BJ, Weir MR, Bakris GL, *et al.* Characterization and implications of the initial estimated glomerular filtration rate 'dip' upon sodium-glucose cotransporter-2 inhibition with empagliflozin in the EMPA-REG OUTCOME trial. Kidney Int 2021; 99(3): 750-62.
[http://dx.doi.org/10.1016/j.kint.2020.10.031] [PMID: 33181154]

[139] Adamson C, Docherty KF, Heerspink HJL, *et al.* Initial decline (Dip) in estimated glomerular filtration rate after initiation of dapagliflozin in patients with heart failure and reduced ejection fraction: insights from DAPA-HF. Circulation 2022; 146(6): 438-49.
[http://dx.doi.org/10.1161/CIRCULATIONAHA.121.058910] [PMID: 35442064]

[140] Krishnan A, Shankar M, Lerma EV, Wiegley N. Sodium Glucose Cotransporter 2 (SGLT2) Inhibitors and CKD: Are You a #Flozinator? Kidney Med 2023; 5(4): 100608.
[http://dx.doi.org/10.1016/j.xkme.2023.100608] [PMID: 36915368]

[141] Baigent C, Emberson JR, Haynes R, *et al.* Impact of diabetes on the effects of sodium glucose co-transporter-2 inhibitors on kidney outcomes: collaborative meta-analysis of large placebo-controlled trials. Lancet 2022; 400(10365): 1788-801.
[http://dx.doi.org/10.1016/S0140-6736(22)02074-8] [PMID: 36351458]

[142] Chen L, Xue Q, Yan C, *et al.* Comparative safety of different recommended doses of sodium–glucose cotransporter 2 inhibitors in patients with type 2 diabetes mellitus: a systematic review and network meta-analysis of randomized clinical trials. Front Endocrinol (Lausanne) 2023; 14: 1256548.
[http://dx.doi.org/10.3389/fendo.2023.1256548] [PMID: 38027214]

CHAPTER 16

Dysbiosis in Acute Kidney Injury and Chronic Kidney Disease

Laura Elena Zamora- Cervantes[1] and **Enzo C. Vásquez-Jiménez**[1,*]

[1] *Department of Nephrology, Hospital Juárez de México, Gustavo A. Madero 07760, Mexico City, Mexico*

Abstract: During acute kidney injury (AKI) and chronic kidney disease (CKD), dysbiosis is induced by mechanisms that alter intestinal homeostasis, leading to a persistent proinflammatory response. This alteration in the intestinal microbiota may regulate immunity, inflammation, and nutrition in patients with AKI and CKD. However, the therapies proposed to reestablish the microbiome balance remain limited and have not shown a benefit. It is possible to use different strategies to modulate the gut microbiota balance to improve kidney function in different renal diseases. Therefore, strategies can be used in combination with available treatment. Nevertheless, it is important to note that individual factors, comorbidities, medications, diet, and lifestyle limit current therapies. Thus, personalized strategies are needed, along with continued research, to achieve outcomes by altering the microbiome and its effects on the progression of kidney disease.

Keywords: Acute kidney injury, Chronic kidney disease, Gut microbiota, Microbiome, Prebiotics, Probiotics.

INTRODUCTION

Epidemiology of AKI and CKD

Acute kidney injury (AKI) and chronic kidney disease (CKD) are considered a continuum in the course of the disease and a failure of the adaptive mechanism after injury. The presence of either of these two entities is associated with high morbidity and mortality [1]. CKD affects more than 10% of the general population and affects more than 800 million people; in 2019, it was estimated that approximately 1.43 million people died from CKD [2]. Even if the estimated mortality of AKI improved compared to that in previous years, from 23% to 17.5% in those who did not require replacement therapy (2013 to 2020), 11.6% of

---

[1] Corresponding author Enzo C. Vázquez-Jiménez: Department of Nephrology, Hospital Juárez de México, Gustavo A. Madero 07760, Mexico City, Mexico; E-mail: enzo.vas.ji@gmail.com

Rafael Valdez-Ortiz, Katy Sánchez-Pozos, Ana Carolina Ariza & Enzo C. Vásquez-Jiménez (Eds.)

survivors were diagnosed with CKD upon discharge, and 24 months later, this percentage increased to 20.7%, with a 36.7% increase in mortality [3].

Both entities have common denominators, such as diabetes, and classic cardiovascular risk factors, such as obesity, hypertension, and dyslipidemia. However, the role of changes in the microbiome or dysbiosis is beginning to be a topic of interest in kidney pathology.

Microbiome and its Functions

The microbiome is composed of a community of microorganisms (microbiota) that cohabit in a specific microenvironment. Approximately 50% of the fecal mass is composed of bacteria, mainly *Firmicutes, Bacteroidetes, Actinobacteria, and Proteobacteria* [4].

The gut microbiota plays a role in the regulation of immunity, inflammation, and nutrition, mainly through the following mechanisms:

- Lymphocyte regulation promotes CD4$^+$ T-cell differentiation to balance Th1 and Th2 populations, which maintains the balance of Th17 cells that secrete different cytokines, such as IL-17F, IL-21, IL-22, IL-23, and TNF-α, and produces an increase in IL-10 and IL-18 (GPR109A), resulting in an anti-inflammatory response.
- The production of short-chain fatty acids, which are the end products of the fermentation activity of the microbiota. With greater kidney relevance, the GPR109A receptor, which has anti-inflammatory activity and is implicated in gut homeostasis, is the GPR43 receptor, which induces the activation of FOXP3, resulting in cellular differentiation, in addition to rennin secretion, since it is expressed in the afferent arteriole and the juxtaglomerular apparatus, as well as the OLFR78 receptor [5 - 7].
- It also maintains homeostasis between the intestinal epithelial cells of the gastrointestinal tract by maintaining the intestinal barrier's permeability and polarity for lipid diffusion, preventing the passage of endotoxins [8, 9].

When a disturbance occurs in gut microbiota, it is known as dysbiosis. This disturbance includes the loss of beneficial organisms, the overgrowth of harmful organisms, and the loss of microbial diversity [10].

Altered Pathways in AKI and CKD

Upon the onset of renal damage, there is an extension phase, which, depending on adaptation or maladaptation, results in repair or progressive renal sclerosis [1].

Regardless of the process, various mechanisms that induce hypoxia are triggered, activating different pathways [11 - 13]:

- Cellular responses of neutrophils, macrophages, and T lymphocytes produce the secretion of proinflammatory cytokines and adhesion molecules, generating nitric oxide and reactive oxygen species by endothelial and mesangial cells, podocytes, and tubular cells.
- Sustained and exaggerated activation of the Wnt/β-catenin pathway, with continuous stimulation of vascular endothelial growth factor (VEGF) and transforming growth factor β (TGF-β).
- Cellular senescence occurs in response to the activation of JNK (c-Jun N-terminal kinase) when renal tubular cells enter the G2/M phase. This allows them to resist apoptosis and secrete cytokines such as IL-6 and IL-8, which promote an inflammatory state.
- Fibrosis following mesangial expansion leads to collagen deposition with increased myofibroblasts and pericytes.

Role of Dysbiosis in Kidney Disease

A change in the microbiota composition may alter intestinal homeostasis (dysbiosis), promoting disturbances in cardiovascular and renal systems and the progression of various diseases, such as AKI and CKD [14, 15]. In CKD patients, it may induce greater dysbiosis. These alterations in the microbiota occur mainly through three mechanisms:

- The expansion of pathobionts (low amounts of commensal bacteria with harmful effects when outnumbering other commensals) can be triggered by various factors, such as genetics; changes in macronutrients, such as diets high in preservatives, which promote the overgrowth of proteobacteria; low-fiber diets that alter fermentation and reduce short-chain fatty acids due to shifts toward *Bacteroides* spp., *Akkermansia muciniphila*, and *Prevotella spp.*; and inflammatory states, such as obesity, which are associated with an increase in the *Firmicutes/Bacteroidetes* ratio [16 - 19].
- Leaky gut, which induces changes in proteolytic fermentation and short-chain fatty acid production, disturbs the junctions of intestinal epithelial cells, allowing more metabolites, including uremic toxins and lipopolysaccharides, to cross through. This latter leads to a subsequent proinflammatory response [20].
- Microinflammation subsequent to the release of lipopolysaccharides from gram-negative bacteria, such as proteobacteria. This causes the migration of macrophages and the nuclear transcription factor kappa B (NF-κB), leading to the synthesis of TNFα, IL-1, IL-6, and IL-8, thus inducing a persistent proinflammatory state [21].

Dysbiosis and Progression Mechanisms of AKI and CKD

Hypoxia

In a symbiotic situation, low oxygen concentrations are ideal. Short-chain fatty acids activate hypoxia-inducible factor (HIF-1), which results in hydroxylation to form the HIF1α complex, which triggers the formation of mucin lining the intestinal epithelium membrane [22]. However, during dysbiosis, there is an overgrowth of aerobic colonies, such as *E. coli, Shigella, Salmonella, Helicobacter,* and *Pseudomonas,* over anaerobic colonies, such as *Bacteroides* or *Lactobacillus.* Along with vascular dysfunction, a high oxygen demand leads to a chronic hypoxic state, which promotes the transcription of the antisense HIF1A-AS2 factor that stabilizes the hydroxylation of HIF1. These events activate the production of reactive oxygen species, leading to NF-κB-induced transcription that stimulates the synthesis of proinflammatory molecules that promote a proinflammatory state and an apoptotic response. In addition, vascular and tubular remodeling is induced by the activation of adhesion molecules and endothelial growth factors, which stimulate interstitial fibrosis and mesangial expansion [23, 24].

Mitochondrial Axis

Short-chain fatty acids can arrest the mitochondrial inflammatory response by stimulating peroxisome proliferator-activated receptor gamma coactivator 1-α (PGC-1α) or by producing antioxidants that prevent NF-κB activation, with cytoprotective and anti-inflammatory activity identified in *Lactobacillus rhamnosus* and *Bacillus LBP32* [25]. Once there is an increase in pathobionts in inflammatory states such as AKI and the hypoxia produced, there is an increase in formyl peptide receptors (a type of G receptor) in macrophages. This triggers adhesion pathways and superoxide production, leading to increased free radical production, NF-κB activation, and fibrosis progression in renal tubular cells [26].

Cellular Imbalance

The microbiota maintains homeostasis by increasing type 2 immune and regulatory responses that are able to inhibit T-cell proliferation and cytokine production. However, in dysbiosis, an imbalance in these populations has been observed. Bacterial translocation promotes a proinflammatory state with increased Th1 cells, M1 macrophages, and dendritic cells, as observed in the initial stages of AKI [27]. This leads to the secretion of proinflammatory cytokines, such as IL-12 and IL-6, altering the differentiation of naive CD4+ T cells and B-cell maturation, resulting in a pattern change similar to that observed in patients with CKD, with a 50% decrease in native CD4+ T cells but a 34% increase in memory CD4+ T cells, resulting in continuous cytokine production, especially that of IL-17 (Fig. **1**) [28].

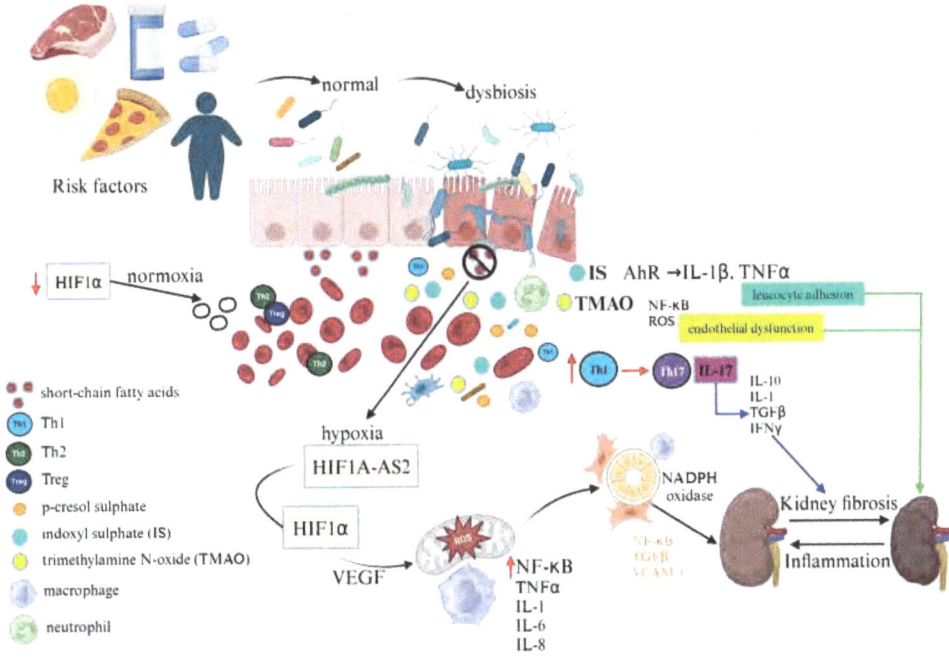

Fig. (1). The gut renal axis.

Uremic Toxins

As the abundance of proteolytic bacteria, such as *Fusobacterium* and *Citrobacter,* increases, the fermentation products change to indoles, ammonia, amines, and phenols rather than short-chain fatty acids, leading to the accumulation of indoxyl sulfate (IS), which, through the aryl hydrocarbon receptor (AhR) pathway, induces the production of IL-1β and TNF-α by monocytes and CX3CL1 in endothelial cells to recruit CD4+ T lymphocytes and NF-κB. The accumulation of p-cresol sulfate inhibits the production of IFN-γ, reducing Th1 lymphocyte and IL-12 production, and the direct production of trimethylamine N-oxide (TMAO), which has been associated with atherosclerosis and renal disease progression, by increasing the population of scavenger macrophages, leading to increased LDL accumulation, intracellular Ca+ release, oxidative stress generation, activation of TGF-β and VCAM-1, and stimulation of the renin-angiotensin-aldosterone system [29 - 31].

Alternatives for Reestablishing the Microbiome Homeostasis

Different therapies have been tested to reestablish the equilibrium state of the microbiome since diet changes with increasing fiber, inhibiting bacterial colonies, and decreasing endotoxin absorption through probiotics, prebiotics, or symbiotics in response to monoclonal therapy. Most of these studies are experimental or vary greatly due to population characteristics. Prebiotics are defined as the fraction of non-digestible carbohydrates (oligo and polysaccharides) contained in foods (mostly vegetable sources) that can stimulate the growth of microbiota, such as *Lactobacillus* and *Bifidobacterium,* with subsequent stimulation and production of short-chain fatty acids and re-establishment of the intestinal epithelium [32]. Probiotics are viable bacteria of the microbiota, most of which include *Lactobacillus* or *Saccharomyce*s, to reestablish homeostasis, while symbiotics are a combination of prebiotics and probiotics to increase microorganism survival [33].

Several studies have assessed the effect of probiotics, prebiotics, or symbiotics in patients with CKD. According to a meta-analysis by Zheng et al., from 2000 to 2019, as shown in 13 randomized clinical trials, probiotics, prebiotics, or symbiotics have only helped to reduce inflammatory parameters, which in theory would induce an improvement in kidney function. Among the evaluated markers were the levels of indoxyl sulfate, C-reactive protein, total antioxidant capacity, and glutathione [34]. Microbial therapies significantly reduced C-reactive protein, lipoperoxidation, and lipid levels and increased antioxidant capacity. Therefore, the authors suggest that prebiotics, probiotics, and symbiotics can improve inflammation, oxidative stress, and lipid profiles in patients with CKD. Nonetheless, these results must be taken with caution because the heterogeneity in the studies considering the type of therapy, duration, diet, patient characteristics, and presentation has prevented other conclusions (Table **1**).

Table 1. Prebiotic, probiotic, and symbiotic evidence in kidney disease.

Study	Targets	Population	Agents	Methods	Outcome	Conclusion
Viramontes *et al.* (2015) [35]	Assess the effect of symbiotics on gastrointestinal symptoms and inflammation markers in HD.	HD	Symbiotic: inulin, *Lactobacillus acidophilus* y, *Bifidobacterium lactis* 1.1- 1.2 g/kg/d for 2 months.	A randomized, double-blind, placebo-controlled trial in CKD with GI symptoms who	Reduction of GI symptoms such as nausea and heartburn, nonsignificant trend to CRP reduction	Safe therapy for the reduction of GI symptoms

(Table 1) cont.....

Study	Targets	Population	Agents	Methods	Outcome	Conclusion
Guida *et al.* (2017) [36]	Assess the effect of symbiotics on p-cresol reduction	Kidney transplant >12 months without rejection	Symbiotic: *Lactobacillus plantarum, casei, rhamnosus, Bifidobacterium, Streptococcus thermophilus* + inulin 5 g t.i.d for 30 days	A randomized, double-blind, placebo-controlled trial in kidney transplant without rejection or infection for 3 months	n=29, reduction of 40% at 15 days of p-cresol, of 33% on day 30, p<0.0; without change in renal function	Symbiotics are effective in reducing uremic toxins such as p-cresol
Kooshki (2019) [37]	Assess the effects of symbiotics on inflammation, oxidative stress, and lipid markers in HD	HD	100 mg *Lactobacillus* q.d. for 8 weeks	A randomized, double-blind, placebo-controlled trial in HD patients	n=50, CRP and MDA decreased from 6.3 to 4.3 and 2.7 to 1.9, respectively, p= 0.01 (no mention of CI)	Supplementation with symbiotics improves CRP and MDA levels in HD patients
McFarlane *et al.* (2021) [38]	Assess the effects of symbiotics on 3-4 CKD in cardiovascular function, indoxyl sulfate, and p-cresol levels	CKD 3-4(GFR 15-60 ml/min/1.73m²)	Synbiotics: *Bifidobacterium* and *Blautia spp*	Randomized, double-blind, placebo-controlled trial in CKD 3-4, 2017-2018	n=68, change in microbiota *Bifidobacterium* spp. *and Blautia* spp., no change in cardiovascular structure or uremic toxins levels	Long-term symbiotic supplementation was feasible and acceptable for CKD patients and modified the GI microbiome
Yang *et al.* (2021) [39]	Asses the renoprotective effect of probiotics in AKI	Mice with AKI ischemia-reperfusion	Probiotics: capsules *of Bifidobacterium bifidum BGN4* q.d. for 2 weeks	Experimental in mice with induced AKI	Decrease in the expansion of enterobacteria, reduction of IL-17A, and increase in Treg.	Decreased severity of AKI after BGN4 by increase in Foxp3 and reduction in IL-17A
Chávez *et al.* (2023) [40]	Asses the probiotic effect on KFR (creatinine <0.3 of baseline)	AKI- sepsis	1080 mg *Streptococcus thermophilus, Lactobacillus acidophilus, Bifidobacterium longum*/q.d for 7 days	A randomized, double-blind, placebo-controlled trial, 2019-2022	n=92, compared with placebo KFR had an HR 0.93 (CI 0.52-1.68, p=0.81); mortality at 6 months with HR 0.56 (IC 0.32-1.04, p=0.06), urea decrease 154-80 mg/dl, p=0.04	Probiotics for seven consecutive days did not increase the probability of KFR

Hemodialysis (HD); acute kidney injury (AKI); kidney function recovery (KFR); chronic kidney disease (CKD); C-reactive protein (CRP); malondialdehyde (MDA); hazard ratio (HR); gastrointestinal (GI); t.i.d. thrice a day; q.d. once a day.

Another potential therapy is the administration of AST-120 adsorbent carbon spheres. The strong binding of AST-120 to proteins of some uremic toxins, such as IS and TMAO, leads to subsequent gastrointestinal sequestration. There are controversial studies about the use of AST-120 in renal disease. In the EPPIC study, Schulman *et al.* evaluated the effect of AST-120 on the progression of CKD in 2035 patients with creatinine levels ranging from 1.5 to 5 mg/dL. The authors observed only a trend toward a more gradual progression (189 weeks vs 124), although this difference was not significant. Thus, the benefit of AST-120 in this study was marginal [41]. In a more recent meta-analysis and systemic review, AST-120 was evaluated as a strategy for lowering protein-bound uremic toxins (indoxyl sulfate and p-cresyl sulfate) associated with increased morbidity and mortality. The study included 38 articles, comprising 28 randomized clinical trials, single-arm or prospective cohort studies, and two cross-sectional studies (2,492 CKD patients). Treatment with AST-120 resulted in lower serum levels of indoxyl sulfate and p-cresyl sulfate in CKD patients than the placebo group; however, the heterogeneity of the included studies was high. Hence, well-conducted randomized clinical trials specifically designed to determine the beneficial effects of AST-120 on AKI and CKD are needed [42].

Fecal microbiota transplantation effectively treats severe *Clostridioides difficile* infections by introducing healthy donor bacteria to restore the microbiome. Initially, this procedure characterized intestinal dysbiosis in kidney diseases [43 - 46]. However, studies on the benefit of fecal microbiota transplantation in kidney disease patients are still insufficient. As mentioned above, the uremic toxin products of dysbiosis and proinflammatory molecules are the main mechanisms involved in the deterioration of kidney function. Fecal microbiota transplantation has been applied to restore eubiosis and modulate uremic toxins in patients with kidney disease. In this context, several studies in mouse models of kidney diseases showed that fecal transplantation from disease mice in healthy mice resulted in high levels of circulating uremic toxins, lipopolysaccharide, and, in some cases, proteinuria. These changes were associated with microbiome alterations [43, 47]. The clinical use of fecal microbiota transplantation has been documented in only two studies of CKD patients. Zhao *et al.* showed that 20 weeks of fecal microbiota transplantation from healthy donors to IgA nephropathy recipients significantly ameliorated proteinuria and restored gut dysbiosis [48]. Another study of membranous nephropathy reported that treatment with fecal microbiota transplantation diminished creatine and 24-hour urine protein, and edema and diarrhea disappeared [49]. Therefore, these findings support using fecal microbiota transplantation as a potential biotherapy or bio-coadjuvant for kidney diseases. Currently, there are few registered and monitored fecal microbiota transplantation protocols for patients with CKD, and only one is available in Mexico (NCT04361097).

Furthermore, direct regulation of the immune response mediated by the microbiome is a strategy within innovative therapies that involves trying to mediate the response of Th17 cells and their renal infiltration, the expansion of which may be interrupted by blocking IL-23 with guselkumab, IL-23/12 with ustekinumab, IL-17A with anti-IL-17A antibodies with secukinumab, or monoclonal antibodies against the receptor brodalumab [50].

CONCLUSION

The results of studies on the microbiome in kidney disease support the important role of the gut microbiota in dysbiosis in kidney injury. Moreover, it is possible to use different strategies to modulate the gut microbiota balance to improve kidney function in different renal diseases. Nevertheless, it is important to note that individual factors, comorbidities, medications, diet, and lifestyle limit current therapies. Thus, personalized strategies are needed, along with continued research, to achieve outcomes by altering the microbiome and its effects on the progression of kidney disease.

REFERENCES

[1] Ferenbach DA, Bonventre JV. Mechanisms of maladaptive repair after AKI leading to accelerated kidney ageing and CKD. Nat Rev Nephrol 2015; 11(5): 264-76.
[http://dx.doi.org/10.1038/nrneph.2015.3] [PMID: 25643664]

[2] Cockwell P, Fisher LA. The global burden of chronic kidney disease. Lancet 2020; 395(10225): 662-4.
[http://dx.doi.org/10.1016/S0140-6736(19)32977-0] [PMID: 32061314]

[3] https://usrds-adr.niddk.nih.gov/2023/chronic-kidney-disease/4-acute-kidney-injury

[4] Icaza-Chávez ME. Microbiota intestinal en la salud y la enfermedad. Rev Gastroenterol Mex 2013; 78(4): 240-8.
[http://dx.doi.org/10.1016/j.rgmx.2013.04.004] [PMID: 24290319]

[5] Zheng D, Liwinski T, Elinav E. Interaction between microbiota and immunity in health and disease. Cell Res 2020; 30(6): 492-506.
[http://dx.doi.org/10.1038/s41422-020-0332-7] [PMID: 32433595]

[6] Magliocca G, Mone P, Di Iorio BR, Heidland A, Marzocco S. Short-Chain Fatty Acids in Chronic Kidney Disease: Focus on Inflammation and Oxidative Stress Regulation. Int J Mol Sci 2022; 23(10): 5354.
[http://dx.doi.org/10.3390/ijms23105354] [PMID: 35628164]

[7] Pluznick JL. Gut microbiota in renal physiology: focus on short-chain fatty acids and their receptors. Kidney Int 2016; 90(6): 1191-8.
[http://dx.doi.org/10.1016/j.kint.2016.06.033] [PMID: 27575555]

[8] Zhou A, Yuan Y, Yang M, *et al.* Crosstalk Between the Gut Microbiota and Epithelial Cells Under Physiological and Infectious Conditions. Front Cell Infect Microbiol 2022; 12: 832672.
[http://dx.doi.org/10.3389/fcimb.2022.832672] [PMID: 35155283]

[9] Cereijido M, Contreras RG, Shoshani L, Flores-Benitez D, Larre I. Tight junction and polarity interaction in the transporting epithelial phenotype. Biochim Biophys Acta Biomembr 2008; 1778(3): 770-93.
[http://dx.doi.org/10.1016/j.bbamem.2007.09.001] [PMID: 18028872]

[10]   DeGruttola AK, Low D, Mizoguchi A, Mizoguchi E. Current understanding of dysbiosis in disease in human and animal models. Inflamm Bowel Dis 2016; 22(5): 1137-50.
[http://dx.doi.org/10.1097/MIB.0000000000000750] [PMID: 27070911]

[11]   Xiao L, Zhou D, Tan RJ, *et al.* Sustained Activation of Wnt/β-Catenin Signaling Drives AKI to CKD Progression. J Am Soc Nephrol 2016; 27(6): 1727-40.
[http://dx.doi.org/10.1681/ASN.2015040449] [PMID: 26453613]

[12]   Schmitt R, Melk A. Molecular mechanisms of renal aging. Kidney Int 2017; 92(3): 569-79.
[http://dx.doi.org/10.1016/j.kint.2017.02.036] [PMID: 28729036]

[13]   Stenvinkel P, Chertow GM, Devarajan P, *et al.* Chronic inflammation in chronic kidney disease progression: Role of Nrf2. Kidney Int Rep 2021; 6(7): 1775-87.
[http://dx.doi.org/10.1016/j.ekir.2021.04.023] [PMID: 34307974]

[14]   Almeida C, Barata P, Fernandes R. The influence of gut microbiota in cardiovascular diseases—a brief review. Porto Biomed J 2021; 6(1): e106.
[http://dx.doi.org/10.1097/j.pbj.0000000000000106] [PMID: 33490701]

[15]   Saranya GR, Viswanathan P. Gut microbiota dysbiosis in AKI to CKD transition. Biomed Pharmacother 2023; 161: 114447.
[http://dx.doi.org/10.1016/j.biopha.2023.114447] [PMID: 37002571]

[16]   Levy M, Kolodziejczyk AA, Thaiss CA, Elinav E. Dysbiosis and the immune system. Nat Rev Immunol 2017; 17(4): 219-32.
[http://dx.doi.org/10.1038/nri.2017.7] [PMID: 28260787]

[17]   Hrncirova L, Hudcovic T, Sukova E, *et al.* Human gut microbes are susceptible to antimicrobial food additives in vitro. Folia Microbiol (Praha) 2019; 64(4): 497-508.
[http://dx.doi.org/10.1007/s12223-018-00674-z] [PMID: 30656592]

[18]   Koh A, De Vadder F, Kovatcheva-Datchary P, Bäckhed F. From dietary fiber to host physiology: short-chain fatty acids as key bacterial metabolites. Cell 2016; 165(6): 1332-45.
[http://dx.doi.org/10.1016/j.cell.2016.05.041] [PMID: 27259147]

[19]   Raoult D. Obesity pandemics and the modification of digestive bacterial flora. Eur J Clin Microbiol Infect Dis 2008; 27(8): 631-4.
[http://dx.doi.org/10.1007/s10096-008-0490-x] [PMID: 18322715]

[20]   Bryniarski MA, Hamarneh F, Yacoub R. The role of chronic kidney disease-associated dysbiosis in cardiovascular disease. Exp Biol Med (Maywood) 2019; 244(6): 514-25.
[http://dx.doi.org/10.1177/1535370219826526] [PMID: 30682892]

[21]   Escárcega RO, Fuentes-Alexandro S, García-Carrasco M, Gatica A, Zamora A. The transcription factor nuclear factor-kappa B and cancer. Clin Oncol (R Coll Radiol) 2007; 19(2): 154-61.
[http://dx.doi.org/10.1016/j.clon.2006.11.013] [PMID: 17355113]

[22]   Van Welden S, Selfridge AC, Hindryckx P. Intestinal hypoxia and hypoxia-induced signalling as therapeutic targets for IBD. Nat Rev Gastroenterol Hepatol 2017; 14(10): 596-611.
[http://dx.doi.org/10.1038/nrgastro.2017.101] [PMID: 28853446]

[23]   Downes N, Niskanen H, Tomas Bosch V, *et al.* Hypoxic regulation of hypoxia inducible factor 1 alpha *via* antisense transcription. J Biol Chem 2023; 299(11): 105291.
[http://dx.doi.org/10.1016/j.jbc.2023.105291] [PMID: 37748649]

[24]   Liu L, Xu W, Kong P, Dou Y. The relationships among gut microbiota, hypoxia-inducible factor and anaemia with chronic kidney disease. Nephrology (Carlton) 2022; 27(11): 851-8.
[http://dx.doi.org/10.1111/nep.14064] [PMID: 35603584]

[25]   Diao Y, Xin Y, Zhou Y, *et al.* Extracellular polysaccharide from Bacillus sp. strain LBP32 prevents LPS-induced inflammation in RAW 264.7 macrophages by inhibiting NF-κB and MAPKs activation and ROS production. Int Immunopharmacol 2014; 18(1): 12-9.

[http://dx.doi.org/10.1016/j.intimp.2013.10.021] [PMID: 24201081]

[26] Saranya GR, Viswanathan P. Gut microbiota dysbiosis in AKI to CKD transition. Biomed Pharmacother 2023; 161: 114447.
[http://dx.doi.org/10.1016/j.biopha.2023.114447] [PMID: 37002571]

[27] Noel S, Mohammad F, White J, Lee K, Gharaie S, Rabb H. Gut microbiota-immune system interactions during acute kidney injury. Kidney360 2021; 2(3): 528-31.
[http://dx.doi.org/10.34067/KID.0006792020] [PMID: 35369013]

[28] Lee TH, Chen JJ, Wu CY, Lin TY, Hung SC, Yang HY. Immunosenescence, gut dysbiosis, and chronic kidney disease: Interplay and implications for clinical management. Biomed J 2024; 47(2): 100638.
[http://dx.doi.org/10.1016/j.bj.2023.100638] [PMID: 37524304]

[29] Korpela K. Diet, microbiota, and metabolic health: trade-off between saccharolytic and proteolytic fermentation. Annu Rev Food Sci Technol 2018; 9(1): 65-84.
[http://dx.doi.org/10.1146/annurev-food-030117-012830] [PMID: 29298101]

[30] Tang Z, Yu S, Pan Y. The gut microbiome tango in the progression of chronic kidney disease and potential therapeutic strategies. J Transl Med 2023; 21(1): 689.
[http://dx.doi.org/10.1186/s12967-023-04455-2] [PMID: 37789439]

[31] Liu H, Jia K, Ren Z, Sun J, Pan LL. PRMT5 critically mediates TMAO-induced inflammatory response in vascular smooth muscle cells. Cell Death Dis 2022; 13(4): 299.
[http://dx.doi.org/10.1038/s41419-022-04719-7] [PMID: 35379776]

[32] Quigley EMM. Prebiotics and probiotics in digestive health. Clin Gastroenterol Hepatol 2019; 17(2): 333-44.
[http://dx.doi.org/10.1016/j.cgh.2018.09.028] [PMID: 30267869]

[33] Abreu-Abreu AT. Prebióticos, probióticos y simbióticos. Rev Gastroenterol Mex 2012; 77 (Suppl. 1): 26-8.
[http://dx.doi.org/10.1016/j.rgmx.2012.07.011] [PMID: 22939472]

[34] Zheng HJ, Guo J, Wang Q, *et al.* Probiotics, prebiotics, and synbiotics for the improvement of metabolic profiles in patients with chronic kidney disease: A systematic review and meta-analysis of randomized controlled trials. Crit Rev Food Sci Nutr 2021; 61(4): 577-98.
[http://dx.doi.org/10.1080/10408398.2020.1740645] [PMID: 32329633]

[35] Viramontes-Hörner D, Márquez-Sandoval F, Martín-del-Campo F, *et al.* Effect of a symbiotic gel (Lactobacillus acidophilus + Bifidobacterium lactis + inulin) on presence and severity of gastrointestinal symptoms in hemodialysis patients. J Ren Nutr 2015; 25(3): 284-91.
[http://dx.doi.org/10.1053/j.jrn.2014.09.008] [PMID: 25455039]

[36] Guida B, Germanò R, Trio R, *et al.* Effect of short-term synbiotic treatment on plasma p-cresol levels in patients with chronic renal failure: A randomized clinical trial. Nutr Metab Cardiovasc Dis 2014; 24(9): 1043-9.
[http://dx.doi.org/10.1016/j.numecd.2014.04.007] [PMID: 24929795]

[37] Kooshki A, Tofighiyan T, Miri M. A synbiotic supplement for inflammation and oxidative stress and lipid abnormalities in hemodialysis patients. Hemodial Int 2019; 23(2): 254-60.
[http://dx.doi.org/10.1111/hdi.12748] [PMID: 30821897]

[38] McFarlane C, Krishnasamy R, Stanton T, *et al.* Synbiotics easing renal failure by improving gut microbiology II (SYNERGY II): A feasibility randomized controlled trial. Nutrients 2021; 13(12): 4481.
[http://dx.doi.org/10.3390/nu13124481] [PMID: 34960037]

[39] Yang J, Ji GE, Park MS, *et al.* Probiotics partially attenuate the severity of acute kidney injury through an immunomodulatory effect. Kidney Res Clin Pract 2021; 40(4): 620-33.
[http://dx.doi.org/10.23876/j.krcp.20.265] [PMID: 34922432]

[40] Chávez-Íñiguez JS, Ibarra-Estrada M, Gallardo-González AM, *et al.* Probiotics in septic acute kidney injury, a double blind, randomized control trial. Ren Fail 2023; 45(2): 2260003.
[http://dx.doi.org/10.1080/0886022X.2023.2260003] [PMID: 37724527]

[41] Schulman G, Berl T, Beck GJ, *et al.* Randomized Placebo-Controlled EPPIC Trials of AST-120 in CKD. J Am Soc Nephrol 2015; 26(7): 1732-46.
[http://dx.doi.org/10.1681/ASN.2014010042] [PMID: 25349205]

[42] Takkavatakarn K, Wuttiputinun T, Phannajit J, Praditpornsilpa K, Eiam-Ong S, Susantitaphong P. Protein-bound uremic toxin lowering strategies in chronic kidney disease: a systematic review and meta-analysis. J Nephrol 2021; 34(6): 1805-17.
[http://dx.doi.org/10.1007/s40620-020-00955-2] [PMID: 33484425]

[43] Li Y, Su X, Gao Y, *et al.* The potential role of the gut microbiota in modulating renal function in experimental diabetic nephropathy murine models established in same environment. Biochim Biophys Acta Mol Basis Dis 2020; 1866(6): 165764.
[http://dx.doi.org/10.1016/j.bbadis.2020.165764] [PMID: 32169506]

[44] Wang X, Yang S, Li S, *et al.* Aberrant gut microbiota alters host metabolome and impacts renal failure in humans and rodents. Gut 2020; 69(12): 2131-42.
[http://dx.doi.org/10.1136/gutjnl-2019-319766] [PMID: 32241904]

[45] Yang J, Kim CJ, Go YS, *et al.* Intestinal microbiota control acute kidney injury severity by immune modulation. Kidney Int 2020; 98(4): 932-46.
[http://dx.doi.org/10.1016/j.kint.2020.04.048] [PMID: 32470493]

[46] Emal D, Rampanelli E, Stroo I, *et al.* Depletion of Gut Microbiota Protects against Renal Ischemia-Reperfusion Injury. J Am Soc Nephrol 2017; 28(5): 1450-61.
[http://dx.doi.org/10.1681/ASN.2016030255] [PMID: 27927779]

[47] Uchiyama K, Wakino S, Irie J, *et al.* Contribution of uremic dysbiosis to insulin resistance and sarcopenia. Nephrol Dial Transplant 2020; 35(9): 1501-17.
[http://dx.doi.org/10.1093/ndt/gfaa076] [PMID: 32535631]

[48] Zhao J, Bai M, Yang X, Wang Y, Li R, Sun S. Alleviation of refractory IgA nephropathy by intensive fecal microbiota transplantation: the first case reports. Ren Fail 2021; 43(1): 928-33.
[http://dx.doi.org/10.1080/0886022X.2021.1936038] [PMID: 34134605]

[49] Zhou G, Zeng J, Peng L, *et al.* Fecal microbiota transplantation for membranous nephropathy. CEN Case Rep 2021; 10(2): 261-4.
[http://dx.doi.org/10.1007/s13730-020-00560-z] [PMID: 33387212]

[50] Baker KF, Isaacs JD. Novel therapies for immune-mediated inflammatory diseases: What can we learn from their use in rheumatoid arthritis, spondyloarthritis, systemic lupus erythematosus, psoriasis, Crohn's disease and ulcerative colitis? Ann Rheum Dis 2018; 77(2): 175-87.
[http://dx.doi.org/10.1136/annrheumdis-2017-211555] [PMID: 28765121]

SUBJECT INDEX

A

Abnormalities 103, 135, 136, 204
 epigenetic 204
 lipid 103
 metabolic 135, 136
Absorption 136, 186
 inadequate 186
 intestinal 136
Acetylcholinesterase activity 180
Acidosis 58, 59, 86, 87, 179
 intracellular 86
 lactic 58, 59, 179
 systemic 87
Acute disease quality initiative (ADQI) 66, 67, 68
Addison's disease 87
Adhesion 100, 165, 167, 217
 cell-cell 100, 167
 cell-matrix 165
 promoting macrophage 217
Akkermansia muciniphila 275
Albumin excretion rate (AER) 163
Alzheimer's disease 256, 257
American Diabetes Association (ADA) 164
American Heart Association 55, 149
Amino acids 5, 6, 7, 78, 127
 branched-chain 6
 cationic 78
 circulating 6, 7
 free 5
 glucogenic 6
 ketogenic 6
 primary 7
 sulfur-containing 78
 transport dibasic 127
Aminoaciduria 82, 84, 180
Aminoglycosides 8, 83, 178, 179, 181
Angiogenesis 19, 206, 207, 237
Angioplasty 179
Angiotensin 69, 96
Apoptosis 22, 25, 28, 189, 275

cellular 189
drug-induced 25
mitochondrial-driven 28
resist 275
triggering 22
Autophagy 26, 183, 217
 abnormal 183
 induced 26
 inhibiting 217
 promoted 26

B

Bartter syndrome 179, 181
Bicarbonate 77, 82, 83, 88, 91, 92
 absorption 92
 administration 82
 concentration 91
 loading 88
 reabsorption 77, 82
 reabsorption threshold 83
Bicarbonaturia 82, 83, 91
Bifidobacterium 278, 279
Bifidobacterium 278, 279
 bifidum 279
 lactis 278
 longum 279
Bioartificial 243
 kidney 243
 renal epithelial cell system (BRECS) 243
Bone disease 41, 88, 214
Bowman capsule 242
Branched-chain amino acids (BCAAs) 6
Brushite stones 137

C

Calculi 84, 130, 132, 133
 detection 132
 radiolucent 130
 renal 84
 urinary 133

www.ingramcontent.com/pod-product-compliance
Lightning Source LLC
Chambersburg PA
CBHW050810220326
41598CB00006B/171